THE QUESTION OF UNWORTHY LIFE

The Question of Unworthy Life

EUGENICS AND GERMANY'S TWENTIETH CENTURY

DAGMAR HERZOG

PRINCETON UNIVERSITY PRESS

PRINCETON & OXFORD

Published by Princeton University Press
41 William Street, Princeton, New Jersey 08540
99 Banbury Road, Oxford OX2 6JX

press.princeton.edu

All Rights Reserved
ISBN: 9780691261706
ISBN (e-book): 9780691261683

British Library Cataloging-in-Publication Data is available

Editorial: Priya Nelson and Emma Wagh
Production Editorial: Jaden Young
Jacket / Cover Design: Chris Ferrante
Production: Danielle Amatucci
Publicity: Alyssa Sanford and Carmen Jimenez
Copyeditor: Karen Verde

Jacket Credit: Photo courtesy of the Archiv der Diakonischen Stifung Wittekindshof

This book has been composed in Arno

Printed in the United States of America

10 9 8 7 6 5 4 3 2 1

CONTENTS

THE QUESTION OF UNWORTHY LIFE

Introduction

THE NAZI "euthanasia" murder program claimed, between 1939 and 1945, the lives of nearly 300,000 individuals, most of them carrying diagnoses of psychiatric illness or cognitive or behavioral deficiencies—an estimated 210,000 in the German Reich and another 80,000 in Nazi-occupied Poland and the Soviet Union. The killing was done by various means: in one of six carbon-monoxide-fueled gas chambers; by mass shootings; or by medication overdose, poisoning, or systematic starvation. Hitler would call a halt to the initial gas chamber (so-called T4) phase of "euthanasia" in the wake of Catholic bishop Clemens August von Galen's internationally resonant sermon of August 1941 eloquently decrying the killings.[1] Yet 121 men who had gotten their training and practice in murdering people with disabilities would soon find themselves transferred to Nazi-occupied Poland to assemble the Operation Reinhardt death factories of Belzec, Sobibor, and Treblinka. There, with great energy and ingenuity, these men would accomplish a full quarter of that mammoth, six-million-victim crime now collectively referred to as the Holocaust.[2] It was not least by persistent reference to this key detail of sequential chronology and overlap in personnel between the murders of individuals with disabilities and the murders of European Jewry, though also by identifying further connective links between the two mass killing programs, that activists and engaged researchers eventually succeeded in cohering a scholarly and popular consensus that the National Socialist "euthanasia" murders deserved recognition as a genocide.[3]

For an English-language audience, strikingly, invoking this sequential link between "euthanasia" and the Judeocide remains to this day the main means by which the significance of the murders of people with disabilities has been articulated. The late historian and Auschwitz survivor Henry Friedlander at several occasions told the story of being recurrently accosted as he was researching the entanglements between "euthanasia" and the Holocaust, and informed that his was a mistaken approach. "How can you compare Jews with crazy people?," one top-level official within an American Jewish organization had indignantly inquired.[4] Friedlander's own answer to the question that had been posed to him came in the form of his groundbreaking book, *The Origins of the Nazi Genocide: From Euthanasia to the Final Solution* (1995). In the preface, Friedlander explained how, based on his immersion in the primary sources—particularly the records of postwar perpetrator trials—he had come, over the course of the 1980s and early 1990s, to understand the murder of the disabled not merely as a "prologue" to the Holocaust, but indeed as its "first chapter." For Friedlander, moreover, unusual among his scholarly peers for also paying close attention to the persecution and murder of Roma and Sinti, the killing of people with disabilities would come to serve as "the model for all Nazi killing operations."[5] Friedlander's framing of the issues has been broadly persuasive. The US Holocaust Memorial Museum, in its own efforts to integrate the history of "euthanasia" more adequately into its presentation of the history of the Holocaust, on a recently developed web page referred to the "euthanasia" murder program as "in itself a rehearsal for Nazi Germany's broader genocidal policies."[6] Relatedly, in 2020, memoirist Kenny Fries (Jewish, gay, endowed with a physical disability), wrote about the connection of the two mass murder programs in the *New York Times* under the headline: "Before the 'Final Solution' There Was a 'Test Killing'. Too few know the history of the Nazi methodical mass murder of disabled people. That is why I write."[7]

Within Germany, however, in the years around the end of the Cold War, highlighting the interrelationships between "euthanasia" and the Holocaust, no matter how asymmetrical their sizes and even as connections were initially made more by intuitive analogy than by specifying literal links, had served a further crucial function. This was the indispensable assistance such references provided for advancing the—so long rebuffed—cause of disability rights.[8] For, with regard to the abuse and killing of people with disabilities, the more immediate post–World War II decades had seen a (in hindsight truly stunning, then simply crushing) breadth of popular support for the perpetrators, and ongoing shaming of the victims and their families.

While memory politics, care practices, and general public attitudes were complexly imbricated, progress on all fronts was excruciatingly slow, and efforts at advancing recognition of people with disabilities as deserving of equal rights and respect faced vicious pushback. Not just ex-Nazis, with their indefatigably inventive ability to rewrite the immediate past, but also non- or anti-Nazis had considerable difficulty in confronting what had occurred. Few of the physician perpetrators ever faced justice but instead had bright postwar careers, often continuing to function as experts adjudicating myriad issues relating to disability. Prejudice and contempt remained rampant. Well into the post–World War II era, people with all manner of disabilities—physical as well as mental or psychological—were not viewed by their fellow citizens as fully human, and their lives, bodies, and souls were not treated as of equal value. Eugenic thinking, in its quadruple dimensions—a pecking order of human worth, a conviction that intellectual disabilities in particular were primarily the result of heredity rather than random accident or environmental damage, an inflated sense of one's own superiority, and a construal of those deemed inferior as dangerous and disgusting or at best pitiable—persisted largely unchallenged, even when expressed in more carefully modulated forms.

It took into the 1980s–1990s to get not just the "euthanasia" murders taken seriously as a mass crime, but also the approximately 400,000 coercive sterilizations—the majority enacted on individuals designated as "feeble-minded"—to be formally acknowledged as an injustice at all, and the tens of thousands of (often deeply traumatized) survivors offered even the most insultingly meager amount of recognition and recompense.[9] It was not until the post-reunification mid-1990s that a statement insisting that no one may be discriminated against on grounds of disability was put into Germany's Basic Law.[10] And it took just about as long for a novel albeit still fragile agreement to be consolidated that saw as equally entitled also those with the most severe impairments, with all that such a reconceived understanding should entail for the necessary financial and infrastructural investments in educational and welfare-care policy and practices at all levels.[11] It would take into the twenty-first century for acknowledgment of all the crimes against the disabled to be integrated more fully into government declarations and legislation and into the national memorial landscape. Unlearning eugenics proved to be a very long postfascist process, and it remains unfinished. The battle for dignified and respectful treatment in the everyday, including high-quality pedagogical and assistive services, but also the right to be visibly "out" and participating fully in all aspects of communal life, remains ongoing.[12]

As noted, the disabled were not "forgotten" victims, but rather aggressively repudiated ones. Given the tenacious persistence of antidisability hostility into the postfascist decades, inducing identification with the plight of people with disabilities, especially cognitive impairments or psychiatric diagnoses, turned out to be enormously challenging. Activists' effort, in presenting the murders of people with disabilities as the "trial run for the Judeocide"—in the words of journalist Ernst Klee in the pages of the leading national weekly *Die Zeit* in 1990—was by no means just a summary finding based on his and others' meticulous recovery of a wealth of empirical evidence.[13] It was above all an ethically engaged, passionately pursued strategy for *un-dehumanizing the disabled*, for insisting that their suffering should matter.[14]

Yet however effective in that historic moment this strategic effort had been, it would seem important also to acknowledge that crimes against the disabled (or those labeled as disabled) were crimes that should not require being described as precursor to the Holocaust in order to be treated with due gravity. Moreover, the dynamics of antidisability hostility—the recent coinage "ableism" is too weak a word—then and now, were and are not fully comparable to those of other kinds of prejudice and animus. Disability, after all, as "crip" theorists have been at the forefront of pointing out, is quite unlike all other forms of "otherness."[15]

This is in part due to disability's universal potential—it can happen to anyone—and, simultaneously, to the way it is associated with the most profound vulnerability and dependency and thus often experienced as especially threatening or despicable.[16]

For centuries, however, there have been ramifications particular to ascriptions of significant mental impairment or illness, both because these phenomena destabilize the idealized notion of the autonomous subject and, not least and most enduringly, because of the challenge that these impairments have raised for the expectation of being able to contribute labor to one's community, rather than requiring the labor of care and of support from others. Here especially, mental impairments' distinctive intersectionality with issues of class and the rise of industrial capitalism—including those components of class conflict that manifest as inequality, exploitation, and subjugation—become acutely apparent. For as it happens, the overwhelming majority of cases of intellectual disability, just as of psychological impairments, through the more than a century with which this book is concerned, were to be found among the very poor.

Welfare provision and remedial education, such as they existed, were thus, at all times, inseparable from poverty management, and the subjective experience and the corporeal materiality of intellectual disability alike were if not directly caused then at least exacerbated by such poverty-related dynamics as infectious diseases, insufficiencies of nutrition, environmental hazards, institutional contexts, and the violences of neglect and coercion. This meant that all the ensuing culture-wide controversies over attitudes toward and treatment of individuals with intellectual and psychological impairments would long remain inextricable from matters of economics. (The 10—or at most 15—percent of cognitive impairment that regularly did also appear among the more well-to-do was typically explained either as an unfortunate chance exception to the rule of good mental health in the family or as caused by childhood fevers or mishaps. Nonetheless, and notably, almost every large residential institution established in the later nineteenth century would also offer a *Pensionat*—a dormitory with better amenities—and not infrequently the income generated by taking in, for fees, the disabled progeny of the more prosperous classes would help significantly to finance care for the overwhelming majority of residents from underprivileged backgrounds.) No matter the familial background, however, inadequately exploitable labor power or, worse, complete dependency on care, would always be perceived as a problem involving other people's money, effort, and time. And this in turn would prompt a recurrent obsession with justifying any charitable or state investment in care or education as only tolerable if the outcome was some improved "usefulness." The difficulties that were to ensue for any efforts to articulate the rights of people unable to become "useful" were inescapable—and devastating.

When I first began the research for this book, I had many questions. The scholarship on the three professions that saw the topic of intellectual disability as part of their respective remits—religious charity, remedial pedagogy, and psychiatric medicine—is vast, but the fields and their complex interactions are rarely analyzed in a unified way. And, oddly, not much attention has been paid specifically to the ways in which contemporaries, at each juncture, argued over the value of disabled lives.

Why, in the *post*fascist era, had it still been so agonizingly difficult to find compelling language and to enact concrete policies and practices to defend, or even to cherish, the positive value of disabled lives? Were there no *pre*fascist traditions that could serve as orienting resources for postfascist rebuilding? How far back in history, or how far forward, did one have to go to find people who did not hierarchize human worth? What ways of thinking about human beings with the most severe disabilities had been inherited from the nineteenth century, and how did those inherited ideas come under pressure and need to be revised just as residential institutions and remedial schools alike were rapidly expanding in both number and size after the 1890s? When lawyer Karl Binding and psychiatrist Alfred Hoche, authors in 1920 of a book concerning "Permission to Annihilate Life Unworthy of Life" (*Die Freigabe der Vernichtung lebensunwerten Lebens*)—the text that would later serve as the main template for the Nazi "euthanasia" program—called openly for the murder of the "total idiots" in the population, what kinds of counterarguments had religious leaders or remedial educators tried to put forward?[17] And when German eugenicists—even while conceding they could not be sure of the source of cognitive impairments and that their surmises about "recessive" genetic transmission were simply guesses and projections—debated frenetically in the 1920s–1930s whether it was 1 percent or 10 percent or even 20 percent or more of their fellow citizens who were so subpar they should be prevented from procreating, who (if anyone) in their time was audacious enough to point out that their math and their science alike were faulty?[18] Was it impossible in that moment to see not just how cruel but also how completely absurd were the so widely promoted eugenic fantasies that it could even be feasible to extirpate—by sterilization and / or by murder—imperfection in the body politic?[19] And how, eventually, would those fantasies come to be robbed of their power—if they ever have fully been?

Most immediately, the search for answers drew me into confrontation with a peculiarly durable problem: No matter how blurry the boundaries between ascribed classifications, and no matter how much the comorbidities, the proximate or presumed causes, and / or the applied nomenclature varied over time, people labeled by others as in some way cognitively deficient were continually being ranked along a multilevel scale. By the 1880s, a tripartite system had already been established in which those perceived as most severely disabled were referred to as solely "care-cases," while those more mildly or moderately affected were being sorted into categories as either "educable" or merely "trainable"—capable of some, either independent or supervised, labor. Certainly, the diverse origins of impairments were reflected in divergent symptomologies and, inevitably, over the course of a century and a half, both the causes of impairments and the prospects for prevention and treatment evolved. The changes in how intellectual disability manifested proved to be both concretely material—at once biological and shaped by environmental factors—and conceptual. Unquestionably, there were substantive differences between cretinism, chromosomal anomalies, cerebral palsies incurred in the birth process, brain damage–inducing meningitis or encephalitis in the toddler years, cumulative brain impairments due to epileptic seizures, and more general health deficits caused by vitamin and protein deficiencies (many of which resulted in physical impairments and "disfigurements" as well, leading to ample overlap between those called "cripples" and those deemed to have mental impairment). Yet no less consequential, as I was to discover, would be the epistemological reorientations as psychiatric professionals, after a half-century of disinterest, rushed into the domain of intellectual disability in the 1890s once that domain—because of reorganizations in institutional administration and funding—became a potential source of career and income enhancements. Ultimately, however, no single trend but a rather a concatenation of factors, including major demographic and socioeconomic upheavals, could help explain how the turn into the twentieth century found an abundance of individuals, previously unremarkable, being drawn first gradually and then swiftly into an ever-expanding portion of the populace being somehow deemed "abnormal" and increasingly tagged—not solely by men of medicine but also by religious and educational professionals—with such fresh terminological inventions as "psychopathological inferiority" or "moral feeble-mindedness."

Nonetheless, and despite this welter of ever-evolving logics and new incoherencies, there were over the many decades, I learned as well, also recognizable continuities, and these showed up with regularity in ways both trivial and colossal. As a first baseline point: It matters enormously, for instance, that, as recent scholarship has shown, we grasp that, although there was some overlap between those individuals targeted for sterilization during the Third Reich and those chosen for murder, they largely belonged to different subgroups. Factors that strongly increased the likelihood of being chosen for death included incontinence, epilepsy, high care needs, and "incapacity for work" (or in the case of children, identification as "ineducable"). And while among those selected for coercive sterilization there were indeed individuals whose sensory impairments, such as blindness or deafness, had been identified as heritable, the second-largest category among the sterilized, after "feeble-mindedness," was "schizophrenia" (like "feeble-mindedness," a designation that was not just elastic, but very much based in the subjective impressions of the diagnostician and often assumed to overlap with forms of mental debility). With regard to sterilizations too, "educability" and "ability to work" mattered greatly.[20]

A second crucial point emerged as well. For throughout, recognizing the special challenges confronting those striving to make a case for the rights to life—and more, the rights to engaged attention, and to love, joy, and education—of those so significantly impaired that they would have been targeted for death in the Third Reich, I kept searching to recover whatever traces I could find of advocacy on behalf of people with the most significant intellectual disabilities, whether this advocacy was religiously or secularly inspired. Without preempting evidence and analyses that will be put forward in the chapters that follow, one short version of an answer to my many questions is that I did find, in every era, noteworthy individuals who made urgent and creative arguments in defense of the value also of the lives of those who were more severely or multiply disabled or who simply acted, whether in care provision, education, or advocacy, on those convictions. In other words, a genealogy of radical un-dehumanizers can be constructed. They were always anomalies, but they show what was imaginable and doable and they can be resources for us in the future as well. No less revelatory is how varied their motives and styles were. Some borrowed from the languages of the Enlightenment and antislavery movements; some drew from Jewish tradition, many from Christianity; others, in the postwar decades, drew from Marxism or from antiauthoritarian and countercultural secular humanism. Some deployed sentimentality, others irony or searing sarcasm, yet others earnest rationality. And while sincere faith was vital for some, others—in disgust at what they perceived as Christian paternalism, hypocrisy, or malice—adopted a deliberately sacrilegious vulgarity to get their moral message across. One of the purposes of this book is to honor them and restore to the historical record the arguments they made.

A third point, however, is that overall, it would take a full hundred years—from the 1870s, when the Protestant and Catholic "idiot-institutions" first proliferated across the German landscape, to the 1970s, when a new generation of professionals and activists revolted against what they perceived as an abhorrent preliminary postfascist settlement—before a comprehensive integrationist, antihierarchical, and egalitarian vision would be articulated and, in experimental oases in both East and West, put into lived practice. And a subsidiary, related point is that, ultimately, it would be necessary for passionate *secular* defenses of the full and equal humanity of people with disabilities to be formulated before the mainstream of Protestant and Catholic church and charity spokespeople were provoked to rethink their conceptions of human dignity and worth—their "image of the human" (*Menschenbild*), to use the German term—and to reconceive their praxes accordingly. This was all the more sobering a discovery, given the reputation both churches so proudly promoted in the postwar of having been stalwart stewards of the vulnerable who had vigorously protested against the Nazi killings (even as substantial majorities of their residents met their deaths).

One measure of the enormity of the transformation that has been achieved, particularly over the last twenty years, can be found in the self-evidence with which *both* secular *and* religious advocacy and support organizations working with and for persons with disabilities and impairments have come to take as their bedrock premises the twinned ideals of individual self-determination and full social integration (now called inclusion). As the premier Catholic service organization Caritas assures visitors to its website: "As Caritas we have committed ourselves to enabling as much self-determined participation as possible." Caritas advances the ideal of equal entitlement in all realms of life, including work, leisure, and residential setting; refers to individuals with impairments as "experts in their own right" whose wishes and preferences have consistent priority; strives to decentralize disability services so that full immersion in a multiplicity of ordinary life situations can be facilitated daily; and references as a mandatory touchstone the expansive catalogue of rights enumerated in the UN Convention on the Rights of Persons with Disabilities, ratified by Germany in 2009.[21] Relatedly, the Protestant Diakonie, too, proclaims the import of "self-determined participation in our society" for the "7.8 million people" in Germany living with some type of disability; advances the "adventure of inclusive living" in small-scale supported settings also for individuals with a variety of intellectual impairments; promotes "integrated kindergartens" as a boon for children with and without disabilities alike; regularly identifies inadequacies in extant legislation and proposes corrections that will enhance individual access and entitlements; and sees as among its main tasks the elucidation of the UN Convention's foundational principles of "self-determination, non-discrimination, and acceptance of difference and diversity among people."[22] Meanwhile, the premier secular lobby association Aktion Mensch has proven itself in the past decade ever more imaginatively inventive, especially with clever ads on billboards and in social media, in marketing the beauties, for everyone, of a "barrier-free" society in which bodily and mental differences are celebrated, and in which encounters with, learning from, and social engagement on behalf of differently abled others are great sources of pleasure and meaning.[23] What in the 1970s and 1980s initially had been the demands of a tiny insurgent minority of dedicatedly integrationist radicals has at long last become the officially pronounced cultural consensus. But as will become clear, the path to get to this point was arduously long and filled with innumerable obstacles.[24]

Most Germany-focused disability history written these days is social history, and I too have taken social, political, and economic factors into account wherever they are relevant.[25] Nonetheless, this book is, unapologetically, an intellectual history. All through, I considered the methodological questions raised by battles over knowledge and meaning. In this sense, the book also addresses the problem of history-writing, of the relationship between evidence and interpretation. For in the case of animus and brutality toward people with disabilities, the facts themselves were generally neither unknown nor in dispute; the issue was always what the facts *meant*. One of the through lines of the book, therefore, involves the recurring question of how previously consolidated culture-wide terms of debate can finally tip, whether gradually or abruptly, and what constituencies, what constellation of arguments, and what historic contingencies it takes to redirect a national conversation in one direction or another.

How does the previously unthinkable become thinkable—or even come to seem like common sense? How can doubt finally grow about unquestioned, stubbornly held premises? How do originally unrelated agendas get woven into ongoing conflicts about other matters entirely? What new ways of imagining but also new misunderstandings can arise, and with what (perhaps unintended) consequences? In short, among the distinctive features of this book is the way it centers battles over what counts as truth and considers how multiple pasts and presents are continually colliding, reciprocally reconfiguring each others' meanings. The controversies over intellectual disability, human vulnerability, and interdependence, I suggest, provide an instructive case study giving us insight into how ideological conflicts work more generally.

A further distinctive feature of this book is its particular interest in what the Marxist literary critic Raymond Williams once referred to as "structures of feeling." The issue, he argued, in making sense of any era, was that "we must go beyond formally held and systematic beliefs, though of course we have always to include them." The more difficult but important thing to get at, Williams urged, was "meanings and values as they are actively lived and felt. . . . elements of impulse, restraint, and tone; specifically affective elements of consciousness and relationships: not feeling against thought, but thought as felt and feeling as thought."[26] This meant, for me, always again reading the primary sources both with and against the grain, noticing tone and mood, metaphors chosen, passing references, scenes of sudden intensity, and seemingly odd asides.[27] It meant as well taking seriously, as pertinent historically, such diverse phenomena as: fierce rivalry between the professions concerned with disability; mystical assumptions about the relationship between the disabled and the divine; innumerable expressions of regret, frustration, disappointment, resentment, and defensiveness; fantasies about the sexuality of others; and an apparently obsessive preoccupation with parent-blaming. But also, and repeatedly: impressive instances of ardent partisanship and imaginative dedication. This book, in sum, can be read as an experiment in writing an intellectual history of intellectual disability—but one that attends throughout to how facts were framed as well as to how emotions were continually being stirred on all sides.

———

In a radio talk delivered in 1966, the Frankfurt School philosopher and sociologist Theodor Adorno made, in passing, a profound observation, and although he was referring to the Holocaust of European Jewry, the insight remains relevant more broadly: "The inability to identify with others was unquestionably the most important psychological condition for the fact that something like Auschwitz could have occurred in the midst of more or less civilized and innocent people." In this text which has since become iconic, although it is one of the most searching, least self-assured of all his writings, Adorno kept circling around the problem of human nature and the mechanisms that induce people to do harm. He struggled to find words to communicate what he experienced, in a postfascist nation to which he had returned from exile in the United States, as a persisting climate of aggressive competitiveness and chilly indifference to the fate of anyone perceived as "weak"—as he worried, too, that the immense sadistic cruelty that Nazism had unleashed with such apparent ease could all too easily erupt again. Adorno diagnosed a vehement disinterest among West Germans in the national past: a widespread tendency "to avoid confronting the horror . . . [and] even rebuke anyone who merely speaks of it." Adorno urged, instead, that it was actually imperative to let the horror "draw near" (as he put it), to let oneself be affected by engagement with it, and to seek to better understand all that had made the Third Reich possible.[28]

One of Adorno's insights was that the objects for humans' tendency to cruelty were demonstrably displaceable and readily interchangeable, as the trouble lay within the perpetrator and their impulse to cause hurt, and not in any purported characteristic of the victims. "Tomorrow," Adorno observed, "a group other than the Jews may come along, say the elderly, who indeed were still spared in the Third Reich, or the intellectuals, or simply deviant groups." But Adorno was concerned as well that the so indispensable capacity "to identify with others" was apparently a rather limited resource, and it was in this context that he mentioned the importance of educating the public to the point that resistance to Nazism, while rare, had in fact been historically possible. Interestingly, this is the one text in all of Adorno's large oeuvre that references the murders of people with disabilities. Adorno explained: "For instance, one should investigate the history of euthanasia murders, which in Germany, thanks to the resistance the program met, was not perpetrated to the full extent planned by the National Socialists." Yet then he segued immediately to remark that in this particular case, alas, "the resistance was limited to the group concerned" (*der Widerstand war auf die eigene Gruppe beschränkt*) and he went on to conclude, in pessimism and sorrow, that "precisely this is a particularly conspicuous, very common symptom of the universal coldness."[29] Adorno assumed, in short, that in the Third Reich those targeted for killing in the "euthanasia" program had been predominantly non-Jewish members of the German Volk—and it was this belonging to the Volk that was the sole reason any objection at all to their murders had arisen.

Far from seeing "euthanasia" and the Holocaust, then, as sequentially or in any other way *connected,* as activists and scholars twenty years into the future would so strenuously underscore, Adorno assumed a sharp *contrast.* The Christian churches, and the German populace as a whole, had been dismayingly silent with regard to the persecution of Germany's and all of Europe's Jews. Jews were that "other" with whom non-Jewish Germans had manifestly failed to identify.

As it turns out, Adorno had it both right and wrong. Von Galen's sermon and the nationwide commotion it caused had certainly seemed to signal broader identification in the citizenry with the plight of people with disabilities and had appeared to prompt Hitler's halt at least to the first phase of "euthanasia" murders, even as the real motivation for Hitler's formal stoppage of the T4 component of the "euthanasia" program was most likely because he needed the churches' and the public's support for the war on the Soviet Union he had launched only two months earlier. Furthermore, Adorno's lack of awareness that, in the second, decentralized phase of "euthanasia," the death toll would be twice that of the six T4 gas chambers was, as of the mid-1960s and for quite a long time thereafter, an ignorance that was widely shared.[30]

Adorno's partial misunderstandings were, however, highly significant for another reason entirely, for his indecisiveness over whether people with disabilities were outsiders or insiders to the Volk was in itself extraordinarily telling. *Were* popular unrest about and Christian leaders' protest against the "euthanasia" killings in fact examples of that vital ability to identify across group boundaries—to empathize with those marked as "other," to imagine oneself in their place, and to care about their fates—that was (and remains to this day) such a key desideratum for preventing another collapse into barbarism? Or were the disabled (as Adorno presumed) best understood as insiders to the then-dominant in-group, and that was (as Adorno, despondently, implied) the only reason anyone bothered formally to risk advocating on their behalf? To put the question in different terms: Were people with disabilities a rejected "them," or did nondisabled Germans claim the disabled as their "own"— and, if the latter, was it with compassion or with revulsion?

My contention is that the *ambiguity* of the position of those victimized on grounds of cognitive or psychiatric impairment explains so much about the disdain and ferocity to which they were regularly subjected. One of the awful conundrums with which this book is concerned is that while individuals with intellectual disability were all too often demeaned and abjected as an expendable "them," conditions for their education and care did not improve when they came to be perceived as a humiliatingly and infuriatingly large segment of "us." It was, moreover, in this tense situation that the rise of eugenics would prove so multifunctional for its proponents, even as quite a few of those proponents were perfectly well aware of its incoherencies. Eugenics served beautifully as distraction from the extensive collateral damage in a nation undergoing rapid industrialization; it provided flattering, cost-free ego boosts for those lucky enough to be deemed nondeficient; and it offered crudely simplified explanations and readily available scapegoats to focus one's anger when the world seemed unfair. Eugenics, as an explanatory framework legitimating the denigration of individuals deemed disabled, diverted attention from the unremediated socioeconomic inequities and then-untreatable ailments that were the actual causes of the vast majority of disabilities and blamed the victims instead, promoting the flawed premise that intellectual deficiency was biologically hereditary, when in fact it only looked that way because conditions of poverty had been replicating across generations. Fictions and fantasies are no less powerful for being rooted in falsehoods.

This, then, is a book that explores the evolution of historical debates over the value of disabled lives. It is a key argument of *The Question of Unworthy Life* that this topic has relevance for the histories of medicine and psychiatry, theology and religion, welfare and pedagogy, but also for the histories of capitalism and labor and of sexuality and reproduction. Each chapter traces not so much a paradigm shift as a *paradigm struggle*: a conflict over the interpretive framing of facts, and the consequences to be drawn from those interpretations. In arguing with each other over how to think and to feel about—and, in practice, how to treat—fellow citizens with a diverse range of intellectual impairments and psychiatric diagnoses, Germans worked out, over the century and a half since the 1870s, a great deal about their self-understanding as a nation.

1

The Problem of Incurability

Yes, if we still lived in Guggenbühl's time, we would be in a different situation! Then we would be showing you pictures of idiots who, as a result of the labor invested in them, reached the highest levels of human knowledge and skill. But the belief in the curability of idiocy is now a vanquished point of view.

—HEINRICH MATTHIAS SENGELMANN,
DIRECTOR OF THE ALSTERDORFER ANSTALTEN, 1886[1]

HOW WERE those human beings deemed to have intellectual disability spoken about *before* the rise of eugenics—or, as it was called in Germany, "racial hygiene" (*Rassenhygiene*)? We know surprisingly little about this, not least because the historiography, while excellent, has been partitioned.[2] There is extensive and impressive historical scholarship on the dozens of residential institutions for the intellectually disabled founded over the course of the second half of the nineteenth century and into the first decades of the twentieth—the majority of them affiliated with the Protestant and Catholic churches, a handful with the Jewish faith community, and others state-sponsored.[3] There has additionally been outstanding work done on the rise of remedial education (*Hilfsschulpädagogik* or, later, *Heilpädagogik*) across the German lands, as the field began to professionalize from the 1880s on and hundreds of German cities and towns established remedial schools.[4] And there is an efflorescence of superb work on the history of psychiatry in Germany as physicians arrived on the scene belatedly in the 1890s not only to assert expertise with regard to diverse manifestations of mental illness (which had been their concern all along) but also to claim authority with regard to phenomena of cognitive impairment, behavioral disorder, or potential delinquency.[5]

These three bodies of historiography, however, remain to this day strangely separate and disconnected from each other—even though the three sensemaking systems of theology, pedagogy, and medicine that are their foci actually had been continuously arguing with, borrowing from, and ultimately blurring into each other. Indeed, it is in the complex competition and interaction *between* these sensemaking systems that the content and contours of what was already by the 1850s called "the idiot-question" (*die Idiotenfrage*) came to cohere.[6] The very notion of intellectual disability has always been a historically variable, fundamentally unstable concept. Its boundaries are by no means self-evident, but rather were (and remain) continually re-elaborated. Yet it was precisely in the contested terrain of conflict among and between clergymen, teachers, and doctors over the meaning and treatment of intellectual disability that terms of debate were established that ultimately consolidated the othering and intensified the stigmatization of the very human beings that all three constituencies claimed as their professional domain. This is the story this chapter will tell.

One of the great difficulties of a history of ideas about intellectual disability—and of the even more elusive and essential matters of attitudes, emotions, and practices surrounding those so categorized—is that, with very few exceptions, the human beings that are being talked about remain silent in the sources. Sometimes, they can speak to us without words—as for instance in a photo, if we look closely, we may suddenly discern their mutual care and therewith their luminous rebuttal, simply by lived example, to the oblivious disregard in which they were so often held (see figure 1.1). Yet such finds are rare. More typical is that in the (very few) instances when people labeled as intellectually limited are quoted directly or their perspectives are in some other way imagined and represented, it is done to prove either their deficiency or their (however slight) potential. In other words, their voices and

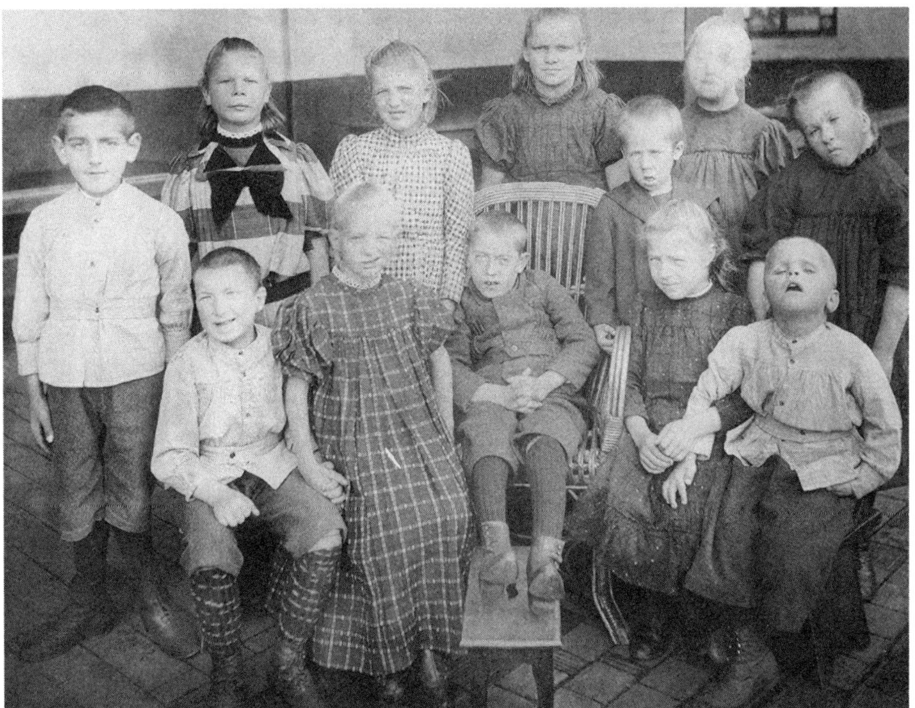

FIGURE 1.1. At the Wittekindshof in 1904. We have so few accounts of institutional residents' experiences from their own perspectives. We can immediately appreciate how finely these children, almost all of impoverished origins, have been dressed for the photographer's visit. A second, closer look, reveals more: Two children hold hands and another two are interlinking arms. They are giving each other care—and therewith communicate to us across more than a century. Archiv der Diakonischen Stiftung Wittekindshof.

perspectives are usually there to sustain an argument being put forward by the experts who do the talking. Nonetheless, even these instances can be quite revealing.

Moreover, it bears emphasizing that there truly was an extraordinary amount of *talking about* people deemed intellectually disabled, and a great deal of that talking was published. Already by the end of the nineteenth century, there were thousands of professional journal articles and dozens of books about every imaginable aspect of the topic of intellectual disability. There were promotional materials to persuade and engage the public and politicians, like fundraising newsletters and annual reports from the residential institutions that already by 1900 housed 20,000 citizens of all ages (and by 1910 housed more than 34,000).[7] There were records of the conferences of the directors of the residential institutions (and subsequently also of remedial schoolteachers and the psychiatrists) as they made presentations and debated with each other over both the causes of intellectual disability and its proper treatment. The source base is substantial.

In Guggenbühl's Time

What happens when we read the nineteenth- and early twentieth-century sources that speak about intellectual disability from *all three* conceptual vantages together, with and against each other? A good starting point for understanding the intricate intersections of religion, pedagogy, and medicine is the case of Swiss physician Johann Jakob Guggenbühl (1816–1863), one of the earliest advocates for educational and therapeutic intervention on behalf of individuals with intellectual disabilities. In 1841, Guggenbühl had founded, near Interlaken in the Swiss Alps, a residential school for children with cognitive challenges. He had maintained that, with fresh mountain air, nutritious food, innovative pedagogy, and the lavishing of sincere love, he could assist children afflicted by "cretinism." (Now known to be caused by iodine deficiency during pregnancy, in the nineteenth century cretinism was one of the major forms in which severe intellectual disability manifested—even as its distinctive visible physical symptoms proved difficult to distinguish from those caused by the many early childhood diseases and vitamin deficiencies so common in conditions of poverty.) All of Guggenbühl's children improved in physical health; some acquired skills in reading, writing, and basic arithmetic; others simply learned rudimentary self-expression. He quickly became an extraordinary inspiration, also internationally. His school, the Abendberg, rapidly became a pilgrimage site. Many national "firsts" in residential intellectual disability education—from the United States to England, Denmark, the Netherlands, and Sardinia—came explicitly to be modeled on Guggenbühl's

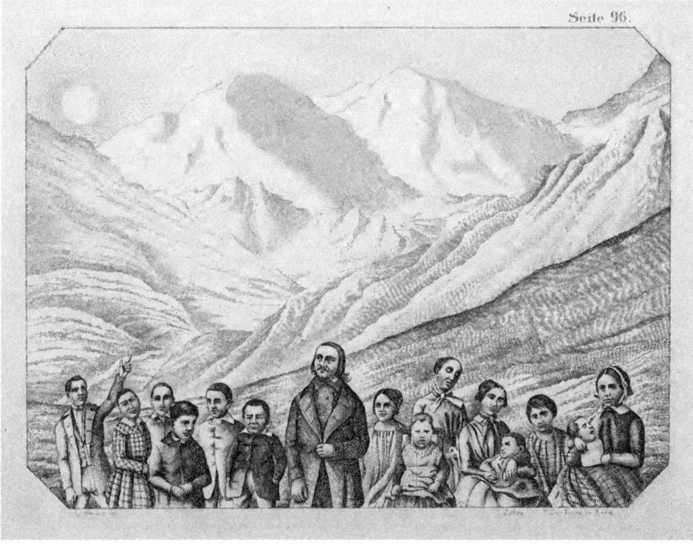

FIGURE 1.2. Dr. Johann Jakob Guggenbühl at the Abendberg with two teachers and a dozen of the pupils, from *Die Heilung und Verhütung des Cretinismus und ihre neuesten Fortschritte* (The Remedying and Prevention of Cretinism and their Latest Advances, Bern 1853). The image is a photogravure print, a precursor process to photography. Guggenbühl wrote that the younger children were not included in the picture because they would not have been able to hold still for the requisite 30 seconds. He announced that he intended to accompany all future accounts of his work with photographic images—"so as to make the condition and the step-by-step development of the children receiving treatment on the Abendberg clearer to the eye than any mere description can." Guggenbühl's aim, in addition to therapeutic treatments (e.g., herbal baths, massages, cod liver oil, music-making, gymnastics, and above all "love and kindness," was "to do battle for the human rights of these unhappy ones"—"in accordance with the model of the English 'Antislavery Society.'"

project. He was made an honorary member of scientific societies from Marseille to St. Petersburg.[8]

Guggenbühl's significance in prompting compassion and motivating practical action cannot be underestimated (figure 1.2). His fervent insistence on the dignity and equality of the disabled was inextricable from his stress on the redeeming effects of genuine affection. For him, "the first requirement" was "to treat the children with love and thereby win their love."[9] He had an explicitly human rights framework—insisting that "the immortal soul is essentially the same in every creature born of woman" and comparing his own efforts on behalf of children with intellectual disabilities to the British philanthropist William Wilberforce's efforts to abolish slavery.[10] In addition, Guggenbühl, in his insistence on seeing the children, no matter how physically and mentally impaired, as profoundly precious, emphasized that those with significant cognitive disabilities also nonetheless possessed a distinctive feeling for the spiritual realm—often even more, he argued, than "healthy" children did.[11] In sum, Guggenbühl was at once a medical professional, a pedagogue, *and* an individual deeply motivated by religion.

However, by the early 1850s, Guggenbühl already faced accusations that he was a self-aggrandizing charlatan or just had a maudlin, overactive religious imagination. As he traveled widely to advance the cause, visitors discovered that in his absence, children had been left in the hands of underqualified staff. Claims of impressive progress made by individual pupils turned out to be overblown, supporting the stance of those who were intent on arguing that "idiocy" could never be remediated and that all educational efforts were futile and an improper allocation of energy and funds. Mocked as especially absurd was Guggenbühl's conviction that disabled children had a particular relationship to the divine.[12] In 1858, after an official investigation by Swiss authorities, the Abendberg would be closed down.[13] He died in ignominy several years later.

Still, Guggenbühl was by no means the only early experimenter in intellectual disability education; there were other remarkable individuals who launched schools or small residential institutions. Whether these were founded by physicians (like Adolf Albrecht Erlenmeyer in Bendorf near Koblenz, or Carl Heinrich Rösch in Württemberg) or teachers, particularly those who had specialized in education for "deaf-mutes" and then adapted their methods for intellectual disability (like Carl W. Saegert in Berlin or Ferdinand Kern in Saxony): They all conceded frankly from the start (as had Guggenbühl) that curing idiocy was impossible, but that with good nutrition and basic hygiene they could achieve improvements in their students' overall physical health, and that with patience and creative educational approaches they could achieve some progress in intellectual abilities and general comportment.[14]

Another early innovator was the French (later American) physician and educator Édouard Séguin.[15]

Many of their ideas, like Guggenbühl's, remain valuable to this day. Among their suggestions: strengthening weak muscles with exercise; stimulating the senses with tastes and smells and sounds; encouraging the exercise of self-expression and will; considering their pupils developmentally, as one would with an infant; providing one-on-one attention and establishing a trusting relationship; turning seemingly meaningless self-stimulating activities into more meaningful and intersubjectively interactive ones; working intensively on relating words not just to pictures but to the concrete objects they named and emphasizing those objects' uses; refusing to isolate the cognitively disabled from nondisabled people; reducing desk learning and spending more time outdoors in nature; and keeping institutions small and family-size, with a teacher and his wife as houseparents, taking in no more than twelve boys and girls and sharing in their daily lives.[16] Nevertheless, later practitioners would view these predecessors as being mostly worthy of dismissal for having had unrealistic expectations.

The backlash against Guggenbühl, the Abendberg, and everything it stood for would be sustained and deeply consequential for the practice of intellectual disability education and care. In all his contradictory infamy, he took on strikingly strong symbolic significance. Ignoring the impressive pedagogical insights of other early pioneers or alluding to them only indirectly (and often inaccurately), commentators well into the 1880s–1890s instead obsessively referenced the Guggenbühl model of how to do intellectual disability care as shorthand for everything that had gone wrong with the entire enterprise. Therefore, that enterprise came to be understood as self-evidently requiring complete reconception. The repudiation of Guggenbühl would become more decisive for the trajectory of intellectual disability care across the German-speaking lands than his original inspiration had been.[17]

Everyone involved as advocates for disability education, training, or care, for decades, appeared to need to accuse *others* of having at one time claimed that they could provide a cure—and self-distancing from the simultaneously embarrassingly overpromising and unabashedly cretin-adoring Guggenbühl was a straightforward way to express this. By projecting onto Guggenbühl a claim about the "curability" of intellectual disability—a claim that, it bears reiterating, neither he nor any of the other early experimenters had made—all subsequent practitioners, no matter their disciplinary background (religious, pedagogic, or medical), felt justified in substituting a new goal. This was the goal of making people deemed cognitively impaired "useful" (*nützlich, brauchbar, tauglich*), rather than a future "burden" on society.[18]

Most remarkably, and however perversely, this substitute goal of usefulness (*Nützlichkeit*) was clung to even as all who invoked it were continually forced to concede that *it too* was never being adequately met. Rather than accepting that some human beings were vulnerable and challenged but that, with engagement and supports, their lives could be ameliorated, the language of "usefulness" would continue to pervade every aspect of debate in and around the residential institutions and remedial schools, even as both continued to grow.

The self-distancing from Guggenbühl and his early experiment high in the Swiss mountains, then, functioned, at a minimum, in two ways. The self-distancing served as a means to tamp down expectations. But then again, by presenting one's own pedagogical ambitions as *both more honest and more modest* than those of this notorious predecessor, expectations could also be raised again and ongoing sponsorship and sympathy secured from politicians and the public alike. And possibly there was a third element. For distinguishing oneself from Guggenbühl allowed the speaker or author to convey just a whiff of ambivalence about the injunction to be loving—especially toward those who were most severely disabled.

The uncritically accepted preoccupation with the goal of "usefulness" would also involve a continual concern with definitions and categorizations and a constant reflex of *hierarchizing* residents and pupils. For, over and over, the children and adults deemed cognitively damaged would be subdivided into three classes according to their alleged educability and / or trainability. This concept of "usefulness" and the practice of sorting became fused, and thereby determined the distribution of individuals either into the residential institutions or the remedial schools.

So too by the 1890s this concept and that practice resulted inexorably in differential treatment and levels of care *within* all the residential institutions. And, first gradually and tentatively, then with great speed, within a quarter of a century, or by 1915 at the latest, the hierarchical valuations would be expressed in terms of deepening alarm over the perceived deteriorating cognitive health of the nation as a whole.[19] By this time, the frame through which intellectual disability was understood had become racialized.

The Rise and Crises of the Institutions and Schools

From its origins in the 1850s, driven by a revivalist piety that understood care for the disadvantaged as the practical side of church duties, the necessary complement to that promulgation of the gospel that came from the pulpit, Protestant charity activism organized under the auspices of the Protestant Inner Mission avidly attended to the needs of the psychiatrically ill, prisoners and ex-prisoners, the alcohol-dependent, and potentially wayward youth perceived to require rescue. Individuals with intellectual disabilities were, as all parties seemed to agree, "the most abandoned among the wretched," "unhappy creatures," "the poorest among the poor."[20] The field of their care was "one of the very last to develop."[21] The ensuing proliferation of confessional institutions that provided a haven for individuals with intellectual disabilities especially from the 1870s on—against, as was continually reasserted, the apparently insuppressible reflexes of ridicule and cruelty of fellow citizens— did a great deal to help to make this theretofore only fuzzily delimited group of the needy acquire contours and content *as* a group in the public imagination.[22]

In the midst of all the enthusiasm for founding and enlarging residential institutions, however, the topic of lack of gratification was peculiarly conspicuous. The Lord Mayor of Frankfurt / Main, Johannes Miquel, welcoming to his city the directors' conference in 1886, noted matter-of-factly in his greeting to the gathering that of all the many arenas in which "active love of humanity and care for our suffering brothers" was flourishing, "surely the care of idiots is one of the most difficult and sacrifice-filled." He went on: "You, sirs, do not consistently experience the delight in amazing results in the healing and further development of those committed to your care that is enjoyed by those who are directors of institutions for the deaf-mute, institutions for the blind, or even the asylums for the insane." Still, Miquel expressed optimism that the newly bounteous proliferation of residential institutions consecrated to care for individuals with intellectual disability—by 1886, more than 4,000 children were being cared for by a staff of 800 in three dozen institutions—did not serve only to "alleviate the suffering of these afflicted ones" and "secure for them an improved physical and mental existence," but "also often in a not inconsiderable way enables a higher development of the individuals concerned, and above all unburdens the tormented families and thereby in all directions spreads blessing."[23]

Two (intertwined) themes in these remarks are noteworthy. One was the alleged difficulty of the *labor* of care. The other was the perplexity regarding the *aim* of care.

With respect to the first point, it was precisely the perceived—or at least perpetually announced—difficulty of leaning in with love and devotion that fostered the conviction among many residential institution directors that deep religious faith was a necessary precondition for the provisioning of care services. The pious orientation was, without question, sincere; worship practices structured daily life and the rhythms of weeks and years; attestations of faith were expected of staff and routinely conveyed to donors and "friends" of the institutions. Nonetheless, admissions of discomfort about the giving of care were (in hindsight disconcertingly, but already in their moment noticeably) frequent even in faith talk. The work could be "heavy, sour, disgusting, often thankless."[24] "It will never be possible to find staff who will at least to some extent do their duty" without an emphasis on "the strengthening of Christian character," and / or if staff were not filled with "God's spirit."[25] This conviction, however inadvertently, held insulting implications for the cared-for. But it had the additional effect of creating a durable association in the public mind between religiosity and nurture of the weak—an association that would become consequential for multiple reasons.

The Protestants were in the lead from the start, and although Catholics followed with some delay—in fact often inspired by religious rivalry, intent on not being outdone—Protestants would continue for decades to dominate the field of care for the disabled, both in sheer numbers and in their vocal role in regional and national discussions and negotiations with government officials. The staff at the Protestant charity institutions was composed largely of deaconesses, unmarried women pledging themselves to lives of faith and service (not irrelevantly, a highly affordable workforce), and a smaller number of deacons, also called "brothers," who were permitted to marry but similarly committed to provision of care for vulnerable populations. Nonetheless, especially the *Kulturkampf* of the 1870s–1880s had the ironic result—as male and female Catholic religious orders were driven out of the education of nondisabled children—of integrating Catholics more deeply into disability services; monasteries and convents were reorganized into residential institutions, and religious orders advertised themselves as well equipped to receive and provide nurture especially for afflicted Catholics.[26] A female Franciscan order in the Rhineland, for instance, promoted their offerings thus in 1883: "In particular, it is our endeavor to give the mentally weak children who are capable of being cured and educated that education and training through which they are put in a position to return to their families as useful or at least quiet members, and to earn their livelihood at least partially through work corresponding to their abilities."[27] The careful phrasings ("who are capable," "useful or at least quiet," "at least partially") would prove indicative.

Here, then, was the problem of the aim of care. Inherent in all the discussion was the assumption—ever frustrated, ever reiterated—that the purpose of the residential institutions was to make their residents "useful." At the same time, apparently there was a constantly felt need to manage public expectation. As early as 1880, an argument had broken out at the residential institution directors' conference over whether the institutions did or did not prepare their residents for independent self-support in the outside world. One pastor-director (from Neinstedt in Saxony-Anhalt) had remarked to his colleagues that the notion "that feebleminded people could be helped in earnest to partake in the struggle for existence and become useful members of society" was not realistic. "After the experiences which we have had in Neinstedt with 300 imbeciles, it is impossible." Or again: "The opinion that imbeciles could be developed into useful members of human society is highly dubious."[28] At this point his peers still expressed vigorous disagreement. But only six years later, the directors agreed collectively to modify their association's mission statement. "The task of idiot-training- and education-institutions is to strengthen and develop further the weakened and restricted mental forces of their charges as well as to make them useful for practical life" was now amended to insert the qualifying words *"insofar as is possible"* before the word "useful" (so as "to prevent misunderstandings among laypeople").[29] In 1894, the teacher-director at a Catholic institution in Essen in the Rhineland estimated that only 5 percent of his residents could be self-supporting on the outside.[30] By 1904, a teacher at the Alsterdorfer Anstalten could reference as a noncontroversial assessment that "only a vanishingly small number of children will be so improved in the institutions that they can return to life in public."[31] Institutionalization, initially designed to be the means to an end of self-support, had within a matter of decades become the end in itself.

Already by 1889, as the residential institution system burgeoned, the habit of sorting and hierarchizing had been formalized. At the top of the hierarchy were those called "feeble-minded" (*schwachsinnig*); these individuals were considered only mildly disabled and hence believed to be properly "educable." In the middling group were those deemed moderately disabled and therefore at least "trainable" (*erziehungsfähig*) in simple work tasks or occupational therapy. And at the bottom of the hierarchy were those defined as most severely disabled, and thereby relegated to being solely "care-cases" (*Pflegefälle*). However, to add to the general confusion, the word "idiot" was for a long time used as an umbrella term to encompass *all* of those deemed cognitively limited. And there would be in addition a continually ongoing recalibration— sometimes a splitting into yet finer subgroupings, sometimes a re-lumping together of categories that had just previously, with considerable effort, been distinguished.[32] Along these lines, for instance, at the top of the hierarchy, commentators worried about the affront implied in the term "feeble-minded," proposing that those who were thought to do better in remedial schools, and to have no need for residential placement, should instead be given the less demeaning moniker "feebly-abled" (*schwachbefähigt*).[33] Or, as the Catholic institution director referred to the higher-functioning ones, these could be labeled the "not-really idiots" (*uneigentliche Idioten*), or simply "poorly gifted."[34]

For those identified as "care-cases" unable to be made in any way "useful," the stigma was strong. These would increasingly be segregated, both in the imagination and literally, into separate buildings or wards. Interest in debating how most effectively to provide them with stimulating and meaningful lives dissipated. The fact of their ongoing existence was increasingly documented primarily in the context of resigned acceptance or defensive regrets about what proportion of them (as much as 30–50 percent) were requiring room in a particular institution, and directors regularly urged that they should be kept apart from the "trainable" others.[35] In an unguarded moment—speaking to an audience on the occasion, in 1889, of the founding of a new preparatory school for deaconesses—one director noted that "spiritual death" (*der geistige Tod*) reigned in the wards harboring those who were most disabled; all the more important, then, he noted, that deaconesses should rotate the care, to avoid exhaustion from this "purely negative labor."[36] And that same year, in another setting, he remarked that he did "not believe that any of us present here would want his institution to be purely a care-institution."[37] By the 1900s, it was unexceptional to find one teacher-director announcing boldly at the directors' conference that it was high time for "a strict cleansing of the training-institutions" to remove "those imbeciles who are solely needful of care" and who could be accommodated "either in the institutions for the insane, or in asylums built specifically for them."[38]

Yet the large middling group of the "trainable" was also perpetually being described as a disappointment. A continually renewed hope and obsession was directed toward guiding those thought to be afflicted with moderate cognitive disabilities into some sort of practical tasks— at the very least, and however tautological the premise, tasks that might helpfully serve the perpetuation of the institution (whether in agriculture or kitchen, sheltered workshops, darning rooms, laundry, or dormitory). By the early twentieth century this in turn would open the institutions to accusations of reluctance to release their charges back to a life in freedom, as those who had become most effective in their labor within the institution became in practice depended-upon—precisely in order to sustain the many in the middling group who could not contribute much and hence would be exceedingly vulnerable on their own.[39]

Or, to put it another way: The less disabled and therewith the more likely to be capable of succeeding, with proper supports, in the outside world, the more valuable for the institution and the more likely to be retained. Work, in short, was not just a marker of value. It could be both therapy and exploitation at once.

Furthermore, due in no small part to the growing custom of retaining residents longer into adulthood, the institutions kept expanding. Institutions that had begun as a small cluster of family-size homes had built up multiple on-site workshops as well as bought up tracts of agricultural land and established entire residential "work-teaching-colonies" (*Arbeiterlehrkolonien*, or simply *Kolonien*). The purpose was to provide supervised labor opportunities for adolescents and adults who had made some gains but were expected to have difficulties supporting themselves independently and—no less important, institutional self-sufficiency being a sincerely held ideal—to help sustain the food needs of the ever-increasing numbers of residents and staff and even ideally to produce items that could be marketed to the public for some small profit.[40] Painfully paradoxical as well was that the very industrial revolution engendering extensive social upheaval and widespread urban and rural poverty was also reducing the number of farmers or independent craft masters who might be willing, in a kind of foster care arrangement, to take in a "simple" apprentice or housemaid after he or she was discharged, at least somewhat "improved" (*gebessert*), from a residential setting.[41] Meanwhile, some institution directors were so concerned about the personal (sexual) safety of their intellectually disabled female institutional "graduates" that they argued for keeping these women institutionalized permanently; this was presented as in the residents' best interest.[42]

In short: First a handful of houses; soon little villages. The Protestant Inner Mission and by the turn of the twentieth century also, though not quite as expansively, the parallel organization of the Catholic Caritas, were building entire counter-worlds to industrial modernity.[43]

The tripartite scheme would remain durable even as the numbers ballooned. In 1889, of the 6,000 residents then in institutions across the German lands, 2,400 were receiving education, 1,850 were being occupied with work-tasks (*beschäftigt*), and 1,700 were "only objects of care" (*sind nur Gegenstand der Pflege*).[44] Already fifteen years later, in 1904, the population of individuals institutionalized on grounds of cognitive difficulty had almost quadrupled—while the proportion of these being educated dropped: 22,949 residents, of whom 5,223 were being taught, 8,276 employed in some kind of occupational therapy or work within their institutions, and 9,450 "solely needful of care."[45]

Meanwhile, and even as initially the institutions had found themselves in rivalry with the remedial schools, the demand for the schools far outstripped the preliminary supply, and town after town launched first remedial classes and soon entire remedial schools. All through the 1880s, at the triannual conferences of institution directors—which some remedial school teachers also attended—there had been unpleasantly frank conversations about perceived competition. Directors—whether they were themselves doctors, pastors, or pedagogues—openly lamented that the remedial schools grabbed up "the better material," "the invigorating elements," leaving the residential institutions with the less capable, more difficult-to-teach pupils.[46] Extended discussions ensued about (as one essay title had it) "which children belong in the remedial schools and which in the idiot-institutions."[47] At times, the directors affirmed with eagerness the possibility of collaboration and averred that pedagogical concerns were shared—indeed, many of the teachers employed at the new schools had gotten their first practical experience working within the institutions—or they admitted that there was need enough to go around for everyone to meet.[48] At other points there was significant anxiety among the directors that their institutions would become entirely "custodial."[49]

The ascendant class of remedial school teachers did not just share the institution directors' habit of hierarchizing, but in asserting to municipal politicians—as well as to their peers who taught typical children—the signal importance of their own novel specialization, they also lamented how strenuous their labors were, and went on to pathologize the very children they aimed to make into their target audience. In the upsurge of professional journal articles and books on intellectual disability pedagogy there was a striking amount of complaint that somehow other teachers were misrepresenting their pupils' achievements, and there were numerous calls for teachers to be forced to demonstrate more honestly how they arrived at their results.[50] One of the more critically self-reflective teachers meditated in an 1898 essay on the urgent desires of remedial teachers for at least "a *mite* of recognition," because "successes" were so sparse and teachers yearned to experience themselves as effective.[51] But as scholars studying the history of remedial pedagogy and its place in the management of the nineteenth-century "social question" have analyzed, leading spokesmen in the emergent discipline of remedial pedagogy went to considerable rhetorical lengths to disparage the remedial school child even as that child was constructed as a "discussion-worthy object"—and even as much of what remedial education was intended to inculcate were the normative values of punctuality, discipline, and obedient work behavior. Thus, for instance, pedagogue Heinrich Kielhorn, addressing the conference of public school teachers in 1887—the first speech to promote to a national audience the idea of a Germany-wide web of remedial schools—pursued a series of steps to call into being a new type of child and a new site located between the custodial institution on the one side and the regular public school on the other. Kielhorn invoked the working-class family as inevitably through ignorance failing a developmentally delayed child, described that "mentally limited" child as more of an "animal-like" rather than "spiritual" being, stressed the vulnerability of such a child to a slide into criminality, but then on the other hand went on to distinguish the "feebly abled" child from the "idiots, imbeciles and cretins" who belonged in residential institutions. Strikingly, in the midst of all the pathologizing, Kielhorn urged his listeners to take inspiration from "Our Lord

Jesus Christ, the teacher of all teachers, who saw how morally and mentally degenerated the people were, but did not turn away from his so deeply sunken people. . . . He reached out his hand and sought to raise up, what lay prostrate so miserably. To us He calls out: Go and do likewise!" Kielhorn mobilized *both* the language of science (alluding to the themes of cultural degeneration and the Darwinian bugaboo of a "struggle for existence") *and* of religious piety.[52]

By the later 1890s, as the field of remedial education was professionalizing, religious language continued to be invoked, albeit in inconsistent ways. In addition, novel allusions to more biological matters appeared in asides. At least two hundred teachers were by the turn of the century self-defining as specialists in remedial education. They organized their own conferences, published in new specialized journals and in book form, promoted various pedagogical approaches, and attempted to assert their rights as qualified experts to regularized pay and pensions as well as class sizes restricted to twenty-five pupils at most (public school classrooms could have as many as sixty).[53] The wrangling over whether particular types of children belonged in residential care or in remedial schools did not stop.[54] But an old theme already voiced in the 1850s in reaction to Guggenbühl—that "idiocy" was simply not remediable with education—was refurbished for the new era. Efforts at adapting pedagogy for those in that vast, vague middling range between the normal and the imbecilic was a fool's errand, as critics delighted in saying.

"Teaching the feebleminded is the field where the teacher can 'run himself ragged' and still achieve hardly anything," an author writing in the flagship journal, *Zeitschrift für die Behandlung Schwachsinniger und Epileptischer*, averred. Like Kielhorn before him, this author clarified that he was not speaking about those "imbeciles" who "only eat and sleep" and whose life flows on "in primitive form," but rather about "the feeble-minded, the half-stupid," that had *some* mental capacities, and were thus, in his view, even more socially dangerous. These more moderately disabled individuals should not be given school instruction, but rather be engaged in practical projects like agriculture. "Instead of spending long years investigating and experimenting with what can with enormous strain for teachers and pupils alike be stuffed into these beings," one should rather think about what *not* to teach them, he proposed. Above all, these people needed constant supervision and certainly should not be permitted to reproduce. What they most needed was "simple work, simple duties, a simple way of life": "Our Lord God has provided well for all. To want to give the feeble-minded freedom and education is to meddle with His handiwork."[55]

Among the attempts at responses, a prominent Dresden-based remedial school teacher, while praising remedial schools as the practical implementation of Jesus's statement, "Whatever you did for one of the least of these, you did for me" (Matthew 25:40), went on to question the rural idyll the author had painted, even as, in his rebuttal, he reinforced the notion that reproduction of the disabled was in fact a major concern. If they were kept illiterate and solely tasked with pasturing the livestock and mowing the meadows, he asked, "Would not the feeble-minded, who have a strong sexual drive, be even more in danger in the rural areas, if we do not do everything humanly possible for them? If we were to take [the author's] point of view, then we'd have to draw the consequences . . . and combat and impede the conceiving of children. . . . This is only possible if the feeble-minded remain to the end of their days in closed institutions." In the remedial schools in Dresden, this teacher continued, hundreds of children had already been educated. "How large the institutions would have to be and how high the costs, if one wanted to move toward a wholly locked-up system!" By providing education in the remedial schools, he asserted, adolescents not only learned functional skills needed to hold down a modest job, but also acquired habits of a moral (i.e., sexually restrained) way of life.[56] This ambivalent defense of remedial education—that it was necessary because it taught good work habits and personal restraint—laid bare the class conflict dimension of the project, even as the provocation to which that defense was directed insisted that education served no purpose. It is no surprise, then, that in 1910 another author would once again raise for general consideration the question, "How shall we deal with the views about the uselessness of teaching the feebleminded?"[57]

And even as the field of remedial education grew dramatically in the first decade of the twentieth century—by 1910, 270 cities and towns had established remedial day schools, in which 25,000 children were receiving instruction—uncertainty about whether to call practical training for work "education" and indecision about the best arguments for justifying education of any kind remained palpable.[58] Also by 1910, 226 residential institutions had become home to 34,400 citizens of all ages. In short, ten years into the twentieth century, as one author surveying the latest statistics was pleased to affirm, close to 60,000 "mentally weak" German citizens were receiving either charity- or government-sponsored services, whether in the form of education, training, or care.[59] Not everyone, however, took this state of affairs as a positive sign of the direction in which Germany was heading.

Racial Hygiene and Death Wishes

While for some commentators, the highlighting of escalating numbers of human beings in need of residential care or remedial schooling functioned as a clarion call to further engaged professional intervention, a number of other observers were starting to conceive of the masses of the needy as a grave menace to the body politic. Nonetheless, a shared language to express the point had not yet fully cohered across disciplinary and ideological divides. The idea that the German "race" as a unified entity might be in danger was just beginning to be debated more broadly. The occasional references to the perils of "reproduction" by individuals with intellectual disability remained scattered. And the notion that intellectual disability was itself a "heritable" condition was by no means fully ensconced.

What characterized the conversation between the 1890s and the 1910s was a paradoxical coexistence of competing frameworks for understanding intellectual disability. A variety of stigmatizing ways of "othering" the disabled (whether these were expressed in long-standing habits of compassion-*cum*-condescension or in more novel economistic-utilitarian or psychiatric-pathologizing terms) were joined by a (first tentative and then dramatic) tendency to articulate hostility to the disabled also in the form of an "us-ing": interpreting the increasing numbers of individuals deemed mentally abnormal as a weakness, or even an illness, *within* the Volk. Most significantly, however, ambivalences long inherent in the projects of both residential care and remedial education were spectacularly exacerbated by very concrete, material pressures. The ensuing transformation in the discourse on intellectual disability was overdetermined. Many different—many utterly uncontrollable—developments came together.

The numbers of people designated as requiring either residential institutionalization or remedial education were booming for multiple reasons. Not only—though also—exponential demographic growth and migration from rural areas to overcrowded urban centers (some cities tripled or even quadrupled in size within a matter of decades, as the overall population surged), but also law and policy changes at the highest governmental levels—initiated by the Prussians and then emulated by other states—directly incentivized institutionalization both by reorganizing funding procedures and by identifying new groups deemed to require it (such as adolescents perceived to be at risk of delinquency).[60] As private philanthropy was no longer adequate and governments accepted greater responsibility for financing disability care, understanding it also as a poverty management tool, an additional policy shift—again pioneered in Prussia—took power away from the pastors (or priests) and pedagogues who for decades had run the residential institutions and conferred it on a rising professional class of psychiatrists.[61] At the time utterly counterintuitive, in view of the fact that physicians in that medical subspecialty had been aggressively disinterested in "idiocy," believing it was in no way related to their remit of "insanity," this decision proved to be extraordinarily consequential.[62] Newly emboldened and seeing an excellent opportunity for extending their research sphere, psychiatrists reversed course and abruptly redefined mental disability as a subset of mental illness—the very move they had for so long resisted.[63] Meanwhile, dozens of residential institutions long involved in intellectual disability care began, again at government encouragement, to target a whole new category of individuals for compulsory institutionalization—"difficult-to-manage" (*schwer erziehbare*) or "neglected" (*verwahrloste*) youth—leading to new pragmatic problems in maintaining discipline but also to increasing cross-professional discussion about the manifold overlaps between poverty, potential for delinquency, behavioral challenges, mental deficiency, and mental illness.[64]

A complex discursive convergence was taking place, as psychiatrists, pedagogues, and pastors or priests came, each via their own circuitous routes, to concur that there were persons situated at the suddenly blurry borders between mental illness, mental disability, and potential delinquency who were their shared concern. Fresh diagnostic labels— including especially the novel coinages of "psychopathic inferiority" (*psychopathische Minderwertigkeit*) and "moral feeble-mindedness" (*moralischer Schwachsinn*)—would bring even more theretofore unattended-to groups of individuals into the purview of residential institutions and remedial schools.[65] The receptiveness among religious charity leaders to an expansion of diagnostic language—even as some explicitly found both the new psychiatric coinages and psychiatrists' superciliousness absurd—would then be partially prompted by the growing numbers of behaviorally challenging adolescents perceived to be hovering at the edge of incipient criminality being drawn into their orbit.[66] Receptiveness would be fueled as well by genuine frustration with the stubborn recalcitrance of mental disability, and hence openness to hearing what physicians might have to say.[67] Yet other currents and pressures were no less significant. These included, on the remedial teachers' part, the urgent desire to sound more "scientific" in their pedagogical approach to their pupils, as they too strove to secure more solidly their own professional status.[68]

Most determinative, however, was the effort by psychiatrists to find a new language that acknowledged the impact of poverty, squalor, malnutrition, alcohol dependency, infectious diseases, and other deleterious environmental conditions on the prevalence of both mental disability and mental illness, but expressed the impact of those conditions in *biologized* terms. It had been universally accepted as basic knowledge that 85 percent of all children with mental disabilities came from the lowest of the lower classes.[69] Whether they pointed to hard physical labor or to malnutrition— especially inadequate protein—for the mother during pregnancy, or to excessive alcohol abuse by both parents (fetal alcohol syndrome had not yet been identified as such, it was fathers' drinking that was considered most suspect—though that too was indisputably correlated with poverty), to the mildew-filled air or contaminated water in unhygienic living conditions, or to the vitamin deficiencies that caused rickets and scrofula, or—most frequently—to the numerous diseases of toddlerhood still untreatable at that time that led to brain infections and thus to permanent neurological disorders as well as crippled limbs: All those who dealt with children with mental disability understood unfavorable environmental conditions as fostering its incidence.[70] As one district school inspector had put it in 1899: "Where do we get our material? Our children may have lived in the past in a room that barely had floorboards and where father, mother, a large number of children, and probably even the chickens stayed."[71] Yet the 1890s had also seen the abrupt ascent of a new line of argument, one in which the dreamed-of aim was no longer the amelioration of poverty, but instead—and even as poverty's deleterious effects were conceded—the eradication of disability through selective breeding and targeted killing.

Denying those with intellectual disability full personhood had been an element of age-old if otherwise mutually incompatible cosmologies. Folk mythology held that elves, trolls, or fairies had taken away a healthy human from its crib and substituted a "changeling" child in its place.[72] Early modern Christianity modified this perspective to propose, as Martin Luther did, that children with intellectual deficits were "possessed by the devil." Upon encountering in 1532 in Dessau a twelve-year-old boy who only "ate, excremented, and screamed," Luther declared that the child should be brought to a nearby river and drowned; disabled children, in his words, were nothing but "a mass of flesh," and lacked a soul.[73] Enlightenment thought, and in its wake nineteenth-century medical science, in their exaltation of rationality, placed the mentally disabled at or lower than the level of animals.[74] Thus, for instance, the prominent progressive German psychiatrist Heinrich Damerow would contend in 1858 (tellingly, the context was a vituperative anti-Guggenbühl diatribe) that all those with cognitive disabilities were "misbegotten creatures," each of them a "nullity." Damerow had introduced a thought experiment in which all cretins would be murdered, just as European settler colonizers bringing Christianity to other parts of the globe had managed to kill indigenous populations with the diseases they imported along with the tidings of the Gospel.[75]

Yet by the last decades of the nineteenth century, freshly inventive conceptual frameworks that justified killing individuals with cognitive impairments would become advanced far more openly and frequently. Expressing "murder-thoughts" was becoming socially acceptable.[76] By the early years of the twentieth century, whether the commentator was a biologist or a feminist activist, a philosopher, a politician, or a poet, the "discussability" of the idea was no longer in question. Two groups especially were foci for lethal fantasies: the long-term institutionalized and the (purportedly malformed) newborn.

The popular dramatist and poet Otto Ernst, for instance, challenged religious institution directors to admit that they themselves had "troubling doubt" about the life-value of individuals with disabilities, and in 1902 he contended with regard to the long-term institutionalized that "Jehovah regrets that he created these" (*Jehova reut es, daß er diese schuf*) (figure 1.3). Ernst proposed bluntly—embedded in flowery iambic pentameter—that God would be most grateful if human beings would take on the task of killing the disabled on His behalf.[77] The prominent women's rights activist Lida Gustava Heymann, for her part, in 1907 unselfconsciously revived the early modern terminology preferred by Martin Luther as she insisted that laws be passed legitimating the killing of "physical and mental cripples," while referring, both implausibly and hyperbolically, to institutionalized individuals as nothing but "mind- and feeling-less masses of flesh without hands and feet" who should be expeditiously "gotten rid of."[78]

There were three main rationales for these death wishes. One was pity, best captured in the aphorisms of Friedrich Nietzsche, who wrote of a disabled infant that it would be "more cruel" to let it live than to kill it.[79] A second important discursive trend was based in cost-benefit utilitarianism, put forth, for example, by Austrian psychologist Adolf Jost, who contended that the life-value of persons with severe disabilities was "not merely zero," but in the "negative" range and that therefore human society had not just the right but "the duty" to give them "this death, as painlessly as possible."[80]

··· 182 ···

Ein Besuch.

In jenem Hause war ich, wo man Tiere
  Bewacht und füttert, welche Menschen
    heißen,
Wo dem gebornen Wahnsinn ein Asyl
Man bietet und den Stumpfsinn zärtlich
    pflegt,
Daß dem Gesunden sich bei seinem Anblick
Vor starrem Schreck das Hirn im Kopfe löst
Und einen eigensinn'gen Wirbel tanzt. —

In jenem Hause war ich, wo der Mensch
Am Boden hockt wie ein verschüchtert Tier.
Die Augen rot und stumpf, die Haare gelb
Wie trocknes Stroh, und schwammig auf-
    gebunsen
Die grauen Wangen —: so sich selbst be-
    geifernd,
Die Zähne fletschend oder äffisch grinsend,
Dann plötzlich wild die ungeschlachten
    Glieder

··· 187 ···

Ins weite Feld der goldnen Zukunftssaaten;
Zum letzten Schlaf berauschest du die Braut,
Wenn schon ihr Geist im Myrtenzauber
    träumt —
So laß mit ernstem Ringen dich erbitten:
Auf diese Stätte einen Tropfen Tod!
Des Todes Wolke laß auf diesen Greuel
Herniederfallen, den du nicht gewollt!"
Denn, meine Brüder im Gebet, gewiß:
Jehova reut es, daß er diese schuf.
Die Bibel lehrt uns ja, daß er bereut.
Er will sich nur von diesem Irrtum nicht
So wohlfeil lösen wie durch jene Flut,
In der er alles Lebende ersäufte.
Wenn aber wir ihn bitten mit der Kraft
Inbrünstigen Gebets, wenn in die Hand
Wir ihm mit allem Schmerz des Mitleids
    fallen,
So muß sich ja sein göttlich Herz erweichen,
Und segnen muß er unsre Hände, wenn
Sie töten, was dem Tod geboren ward.
O seid versichert: Dankend und frohlockend,
Mit heißen Thränen himmlischen Er-
    barmens

FIGURE 1.3. Excerpted passages from a poem by Otto Ernst. "Ein Besuch" (A Visit) works avidly to induce the disgust it claims only to describe, and Ernst mocks as absurd both the Christian faith of residential institution directors and the notion that there might be any meaningful purpose whatsoever in sustaining disabled life. Published in Otto Ernst, *Gedichte*, Leipzig 1902.

Yet no conceptual framework would be more compelling to more people than the racial hygienic, which harkened back to the paradigmatic practice of the ancient Spartans, who left their deformed children to die on Mount Taygetos. Alfred Ploetz, biologist and coiner of "racial hygiene" as the German term for the Anglo-American "eugenics," in 1895 amplified the significance of the ancient Spartans not only by dwelling in detail on their infanticidal practices, but also by presenting them as inspirational in their sexual customs. Pre- and extramarital intercourse were celebrated when these were believed likely to produce strong and healthy offspring. Racial hygienic ideals were thus presented as erotically charged and exciting. Meanwhile, all nurture of the weak and vulnerable was presented as "contra-selective." The innovation of the racial hygienists was to connect conceptually the ancient practice of infanticide with the aspirational ideal that the Germanic people would become—by continually killing off the deformed and weak—beautiful and smart.[81]

In Breitbarth's Time

In 1915, one year into World War I, Martin Breitbarth, rector of a remedial school in Halle and a prominent functionary in the national association of remedial school professionals, published a speech he had given to a citizens' group in the leading professional journal *Die Hilfsschule*. Titled "The Reciprocal Relationships Between Mental Inferiority and Social Misery," Breitbarth spoke of an "impending disaster," "a great danger for the future of our Volk." For him, "the intelligence of the collective and of every individual" (*Intelligenz der Gesamtheit und jedes einzelnen*) was a key factor in German Volk-strength and indeed in Germany's ability already to have "dealt out such heavy losses to those enemies who so greatly outnumber us."[82] The "impending disaster" to which Breitbarth so centrally referred was for him inextricable from the apparent prevalence of German persons deemed to have intellectual disabilities. The text constitutes an entirely derivative, unoriginal compendium of the just-then consolidating perspectives. It remains valuable to examine closely for precisely this reason.

Rather than emphasizing the handicapping effects of impoverishment, Breitbarth's argumentation about the relationships between poverty and disability reversed the long-held understanding of the direction of causation. Blaming the parents for their poor "choice" of living conditions, he stated that the poverty in which so many children with cognitive challenges lived found its "source" specifically in the "mental and moral inferiority" of their parents. The low mental level of the parents, in his view, was *both* the reason for the disproportionate presence of the disabled in the meanest and most unhealthy neighborhoods of his hometown *and* the actual direct biological cause of their children's mental disabilities—*as well as* the reason these parents were incapable of appropriate childrearing. All of this was evidence of "the laws of heredity" (*die Gesetze der Vererbung*).[83] Moreover, rather than treating mental illness and mental disability as unrelated entities, Breitbarth contended that they functioned interchangeably. Instances of mental illness in the extended family were seen as proof-positive evidence for the *hereditary* nature of a mental disability.[84] Furthermore, Breitbarth treated the "colorful variety" of physical disabilities manifested by the children (e.g., nervous disorders, epilepsy, paralyses, crippled limbs, malformations of various kinds) as contributory factors "exacerbating" the children's low mental quality.[85]

In addition, Breitbarth freely intermingled lurid descriptions of the living conditions of the poor with a religiously inflected trope. Again, this placed the blame for poor children's intellectual disabilities squarely on the parents. He described in repellence-provoking minutiae—one might see this as a kind of "poverty porn"—the conditions in Halle's inner city: Five or even six or more people housed in a single room, sometimes including strangers sleeping over (*Schlafgänger*) to help pay for rent, and cooking facilities so filthy one would never want to eat anything prepared there. Breitbarth insisted this description demonstrated "from what wood these unhappy ones are carved, and how in the truest sense of the word they carry the sins of the parents" and, moreover, that "this will largely be the sole patrimony [*einziges Erbgut*] they in turn will transmit to the next generation."[86] Breitbarth warned that if something was not done soon, then this next generation would be entirely given over to crime and yet further misery.

Breitbarth's presentation had two simultaneous albeit contradictory purposes. He made a case for the economic prudence of investing in the building of yet another residential institution. This new facility would hold more than 420 "feeble-minded" individuals and put them to sufficient use in agriculture and gardening to cover the cost of their support. He insisted that this was something of which even the "more inept feeble-minded" should be capable. He compared the necessity of providing wounded veterans with opportunities to experience them-selves as capable again of useful labor with the need to extract labor also from the "mentally inferior."[87]

Yet Breitbarth additionally made a case for culling the ranks of the disabled. His phrasing in this regard was awkward, but his meaning in context was unmistakable. He commented favorably on the high child mortality rates among the poor, and suggested that good-minded people could be of different opinions about whether so many of "this type of German child" (*dieser Typus des deutschen Kindes*) should be kept alive.

> Of course, whether one should under all circumstances be wishing that this type of German child should be kept alive as numerously as possible, by all the means available to medical art and social welfare-care, is a question about which just such people can be divided in opinion who possess a deep understanding of the character of our Volk and from whom one certainly cannot deny, based on their life and work, that they have heart and spirit.[88]

Looking at the families whose offspring attended Halle's sole remedial school, he observed that of 1,814 births in these families, there were only 1,015 living children. Breitbarth concluded: "Personally, according to my experiences, it almost seems to me as if we should be grateful to Nature, which eliminates the less vigorous and less efficient individual early on by way of natural selection."[89] Breitbarth indicated that social policies might be needed to further Nature's work.

However, Breitbarth was quite nebulous about exactly what kinds of action should be taken. But he was completely clear and adamant that the disabled were "from the start on the debit-side of our Volk-life," that while "feeblemindedness can never be eliminated completely . . . reducing it to a bearable amount and eliminating the great danger that it poses to the character of our Volk is a goal that is worthy of the sweat of noble people," and that the danger was both real and great: What was needed, he said, was a "neutralization of the feeble-minded" (*Unschäd-lichmachung der Schwachsinnigen*). Yes, it was the duty of Christians and of human beings in general to carry also the weak and ill, but in addition there was the right to "self-protection and self-preservation":

If we keep away epidemics by various laws and measures, . . . why should we be denied the right to protect the productive part of our people from an imminent rape by the mentally inferior [*einer drohenden Vergewaltigung durch die geistige Minderwertigkeit*]? What tremendous demands the mentally inferior element in our people is already making on the general public, we feel in its full force in this difficult time of war. . . . The feeble-minded, who are almost without exception exempt from any service to the fatherland, make it difficult to provide the people with an abundant supply in view of the scarcity of food and contribute, even if unintentionally, to a reduction of the resistance of the German nation. If with the help of the existing laws it is not possible to make this type of people harmless in our nation for the future, new laws may need to be created.[90]

Breitbarth never did get specific about what those "new laws" should be.[91] But the emotionalized metaphors he chose to create a sense of overwhelming threat would be echoed often by others in the years to follow.

The military defeat in World War I consolidated the trend toward hereditarian thinking even more strongly. Intellectual disability, it turned out, was no marginal matter, of interest only to that minority that was deemed afflicted (was it one in a thousand or one in a hundred? Breitbarth had estimated the latter) and those whose job it was to attempt to make as many members of that minority at least *somewhat* "useful" and "productive."[92] Intellectual disability was relevant for the self-understanding—and, it was increasingly argued, the survival—of the entire nation.

Breitbarth's "The Reciprocal Relationships Between Mental Inferiority and Social Misery" proved to be a transitional text. It retained an older way of conceptualizing disability, calling for increased investment in and commitment to a model of large residential institutions, while it simultaneously adumbrated a newly emerging commonsense in which the hierarchization of human worth and stigmatization of those lower down on the hierarchy was joined by a conviction that health and value were hereditarily transmitted through the generations. Furthermore, even as the deleterious influence of desperate poverty was acknowledged, the urgent conviction communicated was that biological inheritance would always trump the effects of environment and opportunity.

Moreover, the new commonsense redirected attention away from the needs of individuals to a larger collectivity—a racial or ethnic group or nation, in this case the German Volk—whose health as a whole was felt to be compromised by the very *existence* of weaker and ill individuals. In sum, just as the goal of "usefulness" had come in as a repudiation of "curability," so too now the conceptual framework of racial hygiene would replace efforts at training ever-increasing numbers of people for "usefulness" with the new goal of reducing the number of vulnerable people in a given national collectivity. By the 1910s, the mere statistical prevalence of intellectual disability had begun to be constructed as a racial crisis.[93]

Yet the embedding of the phenomenon of cognitive disability into a racialized worldview was not a given. It was an acquired idea, a cultural consensus into which people were socialized. The consequences of that embedding—as well as the ultimate breaking of the consensus—would involve complex processes of learning and unlearning that were to take nearly a century. These processes are the subject of the chapters that follow.

2

Love, Money, Murder

We cannot use any brother who, when he sees a poor epileptic sick person, or imbecile, immediately asks: "Who sinned, this one or his parents?" Rather, we can only use those whose hearts, when they see a particularly wretched person, are overcome with the feeling: *"Oh, you I must love especially."*

—FRIEDRICH VON BODELSCHWINGH, FOUNDING DIRECTOR OF BETHEL, 1902[1]

Our blood be upon you!

—HANS, RESIDENT OF STETTEN, SHOUTING AT THE TRANSPORT PERSONNEL FORCING HIM INTO THE GRAY BUS TO THE T4 KILLING CENTER OF GRAFENECK, 1940[2]

"PERMISSION TO ANNIHILATE Life Unworthy of Life" (*Die Freigabe der Vernichtung lebensunwerten Lebens*) was a slim volume published in 1920—just in the wake of the cataclysm of World War I. Cowritten by a lawyer, Karl Binding, and a psychiatrist, Alfred Hoche, the book has often been invoked when scholars or journalists explain the prehistory of the Nazi "euthanasia" murder program, which is estimated to have claimed nearly 300,000 victims with cognitive disabilities or psychiatric diagnoses in Germany and the lands it occupied during World War II. The "euthanasia" murders are now understood as a genocide—a crime of its own kind, not solely a precursor to but also one intersecting in complex ways with the Holocaust of European Jewry.[3] Far less well studied are the various counter-positions proposed by Christian authors—theologians, pastors, and charity institution directors, most of them active in the Inner Mission, the umbrella organization of all Protestant church welfare work—who, during the years of the Weimar Republic, strove to argue that Binding and Hoche were simply wrong, and that the killing of those Binding and Hoche had demeaningly labeled as "life unworthy of life" should be considered morally *un*acceptable. The Christians, it turns out, had difficulties finding convincing words.

This chapter traces a process of moral and political destabilization and reorientation. In the first decade of the twentieth century, and even while the sprawling network of institutions came under strain as the numbers of residents climbed, the labor of care for the most vulnerable members of society was still being assertively promoted by the directors of the largest charity institutions as truly God's work, a work that also revealed important virtues in those who provided the caring. Aware of the emergence of voices questioning the purpose of care, especially for those residents who were the most dependent, the expansion of the institutions nonetheless continued to be accompanied by celebration of the consecration of each newly constructed building.[4] Yet between the mid-1920s and the early 1930s—well before Adolf Hitler ascended to the position of Chancellor in January 1933—the confidence in that life-sustaining perspective had been seriously eroded. Indeed, the particular argumentative logics advanced by Christian critics of Binding and Hoche reveal profound ambivalence within theological and charity circles: ambivalence about disability as a phenomenon; about individuals with disabilities as human beings; and about the practice of care altogether.

Revisiting the corpus of texts produced in response to Binding and Hoche and seeing there the extraordinary defensiveness Christian charity spokesmen evinced, the specific compromise formations they evolved, and above all their elaborate reworkings of theological concepts to take economic, "biological," and sexual-political concerns into account, in turn gives us original perspectives on important dynamics during the Nazi Third Reich and its immediate aftermath. We certainly

gain new insight into the eagerness with which Protestant charities participated in the Nazis' mass coercive program of "eugenic" sterilizations—
which eventually affected 400,000 German citizens (the Catholics
expressed official disapproval, but ultimately they allowed the sterilizations
to happen as well). We understand more fully the depth of helpless-
ness when charity directors were faced with the implacable ruthlessness
of the Nazi regime's intent to implement "euthanasia" on a mass scale.
And, not least, in view of this impotent ineffectuality, we also come to
recognize more comprehensively what was at stake in the rationalizations, repressions, and reinterpretations of the immediate horrific past
that were produced in the first years after the military defeat of Nazi
Germany in 1945.

Meanwhile, the hierarchizing of gradations of disability that had been
evolving since the late 1880s, as residential institution directors wran-
gled with remedial schoolteachers over who would have the right to
instruct the so-called better material—the not-so-profoundly disabled
individuals—while the "care-cases" and the at best "trainable" but not
fully "educable" were left to the institutions, became ever more significant. So it was not just that through the early decades of the twentieth
century a stark pecking order consolidated among people with disabilities themselves, with individuals who had sensory or physical impairments often adamantly insisting on their superiority to individuals with
cognitive or psychiatric challenges—including, explicitly, with regard
to the newly articulated ideal of "hereditary" health. In fact, the divisions identified *between* those diagnosed with intellectual or emotional-
behavioral disabilities became consequential in ever new ways.[5]

Although the lines continued to be both unclear and unstable, and
the nomenclature varied depending on the whims of the diagnostician
("feebly-abled," "feeble-minded," "imbecile," "idiot," "psychopathically
inferior," "difficult-to-train," "morally feeble-minded"), in practice the
boundaries between three broadly distinguishable groups were freshly
confirmed. To the one side were those with more minor cognitive challenges or only temporary psychiatric or behavioral crises, for the most
part functioning perfectly well, especially in supervised agricultural or
menial mechanical jobs; often, though not always, these were graduates

of the remedial schools. To the other side were the institutionalized. But within this group, too, there was the long-established divide articulated in relation to the notion of "usefulness": between those able to provide labor in and for the institution in some way, and those utterly unable to work (even on something as simple as sorting trash or tearing rags) and who instead required above all the time investment and the labor of care from others (even as that investment and care were, tragically, already all too often minimal). Across the full spectrum of ideological and disciplinary positions, all participants in the debates over the value of "racial hygiene" as a conceptual framework, as over the potential legitimacy (or not) of selective "euthanasia" killings, would base their interventions on these assumed divisions and subdivisions. And while initially "educability" or "work-capacity" (*Arbeitsfähigkeit*) was only one factor in the presumed tripartite gradations of intellectual impairment, it was this theme of work-capacity that would eventually have the gravest implications.

This issue of work-capacity (or its absence) took on heightened urgency in a context of economic crisis in the wake of Germany's defeat in World War I, even as a concomitant upwelling of ideological distortions around the topic of intellectual disability care further confused the national conversation. In what would become by the later years of Weimar and the early Third Reich a much-promoted and media-fueled spiraling of public resentment around the supposedly lavish conditions in which the most severely intellectually disabled people lived—fantastic fictions of "welfare-luxury" (*Wohlfahrtsluxus*) purportedly enjoyed specifically by the *non*working disabled—in actuality hid a far more complicated story.[6] A facility's debt burden; its tax-exempt status; the size of its endowment; the annual level of philanthropic donations; the proportion of private-pay to publicly funded residents; how low the salaries for staff could be kept: All of these matters were existential for the residential institutions, and inevitably reached directly into the corporeal and emotional experiences especially of the most defenseless residents and affected the quality of attentiveness they received. As it happens, a considerable number of larger institutions augmented the small daily per-resident allotments they received from the state with the labor power of the residents. The most economically valuable were the contributions of institutionally affiliated "worker-colonies" (*Arbeiterkolonien*) in which homeless men ("vagabonds") received housing in exchange for agricultural or other land-work. At some institutions, a separate category of youth deemed in danger of delinquency (*Fürsorgezöglinge*), while often perceived as requiring especially strict discipline, could also contribute consistent labor. But a vital additional source was, precisely, the work of the "moderately" disabled residents, even as the labor they provided was presented (and no doubt experienced by many) as both therapeutic and personally meaningful—whether in fields and garden, in the kitchen, laundry, sheltered workshops, or around the grounds. Later, when mass murder was at its height, there were sites at which the entire system—of both care and killing—continued to depend on the labor of these "only moderately" disabled people.[7] How this devastating fact was lost from memory and has yet to be consistently integrated into the scholarship on the histories of eugenics and "euthanasia" is a matter that requires far more research. I will return to it.

Permission to Annihilate

Coming as Binding and Hoche's text did in the wake of the mass carnage of World War I, in which so many had died on the battlefield and the majority of the civilian population too had been exposed to extreme hunger and deprivation and the economy remained ravaged, their insistence that for both *emotional* and *economic* reasons the profoundly disabled should be disposed of gained great public attention and acclaim.[8] The combination of emotions and economics was crucial, as Binding and Hoche played on feelings of revulsion at disability as they also emphasized disability's financial cost. Although the bulk of their text blurred pain relief eventuating in death with deliberate killing and extemporized at length about assisted suicide in the case of terminal illness, the main purpose of the brochure lay in a small subplot. Binding was candid in his view with respect to the group he labeled "incurable idiots." Indignant that "years and decades" of the valuable time and labor of caregivers were being spent on these persons, Binding averred that "I can find neither from the legal, nor the social, nor the moral, nor the religious standpoint any grounds whatsoever not to permit the killing of these humans . . . who arouse horror in almost everyone who encounters them." Hoche, for his part, reinforced this position with mathematical calculations as to the money expended every year on food, clothing, and heating for "the total idiots" (whose numbers he estimated nationally in the tens of thousands, of which he thought "the mentally completely dead" constituted approximately 3,000 to 4,000). In Hoche's view, these people were "ballast-existences" (*Ballastexistenzen*)—nothing but dead weight burdening a struggling society.[9]

Die Freigabe der Vernichtung lebensunwerten Lebens provoked a redirection of the German national discussion. Binding had opened the pamphlet with a direct attack on Christianity for what he deemed *its* cruelty in rejecting assisted suicide. Binding took offense at what he called "the impure idea that the God of love could wish that a person would only be permitted to die after enduring unending bodily or spiritual torments."[10] Religious leaders took notice. This was not just because the rhetorical jab at Christianity was unequivocally directed at them, but for the additional reasons that their institutions were among the primary homes for the class of humans whose right to stay alive was now under attack and that their institutions were indeed—particularly in the immediate aftermath of World War I—in considerable financial stress. But more than that, the very enterprise of Christian charity caregiving itself was increasingly being represented as responsible for the looming death of the German Volk, and not just because it diverted labor power and financial resources, but literally because its tendency to engage in "artificial nurturance" (*künstlich großzupäppeln*) of the less-than-healthy was deemed to be "contra-selective" in a Social Darwinian sense.[11]

Binding and Hoche's proposals were devastating to whatever traces still remained of the sentimental paradigm of care that had animated the work of the Inner Mission from its beginnings, including its leaders' intermittent efforts to deshame and destigmatize even the most acute forms of intellectual disability. At the Alsterdorfer Anstalten in Hamburg, the founding director, Heinrich Matthias Sengelmann, had regularly spoken of the importance of "salvific love" (*rettende Liebe*) and in 1888 had published a comprehensive three-volume guidebook for disability care tellingly titled *Idiotophilus* ("friend of" or "lover of idiots").[12] In addressing fellow directors at the triannual conferences, Sengelmann professed boldly that in the institutions' labor of care: "We are not dealing with 'cases' but with fellow human beings in whom also an immortal soul is alive, even if it is veiled from us."[13] In his poetry in the 1890s, Sengelmann declared that while on earth, people with disabilities were often seen as "trash" (*Kehricht*), God had shown him that these "poorest of the poor" were in fact a true "treasure" (*Kleinode*).[14]

At the legendary and largest institution, Bethel, near Bielefeld, its founder Friedrich von Bodelschwingh, a Pietism-influenced Lutheran pastor, worked yet more tirelessly to alter popular attitudes toward both physical and cognitive handicaps. Bethel's core specialty was epilepsy (not infrequently accompanied by "feeble-mindedness"), but there were also psychiatric wards, and services for alcoholics, hoboes, and "difficult-to-manage" youth, and in his sermons and other writings, von Bodelschwingh wrestled recurrently with the stark and agonizing questions that disability, whether inborn or acquired, posed to an individual and their family. Was it a sign of some moral failing? Was it a test from God? Von Bodelschwingh's own answers were rooted in his particular brand of deeply reverent faith, one feature of which was his conviction that *all* people, himself included, were bound up in sin, as was the whole world, and hence the confrontation with illness was always again a prompt to strive to be even more self-critically penitent.[15] Nonetheless, his most persistent reaction, in the face of any need, was to attempt to alleviate suffering and provide compassionate care in accordance with the ideal of Christian mercy. Indeed, anecdotes recounting his remarkable kindness—or invoking his idea that those being cared for were important teachers for their caregivers—were part of the constantly accumulating lore surrounding Bethel.[16] There was a radical theological egalitarianism inherent in von Bodelschwingh's vision—paternalist as it was in other ways—as he started from a premise of self-abnegation and emphasized the great *privilege* of serving those who were most helpless.[17]

Especially significant, from the point of view of the history of disability, were von Bodelschwingh's efforts to undo reflexive reactions of emotional-physical revulsion at deformation and profound vulnerability.[18] His *Bote von Bethel* (Messenger from Bethel) newsletter (at once a fundraising tool and a pious instruction pamphlet, of which thousands of copies were sent all over the nation) deliberately printed photographs of individuals in his care which he described in the most affectionate and affirmative terms.[19] Moreover, and however mawkishly, he portrayed these individuals, in all their visible nonnormativity, as great inspirations for the healthy—not just, though also, because providing loving care for them brought out the very best values in the nondisabled caregivers, but above all because they themselves were true models in their capacity to express joy and gratitude.[20] Von Bodelschwingh the elder, as did his son Fritz von Bodelschwingh, who gradually took over running Bethel in the years before his father's death in 1910, made a point of refusing to hide from public view those disabled people who would never be able to do any kind of productive work—and made clear that they saw tremendous beauty in them.[21] (See figure 2.1.) It was not an ineffective defense. It provided for funding streams, and for safety and sustenance—and came to serve more generally as an ethical touchstone and model of moral rectitude across the nation and internationally.

Yet World War I marked a turning point. Government rationing led to widespread hunger in the later years of the war, also at many institutions affiliated with the Inner Mission, and tens of thousands of disabled individuals perished from malnutrition (at Bethel the death rate climbed from the usual 4 percent to 16 percent in the final year of the war; at another institution it was close to 20 percent of all residents). At nonreligious institutions, death rates were even higher; at state-run facilities for the mentally ill, one expert estimates, about one-third of patients did not survive the starvation years of World War I; and another author—noting that numerous psychiatric and care institutions repurposed at least some of their wards for wounded soldiers who in turn quite literally received the higher rations that might have otherwise gone to patients—suggests an overall total of more than 140,000 institutionalized residents dead from hunger, infectious disease, and

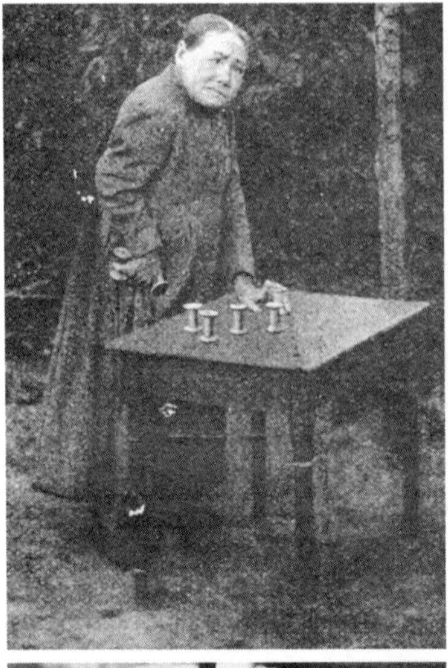
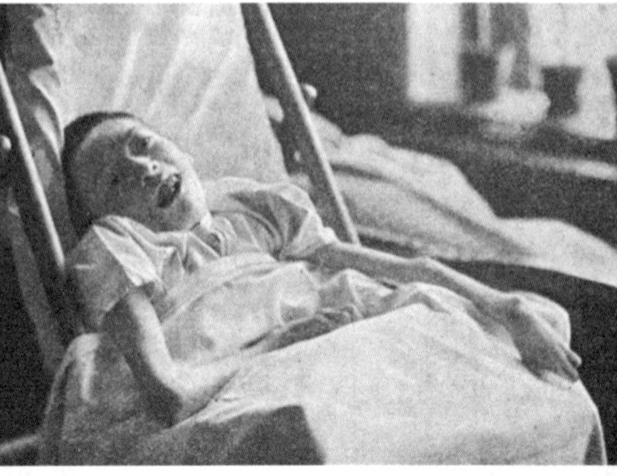
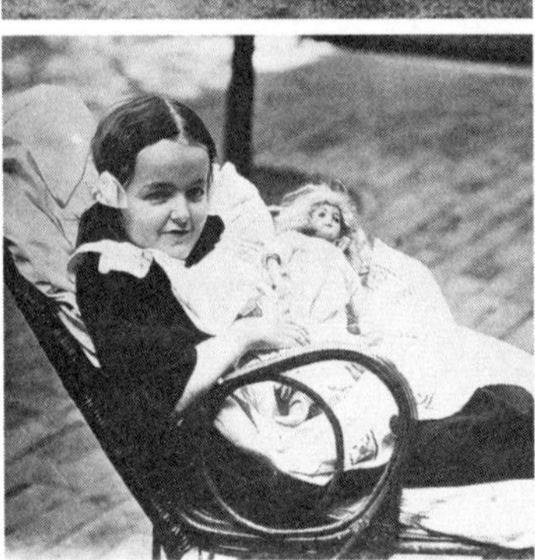
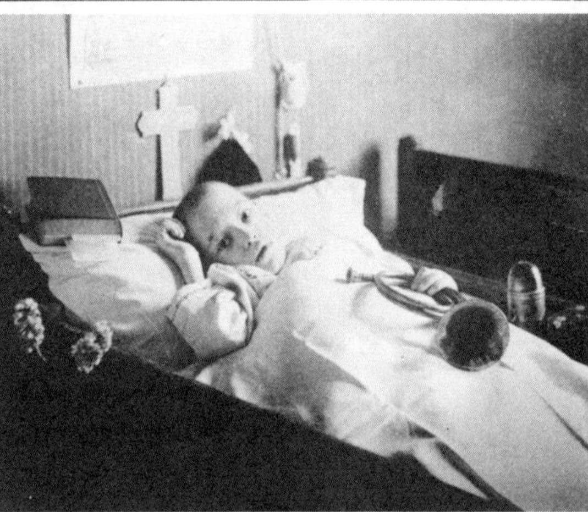

FIGURE 2.1. Photos of much-loved residents Margarete and Christian M. in 1908 and Mariechen and Fritzchen in 1917, all with accompanying narrative portraits, in the *Bote von Bethel* newsletter. Friedrich von Bodelschwingh the elder and his son Fritz von Bodelschwingh evidently went through a transformative learning process between the 1880s and the first years of the 1900s. The heightened emphasis on valuing as especially cherishable those residents who could not contribute any labor was patently a considered, deliberate attempt to counter the ascending trend in denigrating the disabled, in which the unabashed expression of death wishes had become, as of the 1890s, increasingly socially acceptable. © Hauptarchiv der v. Bodelschwingschen Stiftungen Bethel.

inadequate care.[22] Karl Bonhoeffer, first chairman of the German Association for Psychiatry, noted summarily in 1920—in a tone of disconcertedness and worry, not endorsement—that many had privately "almost condoned" the fact that "by these sacrifices" more resources remained for the preservation of the healthy.[23] Binding and Hoche forced such private opinion into print.[24]

Like a Temptation

As Pastor Friedrich Lensch—one of the successors to the *Idiotophilus*-authoring Sengelmann at the Alsterdorfer Anstalten in Hamburg—would summarize the situation as it evolved over the 1920s: "the objections [to keeping the severely disabled alive] can be subdivided into three groups. The first are economic, the second the eugenic type, the third are generally humanitarian." The economic argument—he said in an explicit gesture to Binding and Hoche's concept of "ballast-existences"—could be refuted fairly easily, since Protestant charities like his, he proudly explained, were extremely cost-efficient.[25] The eugenic argument, he averred, had always been a concern of the Inner Mission, since the mid-nineteenth century, and that was precisely why institutionalization was so important, as it kept the disabled out of sexual circulation and provided a source base of subjects for medical research into "feeble-mindedness," in expectation that its prevalence could be reduced in the future. And then there were the so-called humanitarian objections—the notion that the lives of the disabled must be unbearable *for them*. Ultimately, this pastor-director argued that his residents loved life, and that it would be "cowardly" to kill them. But not before he had with rather alarming candor confessed that "Those who tour our institution and perhaps for the first time in their lives stand before this abyss of misery . . . always again, shaken, ask us if one cannot, if only for the sake of the ill ones themselves, liberate them from this life that can after all hardly be called life. I freely admit that I felt no differently when I first came in, and these thoughts also creep up on us again and again, like a temptation [*wie eine Versuchung*]."[26]

His was hardly an anomalous voice. The 1920s saw an outpouring of commentary from theologians, pastors, and Protestant welfare institution directors as they reacted to Binding and Hoche. The possibility of murdering the most severely disabled individuals hovered around the edges of all these conversations. What evolved over the course of the decade was a new way of speaking, a kind of *theo-biopolitics* or *theo-bioeconomics,* one in which religious and moral considerations became confused with financial ones, while issues of biological bodily health or disease got thoroughly re-muddled with questions of guilt and sin, and sin itself became understood in new ways.[27]

Some of the responses to Binding and Hoche took place in personal correspondence, although ultimately they were published in a book with the title "The Problem of Abbreviating Life 'Unworthy' of Life" (*Das Problem der Abkürzung "lebensunwerten" Lebens,* 1925) by Ewald Meltzer, a Protestant doctor who was director of the Katharinenhof, a major institution in Saxony, dedicated to the care of "ineducable feeble-minded children." Meltzer—in the language of the era a "universally beloved father of the imbeciles"[28]—was intent on compiling all possible arguments, both religious and secular, *against* murdering the disabled, but he also catalogued the breadth of arguments in favor. Here we learn of Protestant religious leaders endorsing murder of the most seriously disabled as morally acceptable. We find that a noted religious educator in the Saxon town of Auerbach opined that one could not and should not extrapolate from Jesus's views about mercy for the handicapped as expressed in the Bible to the then-present of the 1920s; he noted that as long as "abbreviating" life was done out of "benevolence" (*Wohlwollen*), it was "not immoral." A theology professor in Heidelberg (known as a conservative biblical Pietist) opined that although a *Christian* may not kill, a *state* may, especially when it came to the more severely disabled individuals whose "soul-life had not been raised above the plant or animal level." And the prominent Protestant professor Arthur Titius in Berlin felt that "the elimination" of such "nuclei" or "sprouts" (*Keime*—he meant severely disabled individuals) "for which the force of human care will not be able to bring them to their destiny-appropriate development" could in fact be "compatible with full love of God and genuine humanitarianism."[29] Although none of these men had close continuous contact with individuals with disabilities, their arguments provided religious legitimation for Binding and Hoche's position.

Commentators who were directly involved in care work, by contrast, were at pains in their texts to declare themselves opposed to killing, or to remind readers that Christianity strictly forbade it. Yet their texts in response to Binding and Hoche, with striking frequency, and peculiarly, amplified rather than challenged a sense of revulsion toward the most severely disabled. Simultaneously, a number of these commentators took the opportunity of public interest in the theme of disability and its supposed high costs to drag in a welter of unrelated subjects, and above all to elaborate a variety of connecting links between sex and sin and disability. Rather than functioning as opposition to Binding and Hoche, then, these responses created an accrual of further negative perspectives on the disabled—and expanded the conversation to include their concerns also about the "moderately" disabled.

Much mid- to late 1920s' response to Binding and Hoche pseudo-scientifically sourced disability as being a *result* of the sexual disorder of Weimar. Binding and Hoche had not mentioned sex; it took their self-defined Christian opponents to introduce, and then keep harping on, the idea that there was—as one author put it—a "connection," indeed "a tight one," "between idiocy and sin."[30] A welfare institution director in Magdeburg (with a doctorate in theology) in 1925 offered as evidence for his own expertise and familiarity with thousands of "abnormals" that "they cannot talk or think . . . they resemble vegetating clumps of flesh whose expressions of life consist in nothing more than eating, drinking, elimination, and sleeping." (In other words, he confirmed in his own words that the severely disabled were indeed "lesser" beings, inferior, gross and disgusting, and also time- and labor-consuming and expensive.) But—raging against couplings and reproduction resulting from "animal rutting" (*tierische Brunst*)—he additionally took the occasion to argue that "the worst sources of lesser-value progeny are those vices of the Volk": "above all alcoholism and sexual aberrations [*die sexuellen Verirrungen*]." Meanwhile, his rationale for why these "lesser-value progeny" should not be "eliminated" was because they would serve as living reminders to their parents to feel "somehow guilty . . . knowing as they do that so much wretchedness is the result of heredity." If the disabled were to be killed, his argument explicitly stated, consciences would be numbed, and then people would just return to producing more disability. According to this director, 80 percent of all "abnormality" was caused by one's "own or others' guilt."[31]

Those who made a point of incorporating some sentimental defense of the severely disabled also joined in the chorus of lament about the only moderately disabled and their purportedly errant ways.[32] As one Berlin-based theologian involved in welfare work observed, even the most severely disabled individuals nonetheless could have a transformative—indeed redemptive—effect on those around them. And at one point he argued that Jesus actually could be more present among the ill than the healthy.[33] Yet for this author, too, the number of "feeble-minded and psychopaths" was "expanding frighteningly," as their sexual "drive-life is stronger." And "the death of the Volk" would soon be "inescapable," for the very existence of welfare care, he further affirmed, was allowing "everything withered, crippled, ailing to keep growing," and then it "combines itself with the healthy, produces sick progeny and causes immeasurable damage."[34] In a Bethel-based publication, a pastor-director from Saxony-Anhalt offered a yet more intricate version of this associative constellation: "If there was no addiction to alcohol . . . , no brothel and no venereal diseases, no overabundance of lust and no submersion in vice—then most of the institutions of the Inner Mission could close their doors" (in other words, they wouldn't have any clients). Again, this was an argument *against* Binding and Hoche, as the author continued: "Because the world is the way it is and because our Volk simply is the way it has become—that is why there are idiots and epileptics and cretins and people ill with venereal diseases and tuberculosis and the cripples and the insane." This author was particularly indignant that "the media-Jews, the dirty-joke-writers and the real estate speculators, the stock exchange jobbers and the whole pleasure-craving populace that knows nothing more than insipid amusements and hot fashions and tawdry wit, all of them should live"— while "the poor newborn children, that have been put into the world by this adulterous generation and which carry the sins of the parents for the rest of their lives" would (if Binding and Hoche's recommendations were to be followed) be put to death.[35]

In this defense of the moral innocence of the disabled, the causal contention could not be more explicit: The purported pervasiveness of sexual dissoluteness and sin was here blamed on Jews (or at least "the media-Jews") among others, and that dissoluteness and sin were proffered as explanation for how disabled people are produced. (So: Sinful sex is the cause of disability.) While there was certainly a kernel of sense and logic in the evidence that venereal diseases could cause birth defects, leaders in the Inner Mission evinced a far more global and diffuse dislike for what they saw as proliferating sexual profligacy.

Compromise Formation

The reconfiguration of theological messaging underway over the course of the 1920s and the developing consensus about the degraded value of disabled lives was to find yet fuller expression in the "Treysa Resolution" of 1931, growing out of a meeting in May of that year at which twenty-two leading figures from the Inner Mission gathered in this small town north of Frankfurt / Main to discuss eugenics and "euthanasia." The lead author was the young physician and population science expert Hans Harmsen, responsible for the health and welfare division of the Inner Mission, but the resolution emerged from the whole group's deliberations (Fritz von Bodelschwingh from Bethel and Friedrich Lensch from Alsterdorf were both present); the results would be published shortly thereafter and would take the form of a kind of Christian charity policy platform. The Treysa Resolution's promulgation was to mark a decisive transition from a version of Protestant charity committed to provision of services for everyone in need to an explicitly eugenic orientation.

Among other things, in response to reductions in per-person subsidies instigated by the budget-strapped Prussian state, along with the generalized crisis unleashed by the Great Depression, the resolution proposed that "differential care" (*differenzierte Fürsorge*) would henceforth be provided to those among their disabled charges who were, due to severe cognitive or psychiatric impairment, unable to engage in any productive labor.[36] In short, and although clearly under significant external duress, these Protestant leaders (ten of them theologians and pastors, nine physicians, one female social worker, one teacher, and one lawyer) would at Treysa formally endorse a hierarchization of human value.

In addition, a succinct version of another of the resolution's conclusions—arguably its main raison d'être—turned out to be a kind of theological compromise formation: *Murder no, sterilization yes* (even as the resolution did propose that sterilizations be implemented only with the consent of the person concerned). Sterilization had previously been rejected by many in the Inner Mission on grounds that an intellectually challenged sterilized female would no longer have a reason *not* to become promiscuous and / or would be vulnerable to male exploitation and rapaciousness, as sexual conservatism had long provided the foundational grid of intelligibility for churchmen's and -women's decision-making.[37] Precisely these concerns were raised over and over again during the extensive discussions in Treysa that preceded the formulation of the resolution.[38]

Under growing pressure to consider murder, however, resistance to sterilizations dissolved. Or, as the Treysa Resolution put it: "We do not want to eliminate the victims of guilt and sin, but to attempt to prevent them." (Worth noting once more here is the blatant implication that disabled progeny was the result of "guilt and sin.") Then again, however, the causation went in the other direction, as one new reason given for the importance of sterilizing was that a body's "God-given functions" might lead to "evil," and hence there was "not only a right, but a moral duty to sterilize out of neighborly love" and—here was a new emphasis on the Volk-collectivity and the future—"out of the responsibility which has been imposed on us not just for the generation that exists already, but also for the coming generation." What Christian "love" meant, in short, had been substantially redefined at Treysa. The language of eugenics, which had initially been received in religious charity circles with some skepticism and reluctance, especially among the older generation, was now being adapted and modified with a view to the efficacious additional reinforcement it might provide for the longed-for restoration of traditional conservative mores. The resolution declared that research revealed "the hereditary factor" (*der Erbfaktor*) to be the source of a "staggeringly large share" of the "mental infirmities" evident among their residents (60 percent was the number mentioned). Yet supplementally, there were once more side swipes at the sexual culture of Weimar. "Brothel-keepers," it was stressed, were "far worse vermin than the physical and mental invalids." And yet, and although Binding and Hoche (cited by name) were repudiated for assuming that there was "no soul-life" among the severely disabled, nonetheless the aversion that Binding and Hoche had articulated against individuals with disabilities was confirmed and re-incited: "Shattering like almost no other thing, the sight of these ailing and miserable beings admonishes the healthy person to keep his body unscathed and pure and to become conscious of his deep responsibility when he founds a family."[39] The case for keeping the disabled alive was that doing so provided a valuable lesson in chastity for the nondisabled.

By 1933, when the Nazis assumed the reins of government and passed their overtly coercive and expansive sterilization law, leaders in Protestant welfare work signed off on it—or even declared that they had been in favor of sterilization all along. (Meltzer even rushed to aver that he favored coercion, and had been dubious about the idea of requiring individual consent.)[40] They began enthusiastically to sterilize, too. At Protestant hospitals and at charitable institutions for the disabled, a regular routine was established, at Bethel for instance with literally a weekly "sterilization day"—and the doctors could hardly keep up.[41] Charity institutions were encouraged to develop card catalogues and clan charts identifying individual and familial vulnerabilities.[42]

This overall trend was not completely inevitable. Not every Protestant immediately got on the pro-eugenics bandwagon. One prominent exception to the newfound zeal—demonstrating that it was at least possible to imagine and sustain alternate understandings of disability as well as of the science of heredity—was Lutheran theologian Paul Althaus at the University of Erlangen. Althaus's case scrambles contemporary assumptions in instructive if perturbing ways. He had in the late 1920s denounced "the Jewish menace to our Volk-character," and in early 1933 placed great hopes in Hitler.[43] Yet in April 1933, he delivered a public lecture in which he not only rejected Binding and Hoche's proposals to kill individuals with severe cognitive disabilities, but also urged caution with sterilization. Althaus expressed repulsion at his contemporaries' fantasies of broad-based sterilization ("eugenic orgies," he called these—indeed the speaker on stage before him favored sterilizing approximately 10 percent of the population), and Althaus highlighted the lack of self-evidence and numerous ongoing enigmas in patterns of hereditary transmission of "feeble-mindedness." He emphasized as well that also the most severely disabled individuals—here he explicitly invoked the residents of Bethel—were evidently capable of joy and of receiving human love. And was this not the very point of life? Althaus further decried the ascendant obsessions with health and strength and the notion of life as above all a "struggle for survival" (*Daseinskampf*), observing that illness could enter any life in an instant, and that "perfectibility" (*Vervollkommnung*) was unattainable and in any event undesirable. Althaus distanced himself utterly from the notion of "unworthy" life by putting the term in quotes in his lecture title, arguing that it was imperative to distinguish between "worth" (*Wert*) and "dignity" (*Würde*), and insisting that "dignity . . . has no gradations" (*Würde . . . verträgt keine Abstufung*).[44]

A different counterexample to the trends of the era was provided by the Bremen-based Protestant physician Karl Stoevesandt, close friends with the anti-Nazi theologian Karl Barth. In an essay published in early 1933, Stoevesandt criticized both eugenics and psychoanalysis as false paths for medicine. Although ultimately he was more indignant about psychoanalysis than eugenics—annoyed at what he took to be Freud's antireligious stance and his overfocus on the unconscious and the libido—he did provide an intriguing original critique of eugenics. Stoevesandt argued that the purposes of medicine as a science were twofold: research and healing. Eugenics, he suggested, was by contrast an ideology, a "worldview" (*Weltanschauung*). It claimed to distinguish between worth and unworth of human life, but from where did it take its measure? Medicine, precisely because it demanded scientific exactitude and the ascertaining of facts, could not provide such an evaluative measure. Meanwhile, he noted, advocates of eugenics perpetually revealed its actually quite *nonscientific* nature in their obsessive preoccupation with matters of money—along with their subjective sensibility:

Thus eugenics is compelled to expose itself, and it does so quite bluntly in all its pronouncements. As the only valid point of view it knows solely the financial one: What do the inferiors cost us? Do they not eat up welfare benefits that would be much better spent on the healthy offspring of families with many children? Are not vast sums wasted on them in institutions and prisons, which we cannot afford in our economic situation? In this way, eugenics, if it can even be called a science, slips in its practical action into being a perception of those who feel themselves to be the healthy ones.[45]

As of 1934, however, Stoevesandt had evolved his arguments. God as the author of creation and revelation had become even more central—as he also proposed that the historic mission of the German Volk was to be the world's conscience with regard to the message of the gospel. But now he praised "the young science of research into heredity" for having uncovered "a wealth of insights into hereditary inequality within a race." He maintained further that "since intellectual inferiority as well as psychological instability . . . are generally hereditarily determined predispositions, largely independent of environmental influences, we can without exaggeration say that what is happening is an undesirable expansion of a particular group within the race." And declaring himself "thankful" that the newly passed sterilization law contained protective checks and balances, Stoevesandt expressed optimism that "over time the race will be able to be cleansed of a series of hereditarily ill lines."[46] It seems that Stoevesandt had been pressured with the threat that he might lose his approbation to practice medicine due both to his challenge to the regime's eugenic policy and his persistence in demonstrating collegiality with "non-Aryan" physicians.[47] If that was indeed the reason, the change of message can be understood even more clearly as acquiescence to an imposed ideological position whose transparent lack of scientific validity he himself had only recently recognized all too astutely.

The majority of Protestants directly involved in disability care, however, immediately and warmly welcomed the Third Reich. In fulsome terms, directors embraced the rise of Nazism, expressing appreciation that—as von Bodelschwingh the younger put it—the new government had effectively "broken . . . the influence of that Jewish liberalism that is totally hostile to the Gospels."[48] "Hitler's strong hand has intervened" and brought to an end the "liberal-Marxist era" which had been "leading to Bolshevism, the Jewish dictatorship"—so Meltzer at the Katharinenhof enthused.[49] Photographs of gatherings of individuals with disabilities, whether accompanied by their caregiving deaconesses amid swastika flags at a sunny festive outing, or with a swastika woven into a hand-made basket in an in-house sheltered workshop, conveyed the climate with special poignancy[50] (figure 2.2). And—while some Protestant spokespeople remained skeptical of coercive sterilization (not least because it would impede their long-standing efforts to get involuntary confinement legislation passed, as sterilization would remove one of the strongest arguments for the need for long-term institutionalization of the purportedly wayward)—once the sterilization law was going into effect, churchmen and charity doctors speaking in the name of Christianity developed yet further *religious* justifications for sterilization.[51] Pastor Lensch in Hamburg was particularly exhilarated that "the much-discussed question of sterilization of the hereditarily ill . . . has been torn away from the materialist motivations of the Marxist era, which mainly defended the idea because the sterilization of patients facilitated an unrestricted pursuit of pleasure (*uneingeschränktes Sichausleben*) . . . . This . . . is why we as Germans and Christians resisted the idea. Now . . . we can honestly welcome the new regulation."[52] And Pastor Ernst Klessmann, affiliated with one of Bethel's auxiliary institutions, asserted in 1934: If there was any past "guilt" for which the Protestant church might self-castigate, it was that it had permitted *too many* hereditarily ill people to marry (and thus reproduce). Joining in the chorus of voices declaring that "the continued existence of our Volk is lethally threatened by the strong expansion of the biologically inferior," cheering that "the liberalistic slogan of the right of the human being to his own body [another reference to Weimar cultural values] has been thoroughly undone by this law," and lauding "much common ground between National Socialism and the gospel," the pastor affirmed "all enthusiasm for the Third Reich and its Führer. . . . God Himself has given this government the power."[53] Along related lines, the head physician from the Protestant

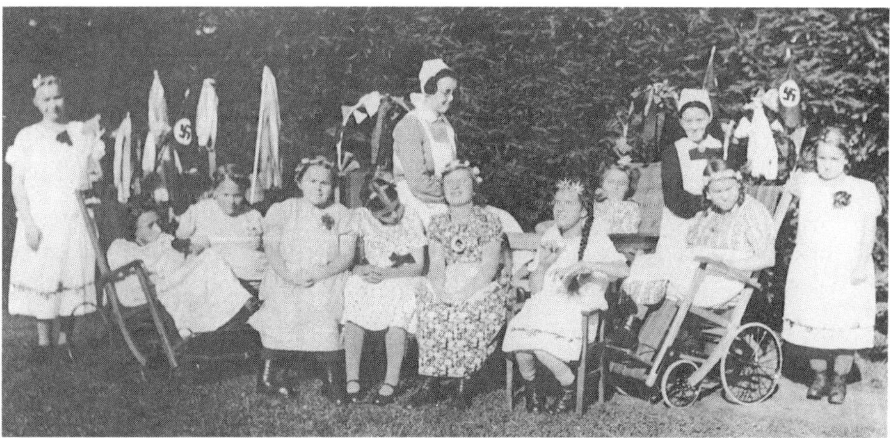

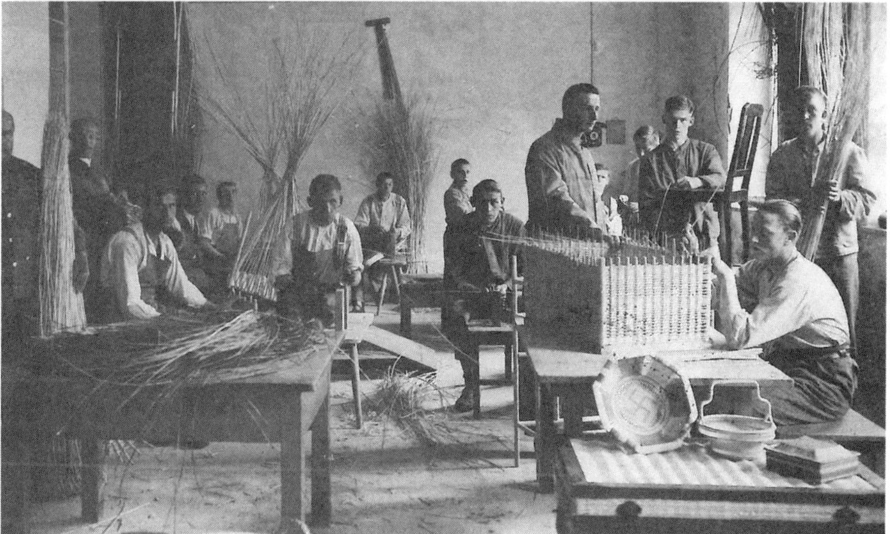

FIGURE 2.2. At the Alsterdorfer Anstalten in Hamburg in the 1930s, and at the Bruckberg branch of the Neuendettelsauer Anstalten in Bavaria in 1935, swastikas were integrated into festivities and crafts. Archiv der Evangelischen Stiftung Alsterdorf; Zentralarchiv Diakoneo Neuendettelsau, Bildarchiv 4004 / 4.

charity institution of Hephata in Treysa delivered a speech to Protestant educators in 1934 in which he continually blended "responsibility before God" with "love for our Volk," blamed "those Marxist-liberal and [Catholic] Center [Party]" politicians for "watching passively as year for year the numbers of mentally inferior people expanded," and explained that "we doctors have before God the calling to help people as individuals and our Volk as a whole" and that this was why he and his peers "had always advocated for eugenic sterilization" due not least to "consciousness of the sacred duty towards our Volk." In addition, he took the occasion to elucidate that "Although in the past one believed that by pairing members of different races, higher-quality offspring would ensue," it had since become apparent that such mixing "with foreign races that are very far from us, like for example the Oriental and Near Eastern, to which the Jews belong, is *as a rule* not possible."[54]

In sum, in their efforts to find reasons not to condone murder, Protestant spokesmen had settled on the effusive endorsement of sterilizations—and so ended up not just eugenicizing theology, but theologizing eugenics. Because they were on the defensive, because they hoped to maintain their cultural status and keep their institutions afloat, but perhaps because they all along had unresolved ambivalences about their own work, the very people who had the disabled in their care cast aspersions on them, and formulated—in the name of Christianity—a novel means of denigrating the disabled. Far from providing a vigorous, robust alternative to Binding and Hoche's cost-benefit arguments and emotional revulsion arguments that demanded killing, Protestant leaders effectively intensified antidisability animus.

Catholics, interestingly, had not felt nearly as directly addressed by Binding and Hoche as Protestants had.[55] There were two prominent Catholic eugenicists in Germany—Josef Mayer and Hermann Muckermann—and both advocated for the reconcilability of Catholic teachings with acceptance of sterilization.[56] Mayer in particular, who liked his role as a renegade, had already with his dissertation of 1926 (which did initially receive the Church's formal approval, although soon investigations challenging that approval were initiated) promoted the idea that (voluntary) sterilization on grounds of mental illness, epilepsy, or mental disability could be morally acceptable, especially if these could be framed in terms of the state's self-defense against a potential national "emergency" (*Notstand*). While Pius XI's encyclical of 1930, *Casti Connubii* (in its pertinent sections authored by the German theologian Franz Hürth, who was utterly hostile to Mayer's line of reasoning), would make Mayer's as well as Muckermann's interventions around sterilizations largely moot, Mayer—who had pronounced pro-Nazi sympathies—would later, during the Third Reich, pseudonymously author a memo that explored situations in which "euthanasia" might be acceptable.[57]

Nonetheless, and on the whole, during the Weimar years, the general attitude that had been communicated to the Catholic faithful and to the wider public alike was that there was nothing to debate; the Church's stance was clear. Life was to be protected from the moment of conception through to a natural death, not least because, a handful of exceptions aside, unlike Protestants, Catholics were well known to reject out of hand any interference with reproduction. A formally articulated compromise position against murder that embraced sterilization was never an option for the Vatican. Catholics did ultimately accommodate the sterilizations even as their bishops registered formal objections.[58] But there was within the Catholic church leadership in Germany no perceived pressing need to make a multidimensional intervention in reaction to Binding and Hoche.

One prominent Catholic, however, did weigh in extensively on Binding and Hoche's call to kill: Franz Xaver Walter, professor of moral theology at the University of Munich. Walter had first entered the conversation with an important article in 1923, and he later returned to the subject in a major book published in 1935. Notably, Walter evinced a great deal more poise and self-assurance than the beleaguered and befuddled Protestants. Already in the early article, his tone was one of calm sarcasm as he mocked the restless eagerness of those demanding the removal of barriers to murder and the way the "euthanasianists" (in Walter's scornful coinage) self-styled as being moved by compassion and high moral ideals.[59] In the book, he went yet further, dismantling as ludicrous—especially in a virtuoso chapter on the "economics" of "euthanasia"—the elaborate mathematical calculations presented by the "euthanasianists" as they highlighted the purportedly enormous expense weighing down the nation and offered as "catnip" for anyone reluctant to embrace their vision the prospect of redirecting all those funds to other, more worthy purposes. Walter was clear that there were far worse "parasites" taking advantage of the labor power of the collective and noted that there was "no causal relationship whatsoever between our situation of economic crisis and the demand for euthanasia." Moreover: "'As bad off as we may be, I am sure we can still carry one useless person for every 15,000.'" Not least, Walter pointed out, to implement "euthanasia" on a broad scale would actually itself be quite expensive; he would certainly be proven correct.[60]

Yet one other constituency did allow itself to be put directly on the defensive by the proliferating warnings that the number of disabled were multiplying unacceptably: remedial school teachers. In the flagship journal *Die Hilfsschule*, authors throughout the 1920s sought to grapple with the accusation that the remedial schools—as one summarized it—"contribute to the maintenance of 'racial cripples'" and, purely by their provision of educational engagement, induced "an effect of a contra-selection" (as they were helping the "less able" portion of the population "to a capacity for life and reproduction it would not otherwise have").[61] The prominent remedial pedagogue Albert Griesinger confirmed in the pages of this journal that teachers at the 875 remedial schools across the nation, serving 68,000 children, were regularly confronted with the accusation that by teaching their pupils to become capable of financial self-support (rather than locking them away in institutions), they were failing in their "racial-hygienic" task of "systematically doing battle against unsuitable breeding." Precisely as he rejected this charge, however, Griesinger bolstered the notion that "the weakest among the mentally impoverished" did in fact live a "life unworthy of life," and that it was not just acceptable but actually a "duty, to prevent these unfit from becoming the ancestors of future generations."[62] Another author, complaining in 1926 that the quality of the pupils in the remedial schools had lately become "significantly worse"—that too often, the children were more "fitting material" for an "idiot-institution"—noted that the recent broad public interest in "discussions about permission to annihilate life unworthy of life," although actually referring to those who were "feeble-minded to a high degree," nonetheless had the additional effect of putting pressure to prove their cost-benefit value also onto the remedial schools.[63]

Meanwhile, at the 1924 "Second Congress for Curative Pedagogy" in Munich, the respected public hygiene expert Ignaz Kaup had already told the assembled teachers that the rising chorus of hysteria claiming that all mental deficiency was being hereditarily transmitted was flat-out false (rather, as Kaup helpfully noted, it simply *seemed* to be transmitted that way because the external circumstances of poverty were replicated across generations)—and yet, Kaup nonetheless offered his unvarnished opinion that the many "minus-variants" in the Volk were indeed an "egregious" financial burden—not least as the nation was being "tormented" by enemy demands for reparations—and "Binding and Hoche's proposal should be supported." Moreover, Kaup counseled, beyond more extensive institutionalization and more efficient utilization of the labor power of residents: "sterilization, after the US model," could be an additional "viable path."[64]

What the contradictory cacophony of commentary reveals is that one could see through the flaws in what was being presented as science and the inadequacy and illogicality of the available recommendations for action, and still end up reconfirming that fellow citizens with mental disabilities were a danger to the health of the nation, whether biologically or economically or both. Meanwhile, Binding and Hoche's terminological coinage, "life unworthy of life," had quite apparently simply entered the national lexicon.[65] And as with Protestant charity spokesmen, so too among remedial school teachers: Sterilization could come to seem a wholly appropriate moral compromise.[66]

In 1933, Gustav Lesemann—chairman of the Association of Remedial Schools before it was absorbed into the National Socialist Teachers' League and (the avidly pro-Nazi) Martin Breitbarth supplanted (the disappointed) Lesemann, who had hoped to maintain his role—published an essay in *Die Hilfsschule* in which he stated that "eugenics and curative pedagogy recognize the absolute value of human life once it exists. They respect it and therefore reject the killing of life unworthy of life." Yet, although he distanced himself from eugenicists' desire to sterilize also those who were only "*possibly* hereditarily ill" and insisted that sterilizations be based on "voluntarism" (*Freiwilligkeit*), he observed that curative pedagogues could support sterilization of the "*definitely* hereditarily ill."[67] Soon thereafter, however, in April 1933, Lesemann, on behalf of the Association, expressed its loyalty to the new regime, glowingly hailed "our universally beloved Volk-Chancellor Adolf Hitler," and promised "the government of the Reich full sympathy and entire trust." At the occasion of the formal self-dissolution of the Association a month later, Lesemann read aloud the text of the "Aryan paragraph" that would drive all Jewish colleagues out of the profession—and the assembled board approved it unanimously. In his words of farewell, Lesemann praised the new era that had dawned ("We stand today . . . under the star of resurgence and resurrection") and urged his peers to declare "a threefold *Sieg Heil!*"[68]

It can come as no great surprise, then, that when the coercive Nazi sterilization law went into effect in January 1934, remedial school teachers were among the groups assigned to identify candidates for sterilization.[69] Efforts by teachers to defend and rescue pupils from this fate appear to have been rare.[70] The connection between being a remedial school pupil and being sterilized became so widely recognized that the remedial schools acquired the pungent and derogatory vernacular moniker "eunuch-institution" (*Eunuchenanstalt*).[71] More than half of their pupils ended up going under the knife.[72]

Unworthy of Life?

The Nazi disability murder project, as it developed momentum from 1939 on, was to have many components: mass shootings and gas vans; thirty "special children's wards"; six T4 gas chambers running from January 1940 to August 1941; a second, "decentralized" phase of killing by medication overdose, poisoning, or deliberate starvation with double the death toll of T4 (figure 2.3). At every stage, it was evident that the murderers' main targets were primarily drawn from those who were long-term institutionalized. Indeed, over and over, the killings that were most brazenly pursued were directed at those requiring labor of care from others, rather than being able to provide labor themselves, even as the bar for what was needed to be allowed to survive was set high.[73] (Thus, for instance, the ability to peel potatoes or mop floors, to weave mats or glue paper bags, was counted as "mechanical" rather than "productive" work, and increasingly deemed insufficient for keeping a person alive.)[74] (See figure 2.4.)

The intricacies surrounding these core economic issues of "work-capacity" and labor power never stopped mattering. This led to countless hallucinatorily grotesque scenes: An administrator at the charity institution of Stetten in Württemberg arguing with deportation personnel at the very door of the gray bus meant to take victims to the gas chamber that he absolutely needed to keep his faithful cook Lina L., otherwise he would be obliged to replace her with "a person of fully sound mind"; he failed.[75] A woman surviving the Pomeranian disability murder center of Meseritz-Obrawalde (as deaconesses who had been obliged to accompany their charges in locked and guarded trains to that site, and then return without them, later discovered) by providing housecleaning services for a physician—possibly one of the perpetrator-physicians—stationed nearby.[76] A man about to be driven into the gas chamber at Grafeneck rescued from this fate by the physician in charge, who decided he needed someone who could regularly polish his boots.[77] Moderately (as opposed to profoundly) psychiatrically ill and / or cognitively disabled residents at the Wiesloch institution near Heidelberg doing all the labor in the kitchen and laundry to sustain care for wounded Wehrmacht soldiers who by that point in the war inhabited the beds freed by an earlier round of killings.[78] A disabled man helping with the corpse-burning in the crematorium at the Kaufbeuren institution in Bavaria—while psychiatrically ill patients at Meseritz-Obrawalde were tasked each morning with collecting the past night's dead on a little wagon to bring them to the morgue.[79] Patients at the Kalmenhof and at Hadamar drawn into the work of killing—compelled, for instance, to hold down by force patients who resisted lethal injections.[80] And a disabled man still living at Hadamar in the 1980s recalling how he had assisted with the digging of mass graves on the hill above the asylum during the decentralized phase of murders there, and was still able to describe exactly the space needed to make the graves the correct size. In the first postwar decades, no one had wanted to hear this man disclose his experience; he was best known in and around the institution's grounds for playing the harmonica[81] (figure 2.5).

Die Gesundung erfolgt durch Gottes GNADE!

Wie groß ist DEINE Stärke,
Wie wunderbar die Werke,
Wie heilig ist DEIN Wort!
Wie ist DEIN Tod so tröstlich,
Wie ist DEIN Blut so köstlich,
    Mein Fels des Heils,
    mein Lebenshort!

Wie reich sind DEINE Gaben!
Wie hoch bist DU erhaben,
Auf DEINEM Königsthrohn!
Es jauchzen, singen, dienen
DIR alle Seraphinen,
    DU wahrer Gott
    und Menschensohn!

Fluch dem Gotte, dem blinden, tauben,
Zu dem wir vergeblich gebetet im Glauben,
Auf den wir vergeblich gehofft und geharrt,
Er hat uns gefoppt, er hat uns genarrt!

Fidi
Patient
Pfleger
Fidi bei der Berufsarbeit – Spritze in'n Arsch!!!

How did Christian charities navigate these nightmares? The entire pathos and complexity of the Protestant Inner Mission's relationship to the Nazi murder of the disabled is encapsulated in the experiences at the asylum of Stetten. Over the course of the fall of 1940, gray buses with male and female transport personnel appeared in the courtyard to cart away, in a series of successive Tuesdays, 323 "feeble-minded" or "epileptic" of the originally 742 residents of the institution, to take them to be murdered in a carbon monoxide T4 gas chamber housed in a garage at the killing center of Grafeneck an hour and a half northwest; another eleven were later killed at Hadamar during its T4 phase; and an unknown number met their deaths in a series of "relocations" during the second, decentralized phase of "euthanasia." The survivors who remained were severely traumatized.[82]

Run since 1930 by the pastor Ludwig Schlaich, an active and well-networked member of the Inner Mission, the atmosphere at Stetten provides a perfect exemplar of the indissoluble blend of compliance and contestation with the government—and ultimately anguishing impossible non-choices—characterizing so many charity institutions in the Third Reich.[83] The Nazi seizure of power was greeted with ardor.

FIGURE 2.3. Sacrilegious, vulgar mockery of a traditional hymn and cartoon drawing from the file of Walter G. (born 1908), a patient admitted to Hadamar in August 1942, during the second phase of "euthanasia," when the gas chamber was no longer being used, and the majority of killings were administered by lethal injection. During this time, Hadamar continued as a psychiatric clinic. Walter G.'s diagnosis was "schizophrenia"; the patient file contains notations about his eagerness to convey his grandiose ideas to Hitler personally, as well as his father's energetic assurances to the Hadamar administration that his son was utterly harmless. The top half of the drawing—in heaven—copies the words of the hymn; the bottom half—in hell—shows a Nazi physician and male nurse injecting a patient, while the text curses God, "the blind, the deaf / To whom we faithfully prayed in vain, / . . . He has deceived us, he has fooled us." With the permission of the police and of Hadamar's head physician, Dr. Adolf Wahlmann, Walter G. was released to his family in January 1943. Dr. Wahlmann himself—as well as nurses Karl Willig and Heinrich Ruoff—were well known among the patients for the frequency with which they killed their patients by injection. Reprinted from Dorothee Roer and Dieter Henkel, eds., *Psychiatrie im Faschismus: Die Anstalt Hadamar 1933–1945*, Bonn 1986, 201.

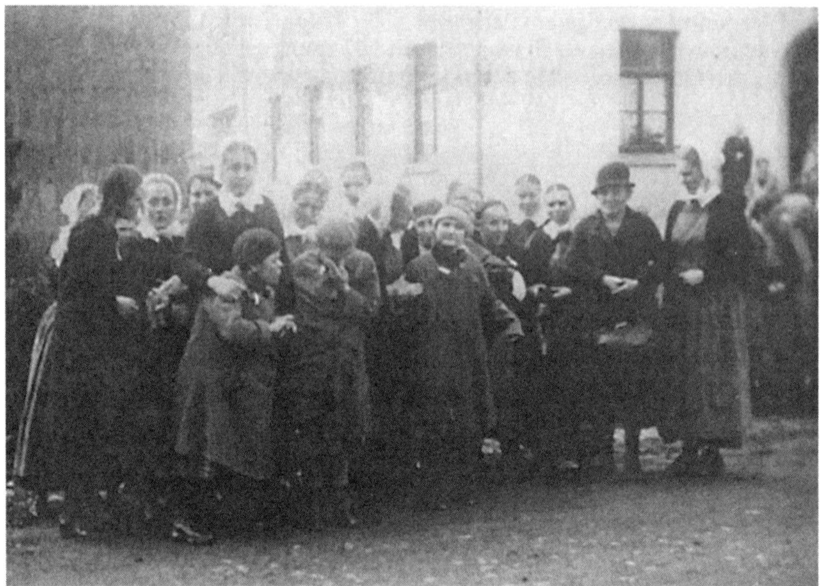

FIGURE 2.4. In May 1944, ninety-eight girls and young women from the Asbacher Hütte, a branch of the Diakonie-Anstalten Bad Kreuznach, are readied for deportation to the psychiatric institution Meseritz-Obrawalde, a killing center. Nearly forty years after war's end, deaconesses from Bad Kreuznach who had lived through the time of the deportations—some of whom accompanied the girls in locked trains to Meseritz-Obrawalde and returned without them—asked the pastor-director Karl-Adolf Bauer to uncover and confront the history of the institution. The ensuing groundbreaking "confession of guilt" (*Schuldanerkenntnis*) formulated by the Diakonie-Anstalten Bad Kreuznach in 1984 was accompanied by this image, the only photograph the institution has with regard to the Nazi "euthanasia" murder program. It was noted, too, that "the girl on the left takes her doll with her on the journey to death." Printed in *Offene Tür* 1 (1985), 5. © Diakonie-Anstalten Bad Kreuznach.

Schlaich did not become a party member, but his deputy did—as did his head doctor, the finance officer, and one of the house-fathers. Schlaich expressly *encouraged* NSDAP (National Socialist German Workers' Party) educational events among his staff; took the staff to Stuttgart to see a Nazi exhibit on Bolshevism; allowed the Hitler Youth and the League of German Girls to use the castle's spaces; gave a lecture already in 1933 stating that "racial mixing" and Jewish-Christian marriages should be outlawed; and both affirmed the Nazi sterilization law

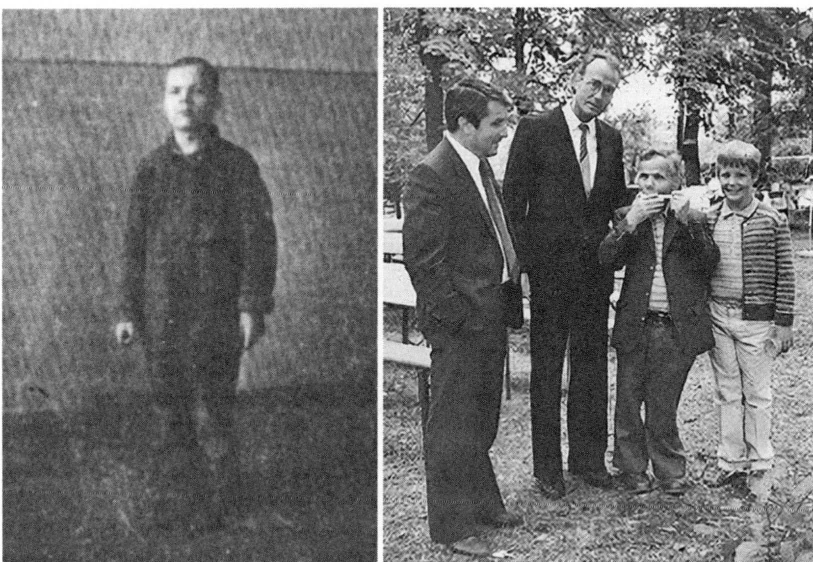

FIGURE 2.5. Heinz Fahr, deported to Hadamar during the second phase of "euthanasia," was immediately forced to work as a gravedigger on the hill above the clinic. Kept institutionalized at Hadamar into the postwar era and frequently leased out as an unpaid laborer who performed garden work for the local priests and the town mayor, he was well known by the townspeople, affectionately referred to as "Heinzje," and remembered above all for his harmonica-playing. The picture on the left, from his (apparently now lost) original patient file, is from the 1930s, reprinted in the book by Gerhard Kneuker and Wulf Steglich, *Begegnungen mit der Euthanasie in Hadamar* (Encounters with Euthanasia in Hadamar, 1985). The picture on the right is from the 1950s and shows him with two other men also named Heinz, along with a young boy from the town. "Die drei Heinze." Archiv Heinz Duchscherer. Kneuker was a social worker while Steglich, a psychiatrist, was the head physician at Hadamar in the early 1980s; both were deeply distressed by the institution's murderous past and the everywhere palpable, unnerving evidence of local disinterest in confronting it. Steglich and his wife Brigitte Schwan-Steglich, also a physician, developed a close and trusting relationship with Fahr and—against considerable opposition from the institution's then-director and regional welfare bureaucrats as well as various town elites— eventually got him discharged and helped him establish a new life in freedom and safety; he lived until 2003.

and implemented it among his charges (184 of them between 1934 and 1940).[84] Aware as early as 1937 that his tax-free status as a charity would be endangered by the fact that he had three Jewish residents (including one man who had lived in Stetten for nearly 60 years), he tried to get them moved out but failed; the old man stayed until he was deported to the gas chamber at Grafeneck with other residents.

And yet—and yet. Schlaich *cherished* his patients. Schlaich expressly, and vigorously, repudiated talk of "use-value" and "productivity." Schlaich argued about the disabled that "through their existence they awaken our love."[85]

Schlaich had been drafted into the Wehrmacht and was not present when the first "reporting forms" were sent to all the Württemberg institutions. Yet when he returned to Stetten and was confronted by the demand to turn over his own beloved patients, he mobilized quickly, entering into grueling and desperate negotiations with the regional authorities that were coordinating the transports, refusing in one case to be present when a staff doctor gave up a group to be deported so the patients would not think he supported the action, mobilizing church leaders to write protest letters at the national and regional levels and writing letters himself (including to Propaganda Minister Joseph Goebbels) that marshalled every imaginable religious and secular argument against murder, urging kin to rescue patients by bringing them home, later bargaining with transport personnel at the door of the buses in hopes of turning them away and saving those he could. He never forgave himself for failing.

Schlaich published an anguished book in 1947. As a historical document, there is nothing like it. *Lebensunwert?* (Unworthy of Life?) is a landmark, milestone text. Muddled in some indicative ways, it is nonetheless an indispensable source. It is a book of sorrow over lives lost and resistance that was insufficient. And it is unique in that it incorporates the voices of victims and survivors and captures their experiences of terror. In these testimonials, what is communicated are the victims' and survivors' deep attachments to their caregivers but also to each other (there are several stories of wanting to die together with friends); and above all their acute awareness of the fate awaiting them. Some can only shriek or sob or try to run. A survivor (in a wheelchair) said: "Who will hide me, who would be my advocate? With me one can see already from far away that I am a useless eater." One woman writes to her family: "When they come and take one by the collar, I sure am not a weakling, that is clear, but I would not believe it if I had not seen it with my own eyes, . . . this is all true, what I am telling, the government no longer wants so many institutions and us they want to be rid of."[86] In another text Schlaich reports on one man—who could not be saved—who shouts to his nurse: "'We'll see each other again in heaven!', but to the personnel that had come for him he screamed in their faces: 'Our blood be upon you!'"[87]

Schlaich demanded recognition for the survivors of the T4 action (and he may have been the first to do so). He declared:

> The psychiatrically ill, the feeble-minded and the epileptics have truly also belonged to *the persecutees of the Third Reich*. Who can deny this? But where is someone, where are the political parties, where the state, that will intercede so that those who have escaped this terrible extermination-action and its terrors can receive reparations? They cannot raise their own voices. They are in the political battles of our days no power-factor that one might fear or that one could leverage on their behalf. That is why no one, also today, just as in the days of the Third Reich, considers them worthy of being paid attention to, to say nothing of fulfilling their rights for justice.[88]

It would ultimately take four decades to make this case that Schlaich had first proposed in 1947: that the sterilizations and the "euthanasia" killings had been crimes—crimes that deserved to be prosecuted, to be memorialized, and to be integrated into the history of the nation. And it would take the efforts of many more activists, advocates, and scholars to bring into view possible alternative paradigms and to model, in concept and in lived practice, what it would mean to consider individuals with disabilities as full human beings.

3

How Does One Recognize a Crime?

Racism does not only mean the discrimination of "foreign" peoples, but also the "perfection" of one's own populace, attempted through discrimination against the "less valuable" within one's own ethnic group.

—HISTORIAN GISELA BOCK, TESTIFYING TO
A COMMITTEE OF THE BUNDESTAG, 1987[1]

IN JANUARY 1946, in the earliest iteration of what would later become Protestant theologian Martin Niemöller's famous poem, "First they came for the Communists," the second group mentioned was not the Jews or the trade unionists, but rather, as Niemöller phrased it, "Then they got rid of the ill, the so-called incurables." Yet before he moved on to talk about other groups, Niemöller inserted this: "I remember a conversation with a person who claimed to be a Christian. He took the view: Maybe it is really right, these incurably sick people just cost the state money, they are for themselves and others only a burden. Is it not the best for all concerned if we get rid of them from our midst?'"[2] Niemöller captured the climate well. In the first postwar years, there was no clear cultural consensus that the murders of the disabled were legally or morally wrong.

This chapter revisits the story of a series of efforts to grapple with the crimes against human beings labeled disabled over the course of the post-1945 period, primarily in the Federal Republic. The story follows two arcs, one running from 1945 through the mid-1960s, the second running from the early 1980s to the 2010s. But what most requires emphasis is the extraordinarily longue-durée impact of that little brochure from 1920 by Binding and Hoche, demanding the "permission to annihilate life unworthy of life." And—this will become yet clearer in the second arc— the even longer reach of that foul moral compromise formulated by Protestant charity men in their efforts to rebut Binding and Hoche, that *theo-biopolitics*, or theologization of eugenics, that sought to meet their opponents halfway. Christians were long complicit in denying full humanity to individuals with disabilities. Only in the 1980s did a complex process of moral and political reorientation begin—crucially involving both emotional-affective and intellectual-conceptual dynamics.

Mistakenness with Regard to Illegality

After a brief initial wave of convictions of doctors and nurses for coordination of or participation in the murders, a trend toward dropped charges, acquittals, amnesties, and more general exculpation marked the years that followed. Various rationalizations evolved to exonerate the killers. Three were especially significant. One was the notion of "collision of duties" (*Pflichtenkollision*), better known in everyday parlance as "in order to prevent worse from happening" (*um Schlimmeres zu verhindern*), in other words: killing some patients in order to save others.[3] A second move involved the German legal concept of "mistakenness with regard to illegality of the deed" (*Irrtum über die Rechtswidrigkeit der Tat*).[4] If the foundational self-defense claim with regard to the murder of Jews was "I was just following orders," the baseline contention with regard to the "euthanasia" killings was "I thought it was legal." A third contention was the argument that Binding and Hoche simply had been correct. A Hamburg court in 1949, while conceding that it was "objectively certain" the accused physicians in the case had killed at least fifty-six children, and that doing so was "objectively illegal," did not only remark that the accused "believed in the legitimacy of their way of acting." Directly invoking Binding and Hoche for support as they dropped the charges, the judges declared as well that they themselves were "not of the opinion that the annihilation of the mentally completely dead and 'empty human shells,' as Hoche had called them, was absolutely and a priori immoral."[5] In a law journal in 1952, an author praised Binding and Hoche for coining the concept of "life unworthy of life" and defended the actions of a doctor in a different case—this one accused of killing 120 children—as "assistance to the Volk, in order to ennoble the Volk and to liberate it from the great sacrifices that the maintenance of the asylums demand."[6] Jurists were not out of sync with the populace.[7] There was tremendous public support for accused physicians, replete with petition campaigns garnering hundreds of signatures demanding amnesty for those few doctors who actually were facing jail time.[8] Walther Schmidt at the Eichberg was one such example.[9] Mathilde Weber at the Kalmenhof was another.[10] The handling of Schmidt's case in the postwar press revealed the perverse inversion of reality with special clarity, as here it was the perpetrator who was lyrically sentimentalized and pitied, not his disabled victims—while the victims were described, in a tone of nauseated aversion, as fantastically, surreally misshapen and monstrous[11] (figure 3.1).

A different set of rationalizations were developed regarding the 400,000 coercive sterilizations. While dismantling the Nazi sterilization courts, the Western Allies (in contrast to the Soviets) had not rescinded the sterilization law of July 1933. The occupiers, in a double misunderstanding, misrecognized the 1933 Nazi sterilization law as not so different from various US state laws—although it was, both in scope and detail, entirely different—while demonstrably rescinding the 1935 Nuremberg Laws (not recognizing those as actually patterned quite directly on the Jim Crow anti-miscegenation legislation regulating relations between Blacks and whites in the US South).[12] The West German Christian Democratic-led government—already quite annoyed about the high cost of reparations that were due to Jewish survivors—was eager to gather expert opinions to justify its refusal to grant recognition or reparations to survivors of the "eugenic" sterilizations.[13] The first paragraph of the federal reparations law (updated in 1956)—itself the result of Western nations' pressure—deemed only those persecuted for

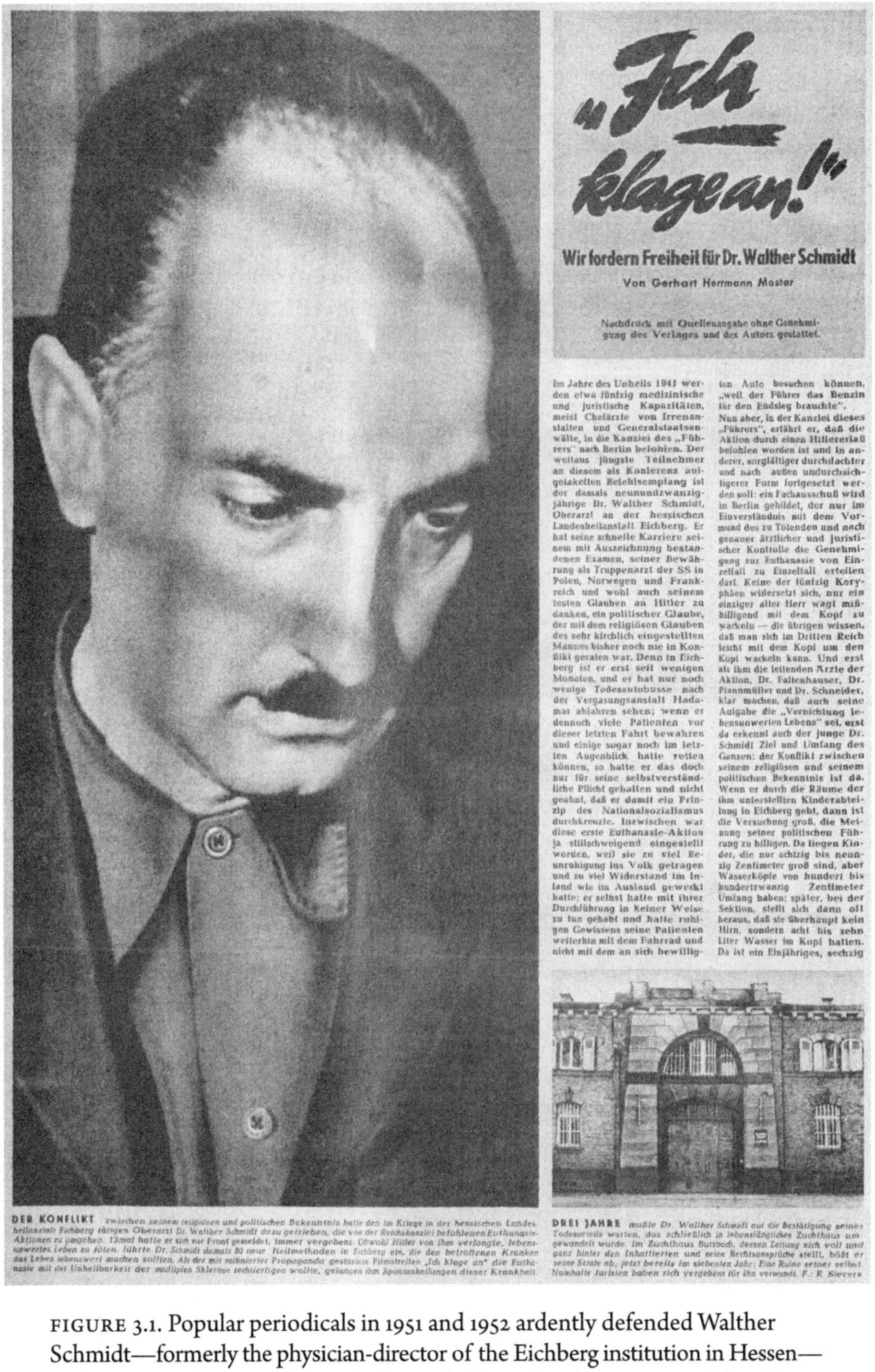

„Ich klage an!"

Wir fordern Freiheit für Dr. Walther Schmidt

Von Gerhart Herrmann Mostar

Nachdruck mit Quellenangabe ohne Genehmigung des Verlages und des Autors gestattet.

Im Jahre des Unheils 1941 werden etwa fünfzig medizinische und juristische Kapazitäten, meist Chefärzte von Irrenanstalten und Generalstaatsanwälte, in die Kanzlei des „Führers" nach Berlin befohlen. Der weitaus jüngste Teilnehmer an diesem als Konferenz aufgetakelten Befehlsempfang ist der damals neunundzwanzigjährige Dr. Walther Schmidt, Oberarzt an der hessischen Landesheilanstalt Eichberg. Er hat seine schnelle Karriere seinem mit Auszeichnung bestandenen Examen, seiner Bewährung als Truppenarzt der SS in Polen, Norwegen und Frankreich und wohl auch seinem festen Glauben an Hitler zu danken, ein politischer Glaube, der mit dem religiösen Glauben des sehr kirchlich eingestellten Mannes bisher noch nie in Konflikt geraten war. Denn in Eichberg ist er erst seit wenigen Monaten, und er hat nur noch wenige Todesautobusse nach der Vergasungsanstalt Hadamar abfahren sehen; wenn er dennoch viele Patienten vor dieser letzten Fahrt bewahren und einige sogar noch im letzten Augenblick hatte retten können, so hatte er das doch nur für seine selbstverständliche Pflicht gehalten und nicht geahnt, daß er damit ein Prinzip des Nationalsozialismus durchkreuzte. Inzwischen war diese erste Euthanasie-Aktion ja stillschweigend eingestellt worden, weil sie zu viel Beunruhigung ins Volk getragen und zu viel Widerstand im Inland wie im Ausland geweckt hatte; er selbst hatte mit ihrer Durchführung in keiner Weise zu tun gehabt und hatte ruhigen Gewissens seine Patienten weiterhin mit dem Fahrrad und nicht mit dem an sich bewilligten Auto besuchen können, „weil der Führer das Benzin für den Endsieg brauchte". Nun aber, in der Kanzlei dieses „Führers", erfährt er, daß die Aktion durch einen Hitlererlaß befohlen worden ist und in anderer, sorgfältiger durchdachter und nach außen undurchsichtigerer Form fortgesetzt werden soll: ein Fachausschuß wird in Berlin gebildet, der nur im Einverständnis mit dem Vormund des zu Tötenden und nach genauer ärztlicher und juristischer Kontrolle die Genehmigung zur Euthanasie von Einzelfall zu Einzelfall erteilen darf. Keine der fünfzig Koryphäen widersetzt sich, nur ein einziger alter Herr wagt mißbilligend mit dem Kopf zu wackeln — die übrigen wissen, daß man sich im Dritten Reich leicht mit dem Kopf um den Kopf wackeln kann. Und erst als ihm die leitenden Ärzte der Aktion, Dr. Faltenhauser, Dr. Pfannmüller und Dr. Schneider, klar machen, daß auch seine Aufgabe die „Vernichtung lebensunwerten Lebens" sei, erst da erkennt auch der junge Dr. Schmidt Ziel und Umfang des Ganzen: der Konflikt zwischen seinem religiösen und seinem politischen Bekenntnis ist da. Wenn er durch die Räume der ihm unterstellten Kinderabteilung in Eichberg geht, dann ist die Versuchung groß, die Meinung seiner politischen Führung zu billigen. Da liegen Kinder, die nur achtzig bis neunzig Zentimeter groß sind, aber Wasserköpfe von hundert bis hundertzwanzig Zentimeter Umfang haben; später, bei der Sektion, stellt sich dann oft heraus, daß sie überhaupt kein Hirn, sondern acht bis zehn Liter Wasser im Kopf hatten. Da ist ein Einjähriges, sechzig

DER KONFLIKT zwischen seinem religiösen und politischen Bekenntnis hatte den im Kriege in der hessischen Landesheilanstalt Eichberg tätigen Oberarzt Dr. Walther Schmidt dazu getrieben, die von der Reichskanzlei befohlenen Euthanasie-Aktionen zu umgehen. 13mal hatte er sich zur Front gemeldet, immer vergebens. Obwohl Hitler von ihm verlangte, lebensunwertes Leben zu töten, führte Dr. Schmidt damals 80 neue Heilmethoden in Eichberg ein, die den betroffenen Kranken das Leben lebenswert machen sollten. Als der mit raffinierter Propaganda gestartete Filmstreifen „Ich klage an" die Euthanasie mit der Unheilbarkeit der multiplen Sklerose rechtfertigen wollte, gelangen ihm Spontanheilungen dieser Krankheit.

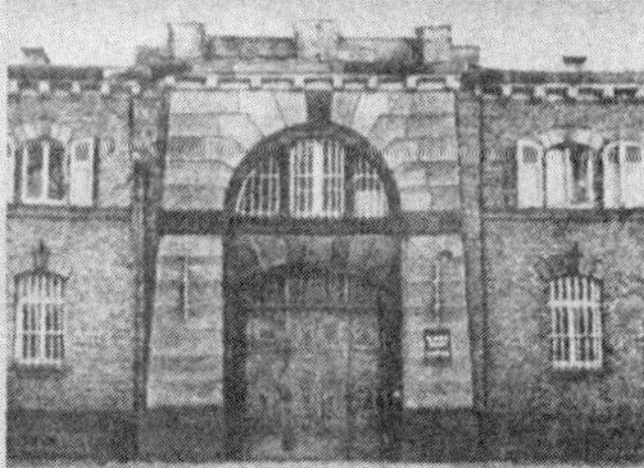

DREI JAHRE mußte Dr. Walther Schmidt auf die Bestätigung seines Todesurteils warten, das schließlich in lebenslängliches Zuchthaus umgewandelt wurde. Im Zuchthaus Butzbach, dessen Leitung sich voll und ganz hinter den Inhaftierten und seine Rechtsansprüche stellt, büßt er seine Strafe ab; jetzt bereits im siebenten Jahr: Eine Ruine seiner selbst. Namhafte Juristen haben sich vergebens für ihn verwandt. F.: R. Sievers

FIGURE 3.1. Popular periodicals in 1951 and 1952 ardently defended Walther Schmidt—formerly the physician-director of the Eichberg institution in Hessen—with canny ingenuity, and urgently demanded his release from prison. Schmidt was both sentimentalized and heroized, while his victims were described in such a way as to elicit the readers' revulsion. *Schwäbische Illustrierte*, August 18, 1951; *Die 7 Tage*, August 1, 1952. As would become more widely known only decades later thanks to the research of journalist Ernst Klee, Schmidt's coworkers at the Eichberg had referred to him mainly by the nickname "mass-murderer" (*Massenmörder*).

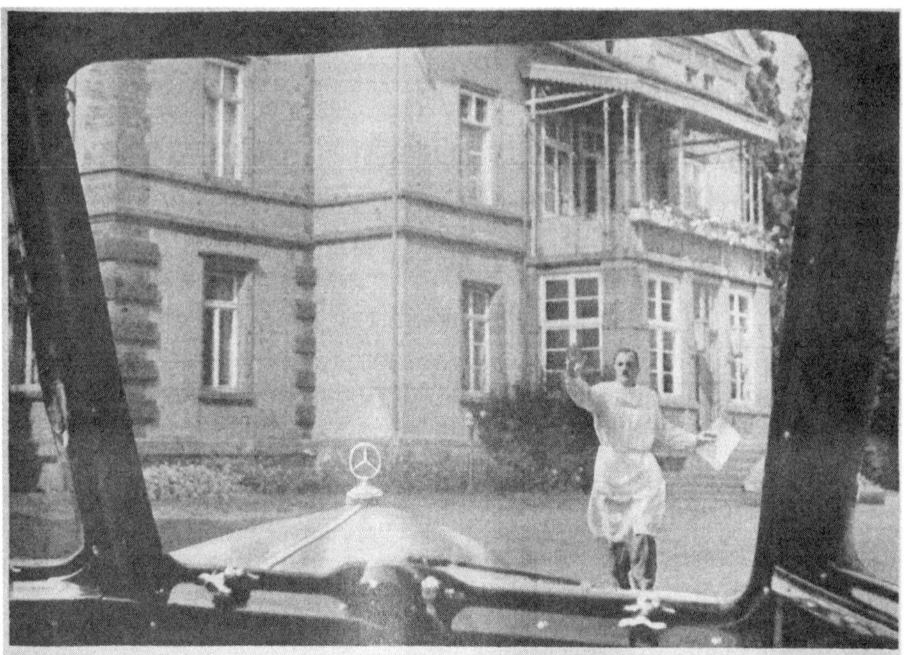

DIE TODESOMNIBUSSE NACH HADAMAR *pflegte Dr. Schmidt nach dem Bericht von Augenzeugen in Eichberg anzuhalten. Der überzeugte Nationalsozialist widersetzte sich auf jede Weise den Euthanasie-Anordnungen. Die Zahl der so allein von ihm geretteten Kranken betrug nachweislich mindestens Zwölfhundert. Trotzdem erfolgte die Verurteilung in Hessen auf lebenslänglich, ein unverständlicher Spruch, der von maßgebenden Juristen in anderen deutschen Ländern, aber auch im Ausland, mit Kopfschütteln aufgenommen wurde. Dr. Schmidt darf im Zuchthaus in der Bibliothek tätig sein, jedoch nicht dem Gefängnisarzt helfen. Das sollen in Hessen irgendwelche Vorschriften verbieten. Sein Mund zittert, wenn er spricht: er ist „fertig". Wenn er nicht bald beurlaubt wird, kann alle Hilfe zu spät kommen.*

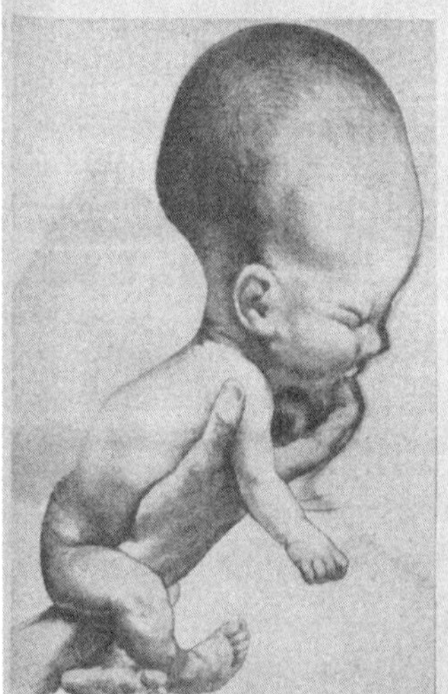

Zentimeter groß, mit einem Kopfumfang von hundertfünfzehn Zentimetern, dessen Stirn ist ein einziges Brandgeschwür, es bedarf zu seiner Wartung einer Schwester, die nur für dieses Wesen tätig sein kann, denn alle drei Minuten muß sie es umbetten: der Kopf zwar ist unbeweglich, aber durch das Strampeln verdreht sich der Hals, die Atemwege werden verlegt, es müßte ersticken. Da liegen Elfjährige, zum Skelett abgemagert, taub, stumm und blind, im eigenen Kot, oft, der Brandgeschwüre wegen, im monatelangen Wasserbad, von Geburt an mit der Sonde ernährt. Ja, die Versuchung ist groß, hier radikal und grundsätzlich Schluß zu machen. Aber der junge Arzt erliegt ihr noch nicht; er sucht zunächst dem furchtbaren Konflikt in seinem Innern zu entfliehen, mitten hinein in den furchtbaren Konflikt da draußen: dreizehnmal meldet er sich zur Front — immer vergebens. Er wird ein Jahr später stellvertretender Direktor und drei Jahre später Chefarzt und Obermedizinalrat, es gibt für ihn keine Flucht.

So stellt er sich denn, stellt sich auf seine Weise. Er muß lebensunwertes Leben töten, fordert sein „Führer", er muß alles Leben erhalten, fordert sein Gott — da sucht und findet er den dritten Weg: er muß lebensunwertes Leben lebenswert machen. Über achtzig damals neue Heilmethoden führt er in Eichberg ein. Von seinem Privateinkommen kauft er teure Apparate. Er geht zur Schock-

Fortsetzung auf Seite 1016

WAR DIE POLITISCHE FÜHRUNG *etwa im Recht? Wenn Dr. Schmidt seine kleinen unglücklichen Patienten in der Landesheilanstalt Eichberg betrachtete, kamen ihm Zweifel an seiner eigenen Einstellung. Der sanfte Tod für hydrocephale (oben) oder taub-stumm-blinde Kinder? Der Arzt erlag in diesem furchtbaren Konflikt nicht der Versuchung, obwohl oft sogar die Eltern den Tod wünschten.*

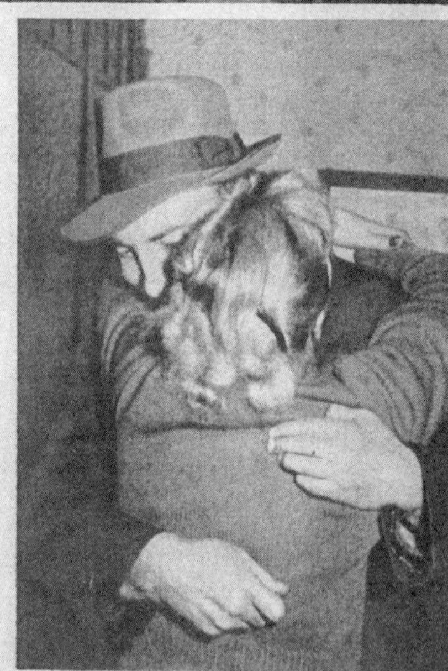

URLAUB AUF EHRENWORT *erhielt Dr. Schmidt Pfingsten 1951: „Dienstag nach Pfingsten melden Sie sich wieder!" wurde ihm im Zuchthaus gesagt. Die Begrüßung mit der Schwägerin bedeutete für den durch lange Jahre der Inhaftierung mitgenommenen Mann eine schwere seelische Belastung. Wie lange wird er noch im Zuchthaus bleiben müssen? Unser Bericht will nur dem Recht dienen, und damit dem Menschen, jedem Menschen. Aus Recht darf nicht Unrecht werden, auch nicht bei Schmidt.*

FIGURE 3.1. (*continued*)

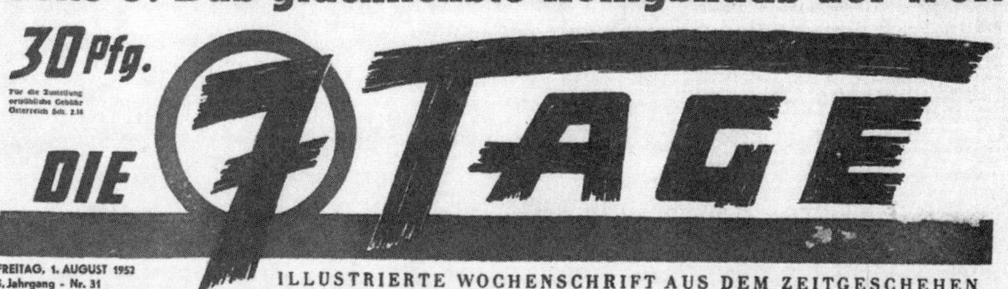

Ein Arzt sitzt im Zuchthaus:

Darüm sterben Tausende!

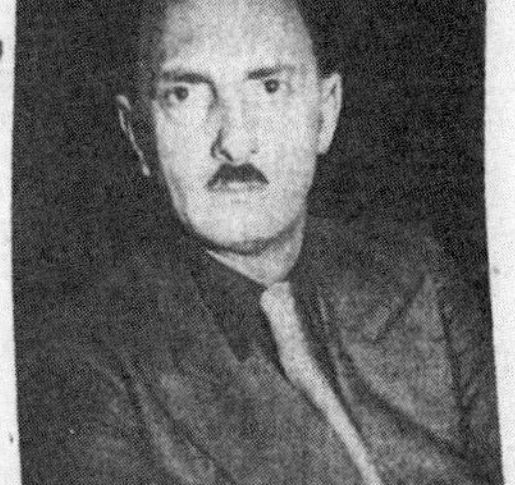

Unheilbar Kranke warten auf Freilassung Dr. Schmidts

In der Bibliothek des hessischen Zuchthauses Butzbach ist ein schmalgesichtiger, blasser Mann tätig. Nach seinem Geburtstag war er am 8. Juli 41 Jahre alt, seinem Aussehen nach könnte er Mitte der Fünfzig sein. Dieser Mann leiht die Bücher an die achthundert Insassen von „Butzbach" aus, jenem Zuchthaus, in dem, abgesehen von einer Handvoll Sträflingen, die hier büßen müssen, was eine unheilvolle Zeit ihnen einmal abforderte, nur Kriminelle untergebracht sind.

Der Bibliothekar ist ein Sträfling, der für Taten bestraft wurde, deren Rechtswidrigkeit erst nach dem Kriege rechtlich festgestellt wurde: Dr. med. Walther Schmidt, einstiger Oberarzt und hessischer Provinzial-Medizinalrat.

Wegen Mordes zum Tode verurteilt und zu „lebenslänglich" begnadigt

Dieser frühere Provinzialmedizinalrat Dr. Walther Eugen Schmidt, geboren am 8. Juli 1911 in Wiesbaden, als Sohn des heute noch in Wiesbaden lebenden Architekten Karl Schmidt, in Haft seit dem 12. Juli 1945, wurde am 21. Dezember 1946 durch die 4. Strafkammer des Landgerichtes in Frankfurt — Az. 4a Js 13/46 — wegen Mordes zu lebenslänglichem Zuchthaus verurteilt. Die Staatsanwaltschaft legte Revision ein und der Strafsenat des Oberlandesgerichtes in Frankfurt am Main hob das Strafmaß am 12. August 1947 auf und verwandelte das Urteil: Dr. Schmidt wurde zum Tode verurteilt! Im Gnadenwege wurde die Strafe am 2. Januar 1949 — also nach 16 Monaten Todeszelle — abermals in lebenslängliches Zuchthaus umgewandelt. 1951 wurde die Strafe auf sieben Jahre Zuchthaus und Ehrverlust reduziert. Dr. Schmidt hat also noch zwei Jahre Haft abzubüßen...

Wer ist dieser Dr. Walther Schmidt? Ein Arzt, wie Zehntausende? Ein Mörder? Ein Gestrauchelter? Ein Unglücklicher?

Er ist ein Arzt, der an der Euthanasie scheiterte. Obwohl er gegen sie war und durch sie selbst vernichtet wurde, Dr. Walther Schmidt ist eine der großen Tragödien unserer Zeit. Er ist einer jener wenigen Ärzte, die, schöpferisch tätig, in einer verblüffenden Kette von Einfällen eine Heilmethode nach der anderen finden. Er hat, neben vielen anderen Therapien, Mittel gefunden:

1. gegen die Multiple Sklerose.
2. gegen die spinale Kinderlähmung.
3. gegen Drüsenerkrankungen.

Dr. Schmidt sitzt jedoch als Bibliothekar im Zuchthaus in Butzbach und gibt Bücher an Mörder, Zuhälter, Diebe, Rückfallbetrüger, Hochstapler, Totschläger und Sittlichkeitsverbrecher aus. Wenn er in zwei Jahren aus der Haft entlassen wird, muß er sich überlegen, was er tun soll. Denn der Ehrverlust verbietet ihm die Ausübung jeglicher ärztlicher Praxis, und es ist die Frage, ob er mit Ehrverlust überhaupt noch im Besitz seines „Dr. med. summa cum laude" ist. Dabei kann dieser Dr. med. Schmidt Zehntausende an Multipler Sklerose Erkrankter heilen, er kann die Spinale Kinderlähmung im Anfangsstadium erfolgreich niederkämpfen, und er kann durch sein Wissen um die Frischhaltung der Hormone Drüsenerkrankungen aufheben.

Ministerpräsident Zinn könnte helfen

Der Ministerpräsident von Hessen, Zinn, der als einziger sofort helfen könnte, hat dem Vater des Zuchthäuslers Schmidt schon vor mehr als einem halben Jahr versprochen, daß er „in Kürze" in positivem Sinne entscheiden werde. An Multipler Sklerose Erkrankte, die diesen Zuchthäusler Schmidt kennen, haben Bittgesuche an den Ministerpräsidenten Zinn gerichtet: Schriften mit dreißig, mit 350, ja mit siebenhundert Unterschriften sind bereits in Wiesbaden vorgelegt worden.

Der SPD-Abgeordnete Arndt, der als Mitankläger 1946 den Richtern zurief: „Wenn Sie diesen Mann nicht zum Tode verurteilen, können Sie Ihre Roben ausziehen", hat sich bei Hessens Ministerpräsident für die sofortige Entlassung des Zuchthausinsassen Schmidt verwandt. Ob es das Gewissen, die Einsicht oder die Unhaltbarkeit eines seinerzeit vielleicht impulsiven Richterspruches gewesen sind, steht nicht zur Debatte. Abgeordneter Arndt hat seine Meinung von 1946 revidiert. Bittsteller, die sich an den Rechtsausschuß des Bundestages wandten und den hessischen FDP-Abgeordneten Dr. Schneider aus Gießen für sich gewannen, haben erneut für Dr. Schmidt interpelliert und sofortige Haftentlassung sowie die Aufhebung der Aberkennung der Ehrenrechte gefordert.

Aus Kassel hat ein an Multipler Sklerose Erkrankter, Schilling mit Namen, eine neue Eingabe eingereicht. Am 7. Juli 1952 haben die Eltern bei Ministerpräsident Zinn einen neuen Versuch unternommen, und schließlich wurde auch in dem gegenwärtig in Wiesbaden laufenden „Eichberg"-Prozeß ein abermaliger Vorstoß zugunsten von Dr. Schmidt gemacht. Das „Wiesbadener Tagblatt" vom 17. Juli 1952 berichtet über den Eichbergprozeß, in dem es um die Wahrheitsbeweise einer Gruppe westdeutscher Journalisten gegen die führenden Ärzte der hessischen Heilanstalt Eichberg geht. Ihnen wurde durch diese Journalisten unterstellt, daß sie sich innerhalb ihrer Anstalt und gegen die Insassen im medizinischen Sinne unkorrekt verhalten hätten. Einer der Angeklagten — darüber berichtete die Wiesbadener Zeitung — erklärte, die Anregung zu der Eichberg-Reportage habe sich aus der Beschäftigung mit dem Fall des früheren Chefarztes Dr. Walther Schmidt ergeben. Die Verurteilung dieses in einen Euthanasieprozeß verwickelten früheren SS-Arztes zu lebenslangem Zuchthaus habe als besonders hart und ungerecht empfunden werden müssen. Im „Wiesbadener Tagblatt" heißt es wörtlich:

Kronzeuge für die Menschlichkeit

„Schmidt genoß trotz seiner Verurteilung eine ungeheure Verehrung im Rheingau. Dieser Name war für uns ein „Sesam öffne dich", sagte einer der Angeklagten. Es habe sich zwar von selbst ergeben, daß die von ihm im Rheingau geführten Gespräche über die aufopfernde und vorbildliche Tätigkeit des Dr. Schmidt zu der Frage führten: „Wie sieht es heute auf dem Eichberg aus?".

Die Tatsache, daß Dr. Schmidt, viele Jahre nach seiner Verurteilung, noch immer als der „gute Geist" einer durch das Euthanasieprogramm Hitlers verrufenen Heilanstalt gilt und heute noch als Kronzeuge für die Menschlichkeit dieser Anstalt genannt wird, zwingt dazu, das Schicksal dieses Mannes in seiner ganzen menschlichen und sachlich-medizinischen Tragik aufzugreifen.

Keiner der nach 1945 inhaftierten und verurteilten Ärzte ist, wie Dr. Schmidt, noch im Zuchthaus. Ein deutsches Gericht hat Dr. Schmidt verurteilt und ein zu diesem Fall eingeholtes Rechtsgutachten besagt, daß nach der heute gültigen Rechtsauffassung gegen den wegen Euthanasie angeklagten Arzt Freispruch auf Grund § 59 des Strafgesetzbuches wegen „Irrtums über die Rechtswidrigkeit der Tat" erfolgen könne. Zwar ist die Frage des Irrtums eines Arztes über die Rechtswidrigkeit des das Euthanasie-Programm anordnenden „Führerbefehls" durch eine bundesgerichtliche Entscheidung bis heute noch nicht fixiert. Es kann aber den Ärzten unterstellt werden, daß sie die „Euthanasie" für rechtmäßig halten mußten und formalrechtlich nicht die Möglichkeit gehabt haben, das Unrechtmäßige ihres Tuns zu erkennen. Umsomehr, als den Ärzten gegenüber nicht nur die Legalität des Führerbefehls betont wurde, sondern auch das Kriegsrecht mit seinen Sonderpflichten sie anhielt, diesen Führerbefehl vorbehaltlos zu befolgen.

Im Frühjahr 1941 wurde Schmidt auf Betreiben des Landesrates Bernotat in Wiesbaden gegen seinen Willen „u. k."-gestellt und zum Oberarzt in Eichberg ernannt. 1942 schied der Direktor der Anstalt, Dr. Mennecke, aus und Dr. Schmidt wurde zum stellvertretenden Direktor bestimmt. Am 1. Januar 1944 wurde er Provinzialmedizinalrat und Chefarzt von Eichberg. Er stand auf diesem Posten, bis ihn die Amerikaner in die Internierung nahmen. Aus dem Internierten-Lager Darmstadt, in dem er Chefarzt des Lagerhospitals war, wurde er dann 1946 in Untersuchungshaft genommen. Ab 21. Dezember 1946 datiert die Strafhaft von Dr. Walther Schmidt.

Als Dr. Schmidt Anfang 1941 wieder nach Eichberg zurückkehrte, hatten Hitler und Bormann die Euthanasie „offiziell" eingestellt. Sie waren auf Grund von Berichten, die der damalige Innenminister Frick vorlegte, zu der Erkenntnis gekommen, daß die Beunruhigung in der Bevölkerung, zusammen mit den Protesten führender katholischer Würdenträger, nicht bagatellisiert werden dürfe. Bormann jedoch hatte lediglich vertagt.

In Eichberg war 1941 auf Anordnung des „Reichsausschusses zur wissenschaftlichen Erforschung und Erfassung von erb- und anlagebedingten schweren Leiden" eine „Kinderfachabteilung" eingerichtet und Dr. Schmidt zu ihrem medizinischen Leiter bestellt worden. Diese Abteilung hatte den Auftrag, neben der rein therapeutischen Betreuung klinische und hirnpathologische Untersuchungen anzustellen.

Führerkanzlei: Euthanasie fortsetzen!

Als Leiter der Kinderfachabteilung wurde Dr. Schmidt im Sommer 1941 mit seinem Chef, Dr. Mennecke, gemeinsam mit allen Leitern der hessischen Landesheilanstalten unter dem Verwaltungschef Landesrat Bernotat, in die Führerkanzlei befohlen. *Dort waren weitere sechzig Fachärzte und Anstaltsleiter anwesend. Die Ärzte wurden von einem Führer-Beauftragten auf die gesetzliche Grundlage der Euthanasie aufmerksam gemacht und unterrichtet, daß die Aktion fortgesetzt werden solle.*

Dr. Schmidt begriff, was geschehen sollte, und versuchte, sofort wieder zur kämpfenden Truppe versetzt zu werden. Alle Gesuche wurden von dem Landesrat Bernotat in Wiesbaden abgelehnt und Schmidt mußte seine Kinderabteilung leiten. In diese Abteilung wurden aus allen Teilen Deutschlands Kinder eingewiesen, die an schweren körperlichen Mißbildungen litten, geisteskrank und effektiv unheilbar waren. Alle diese Kinder wurden mit einer „Behandlungsermächtigung" eingeliefert, die durch den oben angeführten „Reichsausschuß" ausgestellt war.

Dr. Schmidt sah sich vor eine der schwersten Aufgaben gestellt, die es für einen Arzt geben konnte. Er hatte nur noch wenige der berüchtigten Todesomnibusse aus Eichberg abfahren sehen und er hatte, nachweislich, eine Reihe von Patienten, die dem Tode bestimmt waren, vor diesem Tod errettet. Nun aber kommen namhafte Psychiater, die Schmidt als Kapazitäten anerkennt, wie Dr. Faltenhauser (später wegen dreihundert Euthanasiefällen zu drei Jahren Gefängnis verurteilt), Dr. Pfannmüller (tausend Fälle, vier Jahre Gefängnis) und Dr. Schneider (beging 1945 Selbstmord) und verlangen von ihm, daß er „lebensunwerte Leben vernichten" solle.

Wie kommt es zum Tatbestand?

Grübelnd muß Dr. Schmidt in seiner Kinderabteilung sehen, in welch grausenhaften Konflikt er gestürzt ist: Da liegen Kinder, deren Wasserköpfe Umfänge bis zu einem Meter haben ... in diesen Köpfen ist kein Hirn — nur Wasser, bis zu zehn Litern. Jedes dieser Kinder beansprucht volle Pflege. Viele der Kinder liegen stumm und blind, im eigenen Kot, gelähmt. Dann wieder Kinder, die wegen der Brandgeschwüre monatelang in Wasserbädern liegen müssen. Für viele dieser hoffnungslos kranken Kinder liegen Briefe der Eltern vor, daß die Ärzte sie sterben lassen sollen. Auf Grund der „Ermächtigungen" könnte Dr. Schmidt diese Kinder — unter der ihm zuerkannten Rechtmäßigkeit der Euthanasie — sterben lassen. Er tut es nicht. Er sucht den Kindern zu helfen. Er greift schließlich nur ein, wenn er erkennen muß, daß die Kinder ihren Todeskampf beginnen. Im Laufe der Zeit erleichtert Dr. Schmidt etwa dreißig Kindern den Tod; weitere dreißig erhalten durch die Krankenschwester Schörg nach der Weisung von Dr. Schmidt Injektionen.

Das ist der Tatbestand. Er führte zu der Verurteilung Dr. Schmidts. Was Dr. Schmidt getan hat, muß er mit seinem Gewissen abmachen, vor Gott und vor sich selbst, er, der seit seiner Jugend ein gläubiger Christ ist.

(FORTSETZUNG AUF SEITE 2)

Vater und Tochter warten mit gleicher Sehnsucht auf die Freilassung des Butzbacher Sträflings: der Wiesbadener Architekt Karl Schmidt und seine Enkelin. Photos: privat

FIGURE 3.1. (*continued*)

active opposition to Nazism or on grounds of "race, religion, or political worldview" worthy of any restitution.[14] Where did individuals with disability fit in those categories? Two lines of argument rejecting their status as persecutees became key. One strand declared authoritatively that eugenics was internationally recognized *medical science* and had nothing whatsoever to do with "race" or "racism." The other strand—advanced by bureaucrats, doctors, and charity professionals alike—insisted that the sterilizations were *morally right*, caused no great harm or trauma to the individuals affected, and that a great number of those affected were so disabled mentally they did not even really know what had happened to them.

In 1961, at the very first meeting of the reparations subcommittee of the Bundestag at which testimony was heard, several invited experts expressed the view that there might well be both medical and moral questions about the sterilization program. The most systematic and emphatic was Hans Lewenstein, a doctor who had not served on the Nazi sterilization courts and who—although he did not challenge the rectitude of the sterilization law per se—believed these courts had been rife with abuse. He pointed out that "feeblemindedness" and even "schizophrenia" (the most prevalently given diagnoses) were by no means definitively "hereditary," that coercion had been rampant in what was after all a totalitarian state, and that the breakneck speed with which thousands had been sterilized apparently had been motivated not by concern for the welfare of individual families but rather the ideal of "racial refinement of the German Volk."[15] In short, Lewenstein was alert to the "racial" dimension of abuse of the disabled. Others, too, testified that they considered the 1933 law "unjust," or expressed doubts about the correctness of the most prevalently given diagnoses.

Yet Lewenstein and his supporters were drowned out by the louder and more authoritative voices of three physicians who *had* formerly sat on the sterilization courts. The catalogue of illnesses in the 1933 law was "assuredly no National Socialist invention," psychiatrist Helmut Ehrhardt asserted. And: The disabled were in no way comparable to Jews. Giving financial recompense to sterilization survivors would be grossly unfair— an "injustice vis à vis that circle of persons . . . who really were persecuted." Gesturing, moreover, to what he knew was his politician audience's biggest worry—money (while simultaneously reasserting the scientific validity of what had in truth been subjective presumptions on physicians' parts about the heritability of various conditions)—Ehrhardt additionally emphasized just how astronomically prohibitive would be the cost if the government were to have to reevaluate entire clans of German citizens for hereditary defects.[16] Geneticist Hans Nachtsheim, for his part, declared even more firmly that "the hereditary illness law may not be confused or even just lumped together with the National Socialist race laws"; it was, he averred, "an apolitical law." Nachtsheim further discoursed luridly on "products of incest," females with Down syndrome who had multiple children (more prevalent, he proposed, in "a primitive milieu"), and "eugenically undesirable maternities." Certainly, however, Nachtsheim found the "final solution of the Jewish question" decidedly "frightful" (*fürchterlich*)—even as he apparently could not help noting that therewith "one had a method whereby the total extermination of a people made a sterilization superfluous."[17] (It would be discovered many years later that Nachtsheim had conducted pressure chamber experiments on children with epilepsy to test how loss of oxygen could induce seizures, and he had used for his research eyes taken from prisoners murdered at Auschwitz.) Meanwhile, psychiatrist Werner Villinger (he had, it would soon be revealed, been one of the victim-selecting "assessors" in the T4 murder phase) opined that it was "the medical profession" that had "suffered greatly" during the Third Reich, because of the unpleasant compulsion to report candidates for sterilization. Calling attention to research by Danish geneticist Tage Kemp, Villinger went on to position sterilization as an internationally respected medical practice that made "good sense" as it prevented the birth of flawed children.[18] Nachtsheim too would subsequently pick up on the Kemp study, fretting in a 1963 essay that Germans were "falling behind," needing to "at long last free ourselves from the taboo that has lain on eugenics since National Socialism!" and that, alas, in Germany one had to calculate that 2–4 percent of newborns each year would suffer from "inborn feeble-mindedness," whereas Kemp had been able to show that Denmark had managed to reduce its rate to 1–2 percent.[19]

The Finance Ministry was already satisfied. In a file notation made in 1962, one official calculated that if all those who had been sterilized were to receive reparations, 60 percent of the funds would be going to "psychotics, imbeciles, and alcoholics."[20] Also the director of Bethel in those years, Friedrich von Bodelschwingh (the third) had been consulted regarding whether reparations would be advisable. He advised firmly against any restitution, expressing concern that especially "feeble-minded" individuals—"these people who cannot assess such matters"—would just get "disquieted" and "fixated" on the idea "that they must definitely be compensated."[21] A subgroup within the Protestant Inner Mission, zealous in the postwar years to advance its own version of a sexually conservative "personal eugenics," conspired in the early 1960s to find fresh ways to justify—on Christian grounds—a new "voluntary" sterilization law.[22]

The early 1960s saw the renascent discussion of "euthanasia" as well, primarily as a result of two scandals. In May 1962, a woman in the Catholic town of Liège, Belgium, Suzanne Van de Put, killed her thalidomide-injured newborn daughter with an overdose of barbiturates; the case and the ensuing jury trial in November 1962 riveted the international press and public. Also in 1962, former child "euthanasia" doctor Werner Catel—one of the physicians against whom charges had been dropped in that Hamburg case in 1949—published a book, *Grenzsituationen des Lebens* (Liminal Situations of Life), in which he called for the reintroduction, this time openly and legally, of a "limited euthanasia." Two groups were to be targeted: "monstrosities" (i.e., newborns with severe malformations) and "total idiots" (not necessarily newborns, as in these instances it could sometimes take months of repeated examination by a knowledgeable physician to establish incurability); for both categories, Catel assured readers, parental permission for killing was indispensable.[23] What was Catel's expressly invoked inspiration? Again: Binding and Hoche.[24]

Public opinion in Belgium, but also in Germany, was most definitely on Madame Van de Put's side.[25] And arriving as it did into this context of broad-based sympathy for an infanticidal mother, Catel's book and his effort to retool Binding and Hoche for the 1960s garnered more attention than they might have otherwise, and precisely the most aghast reviewers found themselves mightily challenged to spell out compellingly what was wrong with his positions, seeing how much receptivity there palpably was.[26]

Of all Catel's reviewers, Ludwig Schlaich—author of that remarkable 1947 book *Lebensunwert?* (Life Unworthy of Life?) which recorded anguish at the loss of hundreds of his residents from the Stetten charity institution to the Nazi murder machinery, and in 1962 still director there—was the clearest in articulating the emotional-spiritual impasses confronting all Germans. "We should not forget that, apart from a very few men, the overwhelming majority of the German Volk mustered just as little resistance to the 'annihilation of life unworthy of life' as to the 'final solution to the Jewish question' which followed it. We are all in need of the forgiveness of Jesus Christ." Schlaich was less interested in revisiting the past than in getting his fellow citizens to confront the fact that quite apparently there was still widespread popular support for the idea of "merciful deaths." True "'mastery of the past,'" he argued, would require that a genuinely fresh cultural consensus be formed, one in which it would never again be possible for any killer to claim "mistakenness with regard to illegality."[27]

Catel, meanwhile, kept propounding his views. Interviewed by *Der Spiegel* in 1964, Catel not only emphasized that "here we are not talking about humans, but rather about creatures that have merely been begotten by humans, but which themselves can never become humans endowed with reason or a soul." He extemporized at length about prominent Protestant theologians "before the n.s. [National Socialist] time, so in the first third of the twentieth century . . . who were of the opinion that it was not in contradiction with Christian ethics, in the case of subhuman vegetating . . . 'to put an end to what is solely a burden to itself, quite apart from the burdening of others.'"[28] Catel could not have obtained this evidence anywhere but from Ewald Meltzer, whose 1925 book, *Das Problem der Abkürzung "lebensunwerten" Lebens* (The Problem of Abbreviating Life "Unworthy of Life") had been the most important Protestant response to Binding and Hoche's text of 1920.[29] The parameters of conversation, in short, had not shifted since the 1920s—despite the rise and fall of the Third Reich in the interim.

The At Once Unconfident and Capacious Racial Motif

This, then, was the morally disorienting atmosphere within which Hessian state prosecutor Fritz Bauer in 1963 and 1964 was working indefatigably to bring to trial four men who had coordinated the first, T4 gas chamber phase of the adult "euthanasia" program. Dr. Werner Heyde, medical director of T4, was the key defendant, charged with complicity in the murder of 100,000 people; his associates were Friedrich Tillmann, Gerhard Bohne, and Hans Hefelmann. The trial was planned to be bigger than the Frankfurt Auschwitz trial Bauer was conducting simultaneously, an even greater reckoning: this time with mass murder *within* the bounds of the German Reich, and not just with lower-level functionaries as at Auschwitz, but rather with the highest-level organizers.[30]

Bauer and his team prepared an 800+-page indictment that concluded with an extended discussion of none other than Binding and Hoche. Here Bauer aligned himself with Ewald Meltzer's stance that "the proposal to kill idiots or the mentally ill, no matter how profoundly low their level, is to be rejected on legal and ethical grounds." But both the T4 and the children's "euthanasia" programs, the indictment further underscored, had "far exceeded the bounds of that narrowly delimited circle of persons whose killing had been up for debate in the scholarly discussions." And in any event, the supposed ethical motives had not been operative, "but rather pure utility and cost-benefit considerations and perspectives of racial intolerance and arrogance [*rassischer Unduldsamkeit und Überheblichkeit*]." These were the perfidious motives that distinguished murder from manslaughter. Finally, it was patently absurd for the defendants to contend that they believed their actions legal; of all the participants, they knew better than any others—precisely because a then-powerful regime had promised them impunity—how completely illegal the killings had been and remained.[31] These were prudently phrased and compelling arguments.

And then, in February 1964, Werner Heyde hanged himself in his prison cell; Tillmann threw himself (or fell) out of an eighth-story window; Bohne had vanished into Argentina. The trial went forward against just Hefelmann, but his defense successfully characterized him as no longer physically and mentally well enough to stand trial, with a life expectancy of only two more years. (He lived until 1986.) Bauer's indictment was relegated to the dustbin of history.

In a 1965 book, psychiatrist Helmut Ehrhardt—vigorous defender of sterilizations past and future—openly gloated at Bauer's public humiliation. Ehrhardt also and not incidentally mocked Adorno's imperative to "work through the past," noting that Bauer's failure had simply been near-inevitable. He sneered that Bauer and the apparatus he represented had "not exactly [made] it easy for the average educated citizen of the state to understand how it would be better and more right *not* to kill deformed children and the incurably mentally ill sick."[32]

And so matters stood, or stagnated, for the next decade and a half. Bauer died in 1968 under enigmatic circumstances, likely due to accident. The brilliant and bulky indictment Bauer's team had so carefully prepared, along with its vast cache of supporting documents, languished. It would be 1981 before the independent journalist Ernst Klee—more on Klee in a moment—was to turn up unexpectedly at Bauer's former offices to inquire about their whereabouts.[33]

Except, that is, for one remarkable text that appeared in 1965: Gerhard Schmidt's *Selektion in der Heilanstalt* (Selection in the Asylum)—demonstrating that it was already possible at that moment to see through the fog (figure 3.2).While Bauer the prosecutor had been focused on compiling unassailable documentation of legal guilt and, soberly and step by step, working preemptively to refute potential counterarguments likely to be put forward by the defense, Schmidt, a psychiatrist, had no hesitations about taking on directly the moral confusion so apparently rampant among both his professional peers and the wider public. The book had been initially drafted in 1947, based on Schmidt's experience as the first postwar director of the Bavarian asylum of Eglfing-Haar, where he encountered ninety-five emaciated, traumatized survivors ("living corpses," as he later described them).[34] Schmidt had studied closely all the extant in-house documents, including patient records and correspondence with government authorities (everything that had not been burned as American troops were approaching), and interviewed lower-level staff who remembered the many hundreds of murdered patients intimately, by name and by personality. But the manuscript had been actively suppressed by fellow psychiatrists, warning that he should not air dirty linen before an international audience and repeatedly blocking his efforts to get it published—including by physically disappearing the manuscript.

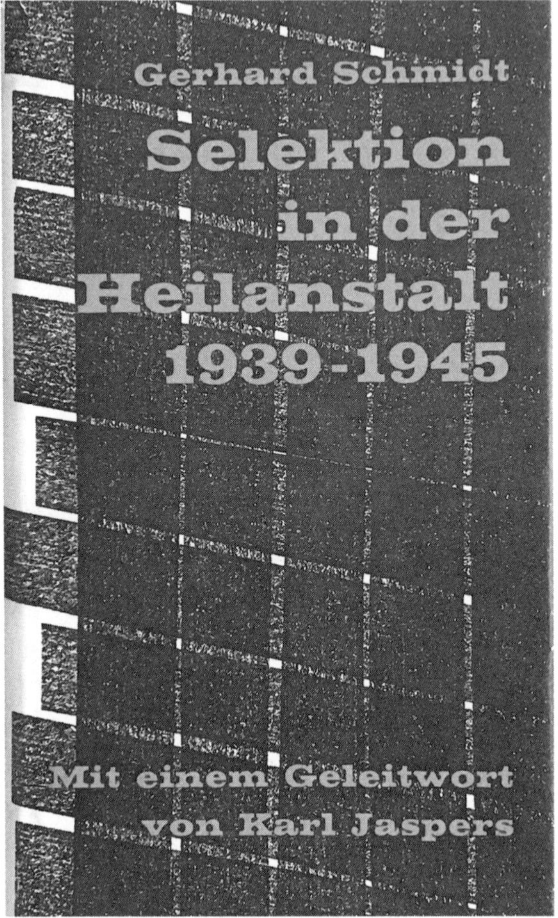

FIGURE 3.2. Cover of the first edition of Gerhard Schmidt, *Selektion in der Heilanstalt* (Selection in the Asylum, 1965)—with a foreword by the psychiatrist-philosopher Karl Jaspers. The manuscript had been completed in 1947, but physician colleagues had campaigned against—and, in some cases, actively thwarted—publication. Their argument was that evidence in the book would embarrass the entire German nation and especially its medical profession.

Only in 1965, in the midst of the heightened media attention surrounding Bauer's failed T4 trial, did a small Protestant press finally bring Schmidt's work into print. And not until 1986, in a changed cultural climate, did Schmidt publicly reveal the arguments that his psychiatrist colleagues had advanced in the early postwar years to suppress the publication. The facts he had assembled, he was told, gave "a hideous and terribly dispiriting impression"; the evidence only made the German people as a whole and in particular the German medical profession look bad. Publication was dangerous, for internationally, the book would cause a "tremendous sensation" and just reinforce the "self-righteousness of all non-National Socialists and all non-Germans."[35]

Because Eglfing-Haar, along with its seven smaller satellite institutions, was one of the sites at which murder by deliberate starvation had been implemented on a mass scale, Schmidt's is one of the few near-to-the-event documents detailing the experiences of victims in the second, "wild," decentralized phase of the "euthanasia" killings. The 1965 book cover immediately accentuated two matters: that in the author's assessment, the murder of the disabled was motivated "solely by the racial ideology of National Socialism," and that (this was an unmistakable allusion to Catel) Schmidt would be forcefully rejecting any more recently circulating ideas that a "'limited euthanasia'" might be reintroduced, "because no delimitation is possible."[36] Yet the book was distinctive for other reasons, too, among them: its style, its analyses, and the acuity of its ethical vision. Schmidt wrote with an elegant clarity inflected by sarcasm, rich with redolent word coinages and sharp observations about the motive forces facilitating the involvement of physicians in mass killing.

In his opening chapter, Schmidt engaged Binding and Hoche at length. He labeled their call for "merciful death" a "smug, arrogant, aggressive" "pseudocompassion" at base motivated by an unacknowledged reflex of dismay or disgust in the face of disability: "Not the incurable are to be cared for, but rather the environment is to be cleansed of the incurable." He dismissed as transparently false the economic arguments claiming that the disabled needed to be killed because their care cost too much. "In the final analysis," Schmidt wrote, the real driving force behind the killing had everything to do with *race*. Or, as he put it: "the at once unconfident and capacious racial motif."[37]

Strikingly, Schmidt dismissed the science of heredity and eugenics as not even deserving of serious engagement as science, but on the other hand a phenomenon very much needing to be engaged as a "complex" (in the sense of a neurosis or psychosis), a "delusion" producing a hallucinated "heredity-demon" (*Erbmar*). (It was no coincidence that Schmidt reached for medieval language to try to convey, simultaneously, the utter un-scientificness and yet also dark magic intensity of hereditarian thinking.) Repeatedly, moreover, Schmidt mocked the faux machismo and "pathos" evident in Binding and Hoche's strident calls for greater "heroism" in leaving behind humanitarian care and becoming comfortable with homicide—as he additionally took recurrent swipes at the idea of the "master-race men" (*Herrenmenschen*).[38] And, perhaps most stingingly, Schmidt pointed out that there was something wholly pathetic about the ambition to kill the disabled—that at bottom it was all about one's own defeat and insecurity and need to feel superior. The central contention of Schmidt's opening chapter was that if Binding and Hoche—those, as he put it, "so oft-invoked key witnesses in the case made for 'permission to annihilate life unworthy of life'"— had a genuinely passionate motivation that they were propounding, it was "at base the benefit to the fatherland, a resurrection-dream for the vanquished and famished postwar Germany of 1920." More important for Schmidt, the insecurity that Binding and Hoche were tapping in the wake of the defeat in World War I continued to be a propulsive force after Hitler came to power. Schmidt already found the sterilization program to be a completely absurd effort to manage "anxiety about the archenemy within the blood." He additionally noted Nazism's general tendency to "escalation." Just as the Nuremberg Laws of 1935 were the precursors to "the gassing of Jewish fellow citizens," so too the sterilization law was a prelude to far worse crimes.[39]

Finally, Schmidt paid particularly close attention to the intricate interconnections between antisemitism and antidisability animus, especially in his analysis of the Nazi propaganda courses held for members of the SS and party functionaries at Eglfing-Haar. The link between the disabled and Jews was not just correlational or contextual; in the phantasmatic Nazi mindset, as Schmidt saw it, the two were inextricable. Reviewing the visual materials in the indoctrination curriculum, Schmidt noticed how Jews and individuals with disabilities were juxtaposed as complementary dangers: "'A worthy representative of the tribe of Juda'

(Fig. 2) and 'an idiot looking retarded' (Fig. 4)," Schmidt observed, "were Reich-propagandistically the two visual poles for racial hatred and racial anxiety [*Rassenhaß und Rassenangst*]." "Hitler's racial insanity" [*Rassenwahn*], in short, had this dual dimension from the start: the external enemy and the internal enemy both needed extirpation.[40] Forty-five years after Binding and Hoche's pamphlet, twenty-five years after the start of the disability murders, and twenty years after the end of the war, this profoundly perceptive analysis had finally found its way into print.

The climate in West Germany in 1965, however, remained strongly resistant to Schmidt's insights. In 1966, another physician—chief doctor at a municipal hospital—took the occasion of yet another unpopular perpetrator trial to write a letter to the court to announce his opinion that "the Autobahn, euthanasia, and eugenic efforts were the best things among Hitler's accomplishments."[41] In 1967, the very fact that a court had actually managed to establish that killing of individuals with disabilities was "murder in the criminal legal sense" was in itself considered newsworthy.[42] Nonetheless, the three doctors in that particular case (between them, they were responsible for 8,000 deaths by gassing) were acquitted—once again on the grounds that they had been unaware of the illegality of their actions and believed the killings were permissible.[43] It would take until the 1980s before the conceptual frames within which the murders and the sterilizations were understood could finally be radically reconfigured.

Belated Working-Through

This is not to say that nothing happened in the interim. On the contrary, and in particular, in the course of the 1970s, there were new parameters of discussion about disability in West Germany being developed by activists in the radical "cripple movement" and by nondisabled individuals who were involved and invested—whether by parenthood, political commitments, and / or pedagogic or psychotherapeutic profession—with the aim above all of reorienting practice in the lived present of disability care. In 1973, the pedagogy professor Jacob Muth, lead author of the federal government's *Recommendation of the Educational Commission for the Pedagogical Development of Children and Youth with Disabilities and at Risk of Becoming Disabled*, surprised everyone by criticizing the segregated system of special education schools and officially advocating that kindergartens and schools begin to integrate children with disabilities into the regular school system.[44] In 1974, the TV channel Zweites Deutsches Fernsehen (ZDF) began airing a series, "Our Walter" (*Unser Walter*), which sympathetically portrayed the travails of a family whose young son Walter—played by the actor Walter Zabel—had Down syndrome, and thereby inaugurated an important shift "from pity for 'worry-children' to enlightenment about discriminations."[45] In 1975—although the process had been underway for several years already—another federally commissioned study, the "Report on the Situation of Psychiatry in the Federal Republic of Germany" (generally referred to in shorthand as the *Psychiatrie-Enquête*), documented "completely inadequate" conditions of overcrowding and understaffing in many residential mega-institutions, and the vast extent of grossly inappropriate "mis-location" (*Fehlplacierung*) of people with intellectual disabilities on psychiatric wards.[46] And all through the 1970s, a new tone became evident in journalism, with a sequence of important media exposés (on radio and in magazines and newspapers) documenting pervasive abuses in homes for "difficult-to-train" youth, in psychiatric clinics, and in charity institutions for individuals with intellectual disabilities alike. There can be no doubt that a passionate ethical defense of the value of disabled lives—whether secularly or religiously inspired—and a basic conceptualization of individuals with learning difficulties or mental illnesses as equally worthy human beings had to arise before a cultural sea change with regard to the past could take place (figure 3.3). It is only against the background of this wider social and cultural ferment on behalf of disabled life that we can begin to appreciate the magnitude of the reorientation of terms of debate about the national past that the 1983 publication of Ernst Klee's magnum opus, *"Euthanasie" im NS-Staat: Die "Vernichtung lebensunwerten Lebens"*, set in motion.[47]

Klee's book, with its 450 densely packed pages of tiny print, much of it reproducing verbatim significant chunks of primary source documents,

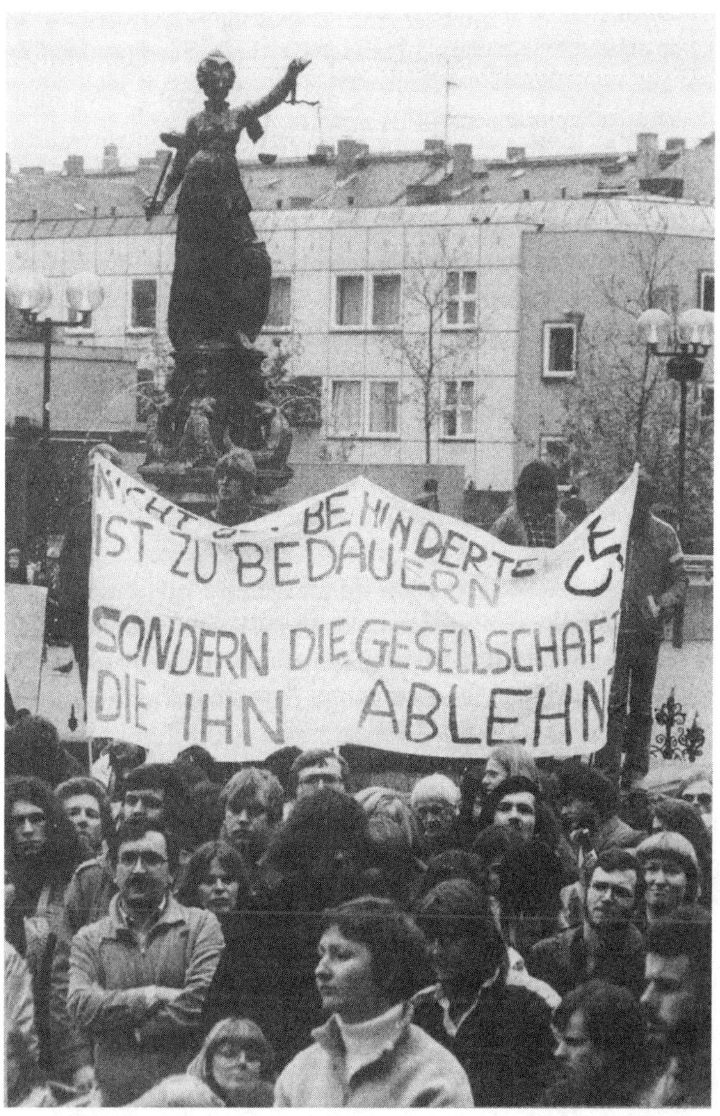

FIGURE 3.3. The first national demonstration of disability rights activists took place in Frankfurt / Main in 1980. The demonstrators protested a Frankfurt / Main court verdict that ordered a travel agency to reimburse a West German woman who had complained that her beach vacation in Greece had been blighted by the sight and sounds of individuals with physical disabilities residing in the same hotel. The banner hoisted above the crowd read: "Don't pity the disabled person; pity the society that rejects him." Photo © 1980, 2017 by Walter Pehle.

along with the book's avid reception across many hundreds of media sites, were only the beginning of what became a multidimensional national conversation—the "working-through," in Adorno's sense, that had been for so long postponed. Klee's method was unconventional in notable ways. All through the book, and while telling a largely chronological story, but without alerting readers within the text to the jumps in time from which his evidence was drawn (that information was embedded in the footnotes), Klee interleaved commentary from the four different temporalities of his source base: 1939–1945; 1945–1949; 1961–1969; 1981–1982. The effect achieved was akin to anthropological "thick description." Especially interesting was Klee's creative repurposing of prosecutorial and trial records, including Bauer's and nearly a dozen others. Klee was not interested per se in proving guilt legally—even as substantiation of legal guilt saturated the documents he included—but rather in capturing tone and sensibilities. This in turn meant giving particular consideration to passing references and unintended slips, and taking rumors, lies, and rationalizations as evidence of meaning-making just as pertinent to our comprehension of the past as expressions of earnest sincerity and conviction.

Facts, in short, mattered greatly to Klee, and he presented an immense accumulation of theretofore neglected data, clarifying the dense abundance of killing sites dotting the landscape of the Reich as well as the prevalence of public knowledge. But so too did the meanings ascribed to those facts offered by the quite variously positioned human beings whose souls or psyches he was auscultating. Klee remained all too aware that in the postwar decades, it had not been the facts of the "euthanasia" murders that were contested. The contentious issue was how to feel about those facts and what conclusions were to be drawn from them.[48]

Two elements were especially significant in prompting a redirection of moral and political discussion. One was that Klee made "euthanasia" corporeally palpable with all one's senses, as he jammed his book with haunting details, conveying as no text had before the horror of the viciousness that had been unleashed against defenseless human beings. These included such memorable images as: the man responsible for running errands for Grafeneck delivering milk from the institution's cows to a nearby dairy, picking up curlers and stocking garters for the female staff, and then in the afternoons running urns of ashes to various post offices; the too-visible flames and unpleasant smell from Brandenburg's ineptly constructed chimney, forcing staff to transition to a daily early morning ritual of carting corpses for burning to a nearby forest edge discreetly away from the city center; the research doctor indignantly complaining that, due to insufficient formaldehyde, "the brains are ruined" of the children with cognitive disabilities he had so meticulously selected for (torturous) premortem examination at Heidelberg University and then postmortem dissection at the Eichberg special children's ward; the diarrhea-green feces floating in the bathwater at the Weilmünster institution in which deliberately starved individuals were lying whose sores were too raw to bed them on (anyway rotted) straw mattresses, while a Catholic priest strove—against official regime regulation, and grateful to be hidden from monitoring authorities by the medical staff—at least to offer these individuals some final gestures and words of consolation; the hallucinatory scene in a Nazi-occupied Silesian town at war's end as bumbling local functionaries struggled and failed to murder surviving psychiatric patients with poison as they had initially planned and instead ended up shooting them as they ran screaming through the hospital corridors.[49] In all these and in innumerable further ways, *"Euthanasie"* was a work of compressed terror.

The second decisive element was Klee's attention to the perpetrators' subjectivities. Klee had made a point of stressing that "the perpetrators, their helpers and helpers' helpers" were "as a rule no slaughter-eager butcher-types, but rather conformist, career-conscious climbers and fellow travelers."[50] But this summary statement was given heft with indicative minutiae: a memo of complaint about an inept colleague at the T4 center at Hartheim apparently unaware about which false "causes of death" were most likely to be plausible; a physician in search of safe haven for his wife and children as German military defeat loomed near, urging a colleague at whose institution he hoped to find refuge simply to kill one hundred forced laborers to make room for his family; or another physician in similar straits proudly summarizing in his letter of inquiry his accomplishments in "emptying" the institutions of entire regions of their residents—and his respondent's offer of a suitable placement as long as he would help there in "reducing the number of the sick, since the institution is bursting to capacity."[51] In supplement and counterpoint, Klee dispersed little bits of revealing personal detail, evidently wagering that incorporating evidence of the perpetrators' indulgence in recreational pleasures in the interstices of their killing labors—from communal music-making to touristic travels, festive indulgence in alcohol, and pursuit of sex and love with fellow staff—was not irrelevant to reader comprehension of the tenor of the times and the mindsets that made mass murdering not just possible but an activity practiced with great verve and independent initiative. Hardly prudish, Klee's point was to challenge the widely held image of a banally obedient desk perpetrator. If these men were banal, it was at the bar, not the desk. Their brazen sense of entitlement and impunity was inseparable from their petty preoccupations with collegial rivalries and the securing of promotions and research funds.[52] But above all, precisely through extensive direct quotation, Klee captured the crass pitilessness of the perpetrators—their hubris, callousness, and utter lack of remorse both before *and* after war's end—the very opposite of the anxiously conflicted or innocently mistaken self-presentations that had later led so many perpetrators to go free.

"Annihilation of Life Unworthy of Life": Klee's subtitle highlighted his mission to produce the definitive counter-text to Binding and Hoche. It is indisputable that Klee saw his efforts as bringing to completion the unfinished business left behind by Bauer's failed prosecution. Whereas Bauer's massive indictment ended with a discussion of Binding and Hoche, Klee's opening chapter revisited the most infamous passages that had been repeatedly referenced over the decades both by their critics and by those continuing to draw inspiration from their message. Indeed, Klee's first chapter title is a quote from Hoche: "An embarrassing image, that entire generations of caregivers are aging away alongside these empty human shells." Klee's greatest fury in that opening chapter, however, focused on the welter of ugly remarks about the disabled in the very texts ostensibly intended as Christian rebuttals to Binding and Hoche's demand to kill. Klee dwelled on how the hapless Christian opponents of Binding and Hoche had affirmed that the disabled were objects of disgust, had denigrated also the "only moderately" disabled and not just the "most severely" disabled, and had mobilized that disgust against the disabled to push their sexually conservative—and frankly antisemitic—message. Klee railed against those Christian leaders who were "only doing the pre-work for the proponents of 'euthanasia,'" and who "with foolhardy ascriptions of guilt (after all, 'idiotic' children are also born to 'pious' pastors' families)," would never be able to "stem the burgeoning impact of the Binding-Hochean euthanasia-manual." Klee further emphasized that the Christian promotion of sterilizations as the compromise solution to the demand to kill gave sterilizations the moral gloss they would not have had otherwise; in sum, he was the first person in the postwar era to note that the Protestant charity leadership had provided *theological* cover to the Nazi sterilization campaign. And he concluded: "I do not present the behavior of the churches in such detail because they sinned more than others. The reason is different: Their stance on sterilization cannot be separated from their conduct during the euthanasia-actions."[53]

For there was one more aspect to Klee's handling of the churches—and although it was only a contrapuntal subplot, it quickly caught the attention of reviewers and journalists: the ambiguities and inadequacies of resistance to the disability murders themselves. Klee had been raised within the Protestant church, had been himself an earnestly faithful believer, and had innocently trusted postwar narratives of Nazi persecution of the churches and of Christian fortitude under duress. It was this trust that was shaken when in the archives, a significant number of church and charity men were revealed to be, however inescapably and sorrowfully so, contaminated by negotiations with the killers. In almost all cases their efforts at protest and protection had been unsuccessful—making their postwar self-revisions and silences at once humanly understandable and (from Klee's perspective, as he did not hide his disappointment) morally dubious.

Klee made clear that no other constituency or organization did more to defend people with disabilities than the churches. He documented the severe pressures and impossible non-choices under which charity directors operated as, whenever they announced noncompliance with government directives, they were threatened with the prospect of closure or takeover of their institutions, or with being arrested themselves—all instances in which their capacity to save even a few of their residents would have been forfeited. He recorded the devastating experience of complete impotence of caregivers and directors when faced with the telltale gray buses at their doors. He listed as many examples of individual acts of refusal (for example declining to fill out the government-mandated patient reporting forms), protest (whether in the form of a letter to the authorities or a statement made by an individual pastor from the pulpit or at a graveside), or protection (changing diagnoses, alerting kin to bring patients home, arguing with the deportation transport staff over an individual resident's health and capacity to work) that he was able to find.[54] Yet Klee's own assessment was one of obvious consternation over misplaced moral emphases when he recorded, in one instance, how nuns at the killing center of Kaufbeuren in the second, decentralized phase of the murders protested vigorously and effectively when female patients were placed on a male ward—but took female patients to another ward where they were to be killed by injection, fully cognizant that the destination was death.[55] He also noted matter-of-factly that Protestant charity institutions had given up their Jewish patients to "relocations" without protest.[56] And Klee was aghast to learn that rather than turning to loud, open protest, church leadership in the environs of the Grafeneck killing center had been caught up in attempting to negotiate with Nazi authorities over the right to provide last rites for those about to be driven into the gas chambers.[57] Taking all the incongruous moments together, Klee certainly leaned toward intemperate moral judgment—evident for example in a pointed subsection headline "Were the churches willing to agree to euthanasia? An inglorious chapter."[58] Outraged defenses of both Catholic and Protestant church and charity leaders were swiftly mounted.[59]

Klee's shock at his own unexpected findings was tangible both in the *"Euthanasie"* book and in subsequent interviews and correspondence.[60] His dismay would motivate him to unearth and expose yet more church malfeasance in the years that followed.[61] Follow-up books concerned the deep involvement of the Protestant and Catholic churches in early endorsement and collaboration with the Nazi regime, and in support of the exterminatory war in the Soviet Union. Klee turned as well to the postwar period, uncovering extensive evidence of clergy, both Protestant and Catholic, being actively solicitous about the fate of accused perpetrators (including of the Judeocide), defending them from prosecution, and in many cases aiding them in leaving the country to escape justice. All this earned him yet more animus from vigorous champions of the churches' reputations—including an accusation from the Vatican that he was promoting "vile propaganda" and "historical falsehood."[62] But it also, from other quarters, earned him more plaudits.[63] Ultimately, in conjunction with a small but growing movement of self-criticism within the Protestant church and an increasing number of studies by professional historians, the ongoing uproar and controversy would force a redirection of the entire discussion of the relationships between church and state under Nazism. Especially moving early signs of changing views were evident in anguished and eloquent "confessions of guilt" offered first by the Protestant charity institution Bad Kreuznach—inspired also by Klee's work—and subsequently by the entire Protestant synod of the Rhineland.[64]

The Right to Be Counted as Persecutees
on Racial Grounds

As Klee had indicated, not just the murders but the "eugenic" sterilizations, too, had to be addressed directly.[65] This meant that the postwar complicity between ex-Nazi psychiatrists and religious leaders in allowing the West German government to continue to refuse recognition to sterilization survivors had to be confronted head-on. As of the mid-1980s, an estimated 88,000 of the original 400,000 sterilization survivors were still alive. Yet disrupting the alliance on sterilizations that existed between ex-Nazis and Protestants was challenging. Everything turned, on the one hand, on the wording of the Federal Reparations Law of 1956, which only acknowledged crimes on grounds of "race, religion, or political worldview" and, on the other, the fact that Protestant church and charity spokespersons had been stubbornly resistant to conceding that they had avidly participated in (as opposed to just reluctantly permitted, as

Catholics had) the violation of the human rights of individuals with disabilities. (Indeed, sterilization of minors—especially girls labeled intellectually disabled—was continuing, due to an ambiguity in the law which seemed to permit parental consent to a sterilization before the age of 18; Protestant charities openly supported this practice. The very idea that involuntary—as opposed to freely chosen—sterilization was a violation of human rights had in no way been concretized.)

The dilemma for advocates on behalf of the survivors was becoming increasingly plain. Activist psychiatrist Klaus Dörner, director of the psychiatric clinic in Gütersloh—conjoining passionate demands for improvements in care for the mentally ill in his present moment with insistence that the "euthanasia" murders in the nation's past be properly mourned and that the needs of sterilization survivors be addressed— had been searching steadily, but largely in vain, for effective language to convince politicians that the survivors deserved both recognition and reparations. In January 1984, Dörner sent a letter to the petition committee of the Bundestag insisting that the 1933 law be recognized as an instance of National Socialist injustice and that those sterilized or killed "on grounds of psychic or mental disability" be recognized officially as victims of National Socialist persecution (this was the first of literally hundreds of letters that Dörner would write to political and religious spokespersons). He requested that *either* a formal new category of recognized injustice be added to the extant reparations law specifically to address the needs of "psychically ill and mentally disabled persons and their kin" *or* that this circle of persons be "subsumed, legally, under the concept of persecution on racial grounds" (figure 3.4). And, regarding

FIGURE 3.4. The first page of psychiatrist Klaus Dörner's letter to the petition commission of the West German Bundestag, January 26, 1984. Dörner called for formal acknowledgment of the "unjust character" of the National Socialist sterilization law of 1933 and—calling attention to the extensive new supporting evidence provided by historian Gisela Bock—urged official recognition as instances of "persecution" (*Verfolgung*) for both the sterilizations and the killings performed on the grounds of "psychic or mental disability." Reprinted from Klaus Dörner, ed., *Gestern minderwertig—Heute gleichwertig?* (Inferior Yesterday—Of Equal Value Today?, 1985).

Prof. Dr. Dr. K. Dörner

An den
Petitionsausschuß des
Deutschen Bundestages
Bundeshaus

5300 Bonn

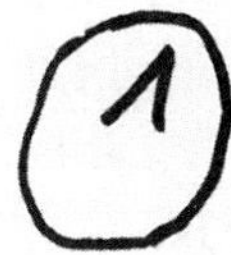

210

Dö/Do   26. 01. 1984

Betr.: Öffentliche Anerkennung des Unrechtscharakters des NS-
        Gesetzes "zur Verhütung Erbkranken Nachwuchses" und Anerkennung
        der Sterilisierung und der Tötung aus Gründen psychischer oder
        geistiger Behinderung während der NS-Zeit als Verfolgung

Sehr geehrte Damen und Herren,

mir ist bekannt, daß seit Bestehen der Bundesrepublik der Petitionsausschuß des Deutschen Bundestages sich immer wieder mit der Frage
der Rechtsstellung der während der NS-Zeit Sterilisierten und ihrer
Familie sowie der "Euthanasierten" und ihrer Familien beschäftigt hat
- jedoch ohne befriedigenden Erfolg. Der letzte Kompromiß, der dank
Ihrer Bemühungen zustande kam, stammt aus dem Jahre 1980 und betrifft
die Einrichtung eines Härtefonds, aus dem sterilisierte Personen bei
entsprechendem Nachweis DM 5.000,-- erhalten können. Die gesetzliche
Basis dafür ist - soweit ich weiß - jedoch nicht das Bundesentschädi-
gungsgesetz, sonder das allgemeine Kriegsfolgengesetz.

Nunmehr hat sich jedoch die Beweislage grundlegend geändert: Es
liegt nämlich jetzt endlich eine umfassende historische Untersuchung
über das NS-Sterilisierungsgesetz vor, die eindeutig nachweist, daß
das "Gesetz zur Verhütung Erbkranken Nachwuchses" von vornherein ein
Unrechtsgesetz war. Es handelt sich um die Habilitationsarbeit der
schon zuvor anerkannten Historikerin Frau Dr. phil. Gisela Bock,
Sybelstr. 13, 1000 Berlin 12. Die Arbeit, die über diese Adresse zu
beziehen ist, trägt den Titel: Zwangssterilisierung im National -
sozialistischen Staat. Untersuchungen zur Rassenpolitik und Frauen-
politik." Die Arbeit ist als Habilitationsschrift beim Historischen
Institut der Technischen Universität Berlin eingereicht.

Aus meiner eigenen gründlichen sowohl psychiatrischen als auch
historischen Kenntnis der Materie kann ich allen wesentlichen Aussagen der angegebenen Arbeit beitreten. Dies Arbeit weist nach, daß das
NS-Gesetz selbst nach der damals gültigen Reichsverfassung ein Unrechtsgesetz war, daß sich mit diesem Gesetz der Staat zum Herrn über
Lebenswert und Lebensunwert gemacht hat; daß das Gesetz somit gegen
die Freiheit des Menschen als auch gegen die Gleichheit der Menschen
verstoßen hat; daß es von vornherein ein Zwangsgesetz gewesen ist;

                                                        ...

the latter option—that Nazi-era violation of the rights of the disabled might at long last, forty years after war's end, properly be construed as a manifestation of *racism*—Dörner expressed the hope that the results of historian Gisela Bock's *Habilitation*—which in early 1984 he had been relieved and delighted to receive in manuscript—could perhaps provide substantive support.[66]

When she began her research in the 1970s, Bock's interest had focused on correcting lingering misunderstandings about Nazi reproductive politics, as she documented that a long-neglected but absolutely critical other side of the coin of the more notorious phenomenon of Nazi pronatalism and the Third Reich's cult of motherhood was a vicious antinatalism.[67] But as she worked through the evidence and developed this argument, she found herself formulating a then wholly new conceptualization of Nazi racism. Or, more precisely: a perfectly well known but perpetually strenuously denied conceptualization of Nazi racism. As Bock's evidence appeared to suggest, Nazi racism had always had two faces and came in two complementary forms: "anthropological" (directed against Jews, Roma, Blacks, etc.) and "hygienic" (directed against those deemed mentally deficient or unstable).[68] Here Bock was echoing a conceptualization advanced so evocatively by Gerhard Schmidt in 1965 when he described the Nazis as motivated by both "racial hatred" (*Rassenhaß*) and "racial anxiety" (*Rassenangst*).[69]

Both types, Bock observed—the hatred directed against those imagined as outsiders to the Volk and the anxiety directed at supposedly deficient insiders—translated something *social*, something culturally constructed and subjectively determined, into (purported) "biology." The "pivotal point" of both, she stressed, was the categorization of people into hierarchies of "worth" and "unworth." The two forms of racism had been mutually, inextricably enmeshed. Eugenics simply was one of the fundamental forms that racism takes. Moreover, she observed, the previously consulted experts' assurances that Nazi science had been up to international standards was completely spurious; throughout, "heritability" was never proven but rather presumed; *social* behavior was what was being measured—but *that* was precisely what made the judgments "racist."[70] And, again echoing Schmidt, Bock emphasized the phantasmatic anxiety-*cum*-arrogance driving the sterilization project. After all, she noted: "The promised 'race,' the 'master-Volk,' was not a given, it was not the real-existing German Volk, rather [the master race] had yet to be produced."[71]

In 1987, as part of Dörner's unremitting crusade to shift politicians' views on sterilization, Bock found herself joining Dörner in front of yet another Bundestag committee which was once again seeking the opinion of ex-Nazi psychiatrist Helmut Ehrhardt, and knowing full well that the refusal of reparations, for decades, had always turned on the ability of the government to define the sterilizations, legally, as not "racial." Ehrhardt resubmitted to the legislators his prior expert reports asserting that sterilizations under the 1933 law had nothing whatsoever to do with "race" and extemporizing in bizarrely luxuriant detail on a case of a schizophrenic who had murdered the object of his sexual-romantic obsession as proof of the extraordinary value of sterilizations. Evidently unable to make his case without insulting those deemed disabled, Ehrhardt insisted that someone "who for years as a racial persecutee sat in a concentration camp and only by chance escaped with his life" would "*by his nature*" have "suffered *totally different* damages than a cognitively severely disabled or psychiatrically ill individual who has lived for 50 years in institutional care and did not even notice that he got sterilized or has long since forgotten it."[72] Clearly irritated at being faced with opposition to his status as eminent authority, in a supplemental expert opinion handed in after the hearings, Ehrhardt complained that Dörner was working "in the style of typical antifa-agitation," while Bock had "added some accents of a trendy feminism," and he declared the efforts of both to be "lacking" in "the most elementary preconditions for historiographical work, for example source-historical analysis." But above all he reiterated his rejection of Bock's central claim about the two forms of racism and their intimate interrelationship: "Prof. Bock and Prof. Dörner convey the impression that in the implementation of the Law for the Prevention of Hereditarily Ill Progeny this was not about sick or disabled people at all, but at best about an 'inferiority' imputed by racists." In his view, supporters of the 1933 law when it was passed may have been overly optimistic about its usefulness for preventing the proliferation of disabilities. But they were most certainly not, he averred yet again, motivated "by any kind of racism."[73]

Meanwhile, and this for the first time ever, two survivors of coercive sterilizations—Klara Nowak and Fritz Niemand—had testified to the assembled politicians about the crushing consequences on their lives of what both had experienced as devastating mutilations. Both had, as it happened, been diagnosed with the extremely elastic category of "schizophrenia," even as the (utterly flimsy) evidence that had been adduced in each of their cases would have made no sense whatsoever to observers in later eras.[74] Nowak spoke for herself but also on behalf of other members of the mutual support and advocacy organization she had just a few months earlier co-founded with Klaus Dörner in the city of Detmold: the Federation of Those Harmed by 'Euthanasia' and Coercive Sterilization (*Bund der "Euthanasie"-Geschädigten und Zwangssterilisierten*).[75] She detailed the traumatic consequences of the operations, from the professional and personal opportunities that had been denied survivors because higher education as well as marriage to the partner of one's choice were forbidden to those sterilized under the Nazi law to the physiological sequelae of the operations, especially for women, and the generalized shame, silence, and enforced social isolation that continued to haunt almost all survivors. "It simply cannot be overlooked," she declared summarily, "that our bodies were maimed by the operation, destroying our further life-development. . . . [O]ur life was curtailed in every way." The contemptuous indifference and "incomprehension" of postwar society compounded the harm. It was, she averred, "shattering," and for the survivors, the injury was also psychological: "Due to the inferiority attributed to them, they suffered considerable wounding during their childhood and adolescence but were not able to compensate for it in their later lives." Niemand, in turn, testified not just about the sterilization itself and the terror, before his valiant mother had successfully obtained his release from the psychiatric ward in which he initially had been placed, that he would be deported to a gas chamber. He additionally described a subsequent set of torments when, in the wake of a second commitment to a psychiatric facility, he had been sent to Meseritz-Obrawalde in Pomerania (now in Poland, but just two hours east of Berlin). This was a major center for "euthanasia" during the second, decentralized phase of killings; here Niemand witnessed the steady arrival of trains full of deportees destined to be murdered by medication overdose and poisoning. Meseritz-Obrawalde resembled a concentration camp in many ways, and in his address to the politicians, Niemand did not hesitate to describe his own role as that of a "forced laborer" (*Zwangsarbeiter*). He knew he would be among the dead if he did not keep up with the demanded assignments: "Here we had to do all kinds of work from early in the morning until late at night: in the gravel pit, unloading wagons with coal—some of it was labor of the hardest kind—and [we were] starving. . . . The selections took place regularly."[76]

Nowak's and Niemand's statements were indispensable in helping listeners to understand the human cost of the sterilizations—even as, in his follow-up memorandum, Ehrhardt was characteristically snide, suggesting that with regard to an individual who was "psychically ill or intellectually disabled" (by implication he was referring to Nowak and Niemand) it would be difficult for a medical "nonexpert" to distinguish between what a person had "experienced himself"—versus what "he had been talked into—perhaps many decades later."[77] But quite apart from Ehrhardt's undercutting skepticism, Nowak's and Niemand's stories did not yet show a way to reconsider legal categories. This is where Bock's intervention specifically as a historian became crucial.

Drawing her evidence not least from the words of leading Nazis, including Adolf Hitler but also several others, in her testimony Bock called attention to how Nazis articulated the interconnections they themselves identified between the two aspects of their race-politics. She further explained that every single one of the sterilizations during the Third Reich had been coerced. Above all, her core concluding message was that "the historical circumstances prove that the victims of National Socialist sterilization politics have the right to be counted as persecutees on racial grounds [in the sense of the reparations law], Paragraph 1."[78]

Leaving aside ex-Nazis and budget-conscious Christian Democrats, Bock's proposition—that all racisms are socially based pseudo-biological arguments—was to be a breakthrough revelation in its moment. For multiple reasons, racism had been inadequately theorized in postwar

West Germany.[79] It is both astonishing from the perspective of our present and indispensable for our understanding of the dynamics of the 1980s–1990s, how *non*obvious Bock's points initially were to German academic historians at the time. But Bock had made her case exceedingly well. Her formulations transformed the historiography of twentieth-century Germany, becoming the gold standard for scholarship—and eventually the accepted framework in numerous memorial projects. Historian Dirk Blasius captured the newly developed consensus especially pithily and assertively in 1994: "'Hygienic' and 'anthropological' racism interlocked [*griffen ineinander*]. Politics with regard to Jews and the politics of eugenic sterilization were the two sides of 'real historical racism' in the 'Third Reich.'"[80] Bock's reconceptualizations also, albeit with a time lag, fundamentally transformed the understanding of West (and then reunited) Germany's political leadership.

While at the moment of the Bundestag hearing, in 1987, the CDU remained resistant to further expenditures, Bock's efforts—in conjunction with the rising chorus of pressure especially from the young Green Party, from an increasingly engaged media, and not least, and importantly, even from the churches (inspired and pushed by Dörner's steady stream of letters and by Klee's ongoing critical exposés of the churches' wartime and postwar records)—brought short- and long-term results for survivors.[81] Most immediately, in May 1988, the Bundestag did formally declare the verdicts pronounced by the sterilization courts due to the 1933 law to have constituted a "National Socialist injustice."[82] After another ten years of ongoing efforts, in 1998, the sterilization verdicts were formally nullified.[83] And although the sterilization law of 1933 itself would not be formally repudiated until 2007, what remains remarkable is that the motion calling for that repudiation—now finally carried by Christian Democrats as well—explained expressly that the 1933 law had emerged from "the hallucinatory racist idea of the 'purification of the body of the Volk.'"[84] Moreover, and at long last adopting what had become self-advocates' and their supporters' most fervent argument, the politicians' 2007 recommended resolution went so far as to designate the sterilization law as the Nazis' "first racial law" (*das erste Rassengesetz*).[85] This all may seem to be solely a matter of semantics. But if so, it was semantics with enormous consequences.

Moreover, the insight that the corporeal violation and methodical slaughter of fellow citizens designated as cognitively or psychically impaired was itself a manifestation of racism was—contra Ehrhardt's confident disclaimers and denials—by no means solely an invention of the 1980s. It remains noteworthy and revealing just how much energy was expended by the opponents of recognition of and restitution for the disabled as persecutees of Nazism into asserting that racism had nothing to do with the coercive sterilizations or the killings. Why did they protest so vehemently? Most strikingly, it remains quite telling that it was consistently the tiny handful of *critics* of the persistence of Nazi attitudes into the early postwar decades—whether jurists like Fritz Bauer and his team, or singularly courageous medical professionals like Hans Lewenstein or Gerhard Schmidt—who saw it as simply, uncontroversially true that hostility toward the disabled was a form of racial arrogance and / or anxiety and named it as such.

The conceptual reformulations articulated by Bock have remained durably consequential. In 2011, the Bundestag finally turned to considering the need for a national memorial to recognize all the various crimes against human beings the Nazis had deemed disabled—the sterilizations, the medical experiments, and the hundredthousandfold murders—in a manner commensurate with the memorials that had been or were being erected in the heart of Berlin for other persecuted and murdered groups.[86] The cross-party motion (Christian, Free, and Social Democrats and Greens) calling for the establishment of such a memorial opened with the—by that point apparently self-evident—statement: "Part of the National Socialist racial ideology was the registration, persecution and murder of people with disabilities and the mentally ill."[87] Ninety years after the astoundingly durable concept of "life unworthy of life" had been introduced, and exactly fifty years after smug ex-Nazis had come up with the formula that negativity toward disability was never racism, the crimes against people with disabilities were finally recognized, also at the highest levels of government, *as crimes*.

4

The Fascism in the Heads

Do you want your children to be wasting away in institutions?—
Answer: No!

—LEBENSHILFE ADVERTISEMENT,
EARLY 1960S[1]

Thus, after the destruction of the fascist state apparatus, the fascism in
the heads remains. . . . A fascism in the heads, which across the FRG
still speaks of ineducability and unschoolability, practices psychosurgery
and electroshock, segregates instead of integrates, in the Frankfurt court
judgment describes disabled people at a vacation resort as an intolerable
annoyance, and is reflected in public opinion in such a way that a
majority finds it better if mentally disabled children die early and 80%
want to deport these children to remote destinations.

—DISABILITY PEDAGOGUE WOLFGANG JANTZEN, 1981[2]

THE PRIOR CHAPTER concerned memory-political battles over the
national past. It took an extraordinary effort, over many decades, for
activists and engaged scholars finally to begin to get the Nazis' hundredthousandfold coercive sterilizations and "euthanasia" murders of
people diagnosed with intellectual disabilities or mental illnesses to be
popularly as well as officially acknowledged as utterly grotesque crimes
whose pursuit had been based both in cynical opportunism and phantasmatic delusions. This chapter turns to a less frequently studied, more

110

elusive topic: the multidimensional battle to transform the present and future everyday lives of people deemed to be intellectually disabled—whether these were adolescent or adult survivors of the Nazi campaign to exterminate alleged imperfection in the body politic, or children with diverse impairments newly born into a post-"euthanistic" nation.

For myriad, overdetermined reasons, for people with intellectual disabilities as for those diagnosed with psychiatric illnesses, the practical situation after 1945 was, with remarkably few exceptions, desolate. Conditions were worse in many ways than they had been before the Nazis had come to power in 1933. The systematic killing had been stopped, but the postfascist settlement witnessed a complicated confluence of longer-term cumulative with theretofore unanticipated new trends. Especially for those who were living in institutions and had—either by luck or capacity to provide some form of labor—managed to elude the murder machinery, the circumstances were especially grim. This was not only because of wartime damages to the physical plant of the institutions and insufficiency of resources in conditions of postwar scarcity. Attitudes and care practices also had become brutalized. Ex-Nazi and formerly Nazi-sympathizing employees were hired back as nurses and wardens, as the perpetual staff shortages persisted.[3]

The elites were no less tainted. All three disciplines that had claimed disability as their domain—psychiatric medicine, religious charity, and remedial pedagogy—were contaminated by entanglement in the crimes. With the precious exceptions of, in each field, a handful of individuals, the leading figures in these professions had not only tolerated Nazi policies with at most feeble objections. They had all too often abetted their implementation, however ambivalently. Even as each guild made its own highly adept moves to construct narratives that absolved the vast majority of its members from any blemish of wrongdoing, the continuities in personnel, in professional practice, and in opinion across the divide of 1945 were strong.[4]

Three dynamics were, however paradoxically, mutually reinforcing. First, there was the long-inculcated, unreflected habit of hierarchizing human worth. This habit had taken shape already in the 1880s–1890s, with numerous institutions shunting a significant percentage of their residents into the category of "care-cases" (*Pflegefälle*), for whom no engaged therapeutic intervention was provided. Second, there was the vicious exacerbation of antidisability prejudices by Nazi propaganda. The effects of the propaganda did not simply evaporate. Rather, the propaganda had the counterintuitive consequence of encouraging rationalization of the crimes in the recent past as having been justified by the inferiority of their victims. Most perversely, the stubbornly lingering efficacy of the propaganda had the effect of making shame and embarrassment that one was even in the business of providing care for people who could not care for themselves continue to adhere to numerous charity facilities also in the postwar (figure 4.1). Meanwhile, prominent spokesmen for the field of remedial pedagogy—freshly rebranded as "special pedagogy"—were thrilled to report in the 1950s–1960s that over the prior decades (implicitly including the Third Reich) the field had successfully expelled "the feeble-minded, imbeciles and idiots" and turned its schools for the (only mildly or moderately) "learning-disabled" into true "achievement-schools" (*Leistungsschulen*).[5]

Third, there was bristling irritation and resentment at international moral judgment on Germany and on Germans, and determination to reassert one's honor and reestablish professional prestige. This dynamic was supplemented with a peculiarly contradictory phenomenon specifically relevant for both Christian churches. On the one hand, the churches insisted publicly on the great bravery that Catholic and Protestant leaders had shown during the Third Reich in protesting the "euthanasia" killings. Indeed, since nothing had been said, at least officially, on behalf of Nazism's Jewish victims, protests on behalf of the disabled functioned synecdochically as essential evidence of Christian opposition to

FIGURE 4.1. One of several powerful photographs accompanying a markedly depressing story about postwar conditions at Bethel published in the popular magazine *Kristall*. In the caption to this picture, "The ill help the ill. The older ones among the patients frequently of their own accord relieve the nursing personnel"—the day-to-day unpaid labor of residents is presented as spontaneous assistance that lightens the burdens of the care staff. Throughout the essay, life for the residents at Bethel is presented as "unhappy" and a "tragedy," and the reporter discusses with director Friedrich von Bodelschwingh III the lamentable—and in the postwar decades apparently increasing—difficulty of finding staff

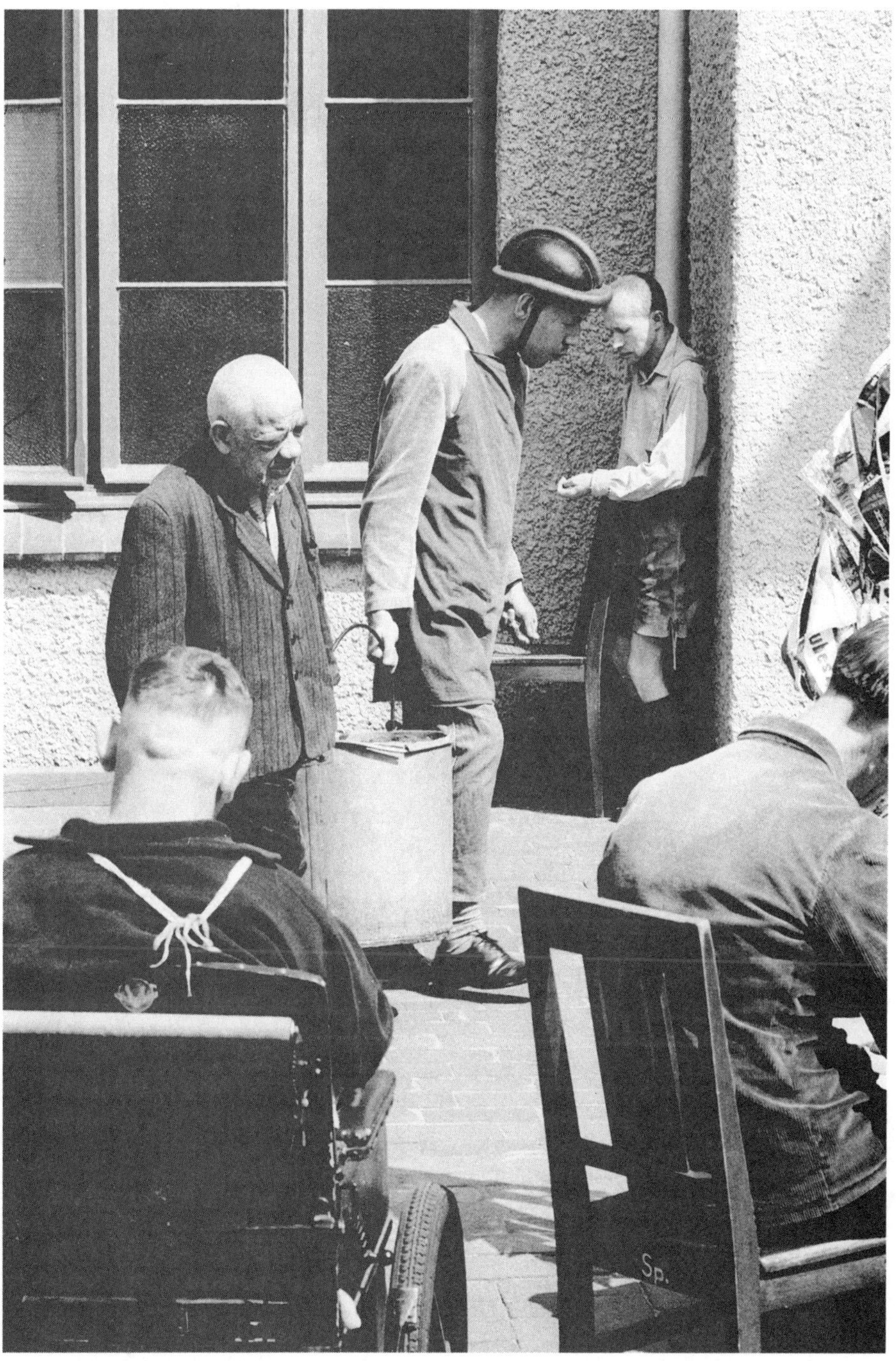

willing to take up "a helping profession" and provide care to people with disabilities. Roger Anderson, "Ein hilfloser Schrei: Kristall besuchte die unglücklichen Menschen von Bethel," *Kristall* 14 (1964). © Archiv Robert Lebeck.

Nazism.[6] On the other hand, and while effectively repressing the tarnished memories of passivity or participation in the deportations of their weakest residents and defiantly unapologetic about their complicity in mass sterilizations, charity institution directors continued to display difficulty in articulating a vigorous defense of the value of disabled lives. Overcrowding and understaffing, labor exploitation of the "fitter" residents coupled with custodial warehousing of those relegated to being solely objects of "care" marked every aspect of daily life in the institutions, and institutional administrators continued to defer to medical experts' ongoing practice of supercilious pathologizing.[7]

In the wider public, not just indifference but active hostility toward the disabled remained an unquestioned norm, and arguably even deepened in the postwar decades.[8] In the autumn of 1969, when villagers from a tiny hamlet in Bavaria, led by their Catholic priest, erupted in brutal violence against the prospect of a residential home for boys with mental disabilities in their region—arguing that "these moron children" (*diese depperten Kinder*) would drive away the tourists they were so eager to attract—they beat the home manager till his kidneys bled and sent the prospective residence up in flames. The story stayed in the national news for a full three years.[9] Yet the predominant messages conveyed in the tellingly incoherent coverage were that although the thuggish "backwoods hicks" had unfortunately lost control of themselves, their concerns were "not entirely unjustifiable" and they were understandably worried that the new young residents would have "an unwholesome moral influence" on the progeny of the locals.[10] The *Frankfurter Allgemeine Zeitung* went so far as to aver that "mentally handicapped children (who may be behaviorally difficult or even criminals?)" could after all be "quite eerie [*ganz und gar nicht geheuer*]."[11] *Der Spiegel*, gratuitously imagining the prospective residents as "hydrocephalics and mongoloids," explained that the villagers had reason to fear that seventy "imbeciles" imported into the area from other parts of Germany might well make "both the horses and the spa guests shy."[12] The cultural consensus that intellectual disability was a matter for disgrace and disgust was simply confirmed.[13]

What would it take to rupture this unchallenged consensus, and to introduce new terms of debate? In 1970s–1980s West Germany, it was in the context of two theretofore unprecedented, initially separate but soon intersecting campaigns—one demanding comprehensive integration of children with all manner and gradations of disabilities into the regular school system, the other a battle to dismantle entirely the residential mega-institutions or at the very least radically reform care within them—that wholly novel notions of justice, dignity, respect, and recognition of full personhood for those deemed to be significantly mentally disabled were formulated. In teacher and caregiver training and in the direct provision of education and care, new ways of being-in-interaction-with those most vulnerable were tried out and continually refined, accompanied by a constantly evolving struggle to find the best, most compelling language to express what needed to change in the hearts of fellow citizens and in social and political structures alike. The aim was to transform practices.

The Nature of Prejudice

There were tremendous hurdles to be overcome. In the course of the 1960s, personality psychologist and professor of special education at the University of Marburg (formerly, during the Weimar era, a remedial school teacher), Helmut von Bracken drew heavily on the social psychological research of Harvard professor Gordon Allport, *The Nature of Prejudice* (1954), to conduct a multiyear national survey of West German attitudes toward the intellectually disabled. His findings were devastating. Close to 70 percent of the general populace took the view—either unreservedly (20 percent) or conditionally (50 percent)—that it "would be good" if a child with mental disability "died young."[14] Further, 75 percent of the citizens took as self-evident that parents must be to blame for their children's mental or learning disability. Beliefs that the cause lay in "heredity" (*Vererbung*)—88 percent concurred here—or "alcohol abuse" (*Trunksucht*) (83 percent) or "incest" (*Inzest*) (75 percent) were most prevalently named (while somewhere between 15 and 20 percent indicated they thought the sources could be "poor childrearing" or "insufficient love").[15] One-third admitted that it would "disturb" them personally if they had to encounter a mentally disabled child in their daily lives, and two-thirds of respondents were of the opinion that children with mental disability should not be raised within their family but rather dispatched to institutions, ideally in "remote locations."[16] For the first time in German history, a social psychological framework developed to analyze ethnic and racial hatred had been adapted and applied to an investigation of the emotions and opinions stirred in the popular imagination by intellectual disability. Smaller studies conducted by other scholars in those same years revealed comparable results, additionally stressing that the opinions pronounced were rooted in "very fixed notions," ideas "which cannot be dislodged by chance, but which would require a great deal of publicity and propaganda to change."[17] What von Bracken found corroborated formally and beyond any doubt what parents already knew from anguishing personal experience.

The extent of the cruelty directed against families of children with intellectual disabilities was overwhelming. Parents whose children still lived at home often hid their children away and avoided taking them into public places during daylight. Many avoided speaking about their children. They were also regularly urged to give up their children to institutions shortly after birth, as medical professionals recommended separation from the child on the arguments that to keep the child at home would be damaging to siblings and stigmatizing for the family more generally. When families did give up their children with disabilities to residential institutions—and poorer families in particular frequently felt they had no other choice—the expectation of the institutions was that families would minimize contact or abandon their children entirely.[18] Again, more than just a tragic continuity with trends in deprecation of the disabled that had existed since the turn of the twentieth century, not just the vituperative animus against the disabled themselves but also the presumption that parents were—whether biologically or behaviorally— to blame had been aggravated exponentially in the course of the Third Reich. Yet at the same time, the long-standing strong empirical correlation between lower-class status origins and the likelihood of being diagnosed with intellectual disability or behavioral disorders persisted, even as, by various random biological events, children with cognitive impairments continued to be born into middle- and upper-class families as well.

It had been in this context that the Lebenshilfe (Life-Assistance), an organization founded by middle-class professional parents in 1958, sought to expand the category of children who could be considered eligible to attend school. (Notably, part of the Lebenshilfe parents' success was due to their strategic collaboration with two prominent ex-Nazi—and in one case, albeit unbeknownst to the parents, ex-perpetrator—medical professionals, whose ongoing high renown and close ties to government leaders facilitated the Lebenshilfe's reformist goals.)[19] The West German school system still followed the guidelines established in a 1938 law which "excused"—but in fact *excluded*—from education children found to be so disabled either physically or mentally that they were deemed unable to participate in a classroom setting.[20] This Nazi law had been the grounds on which more significantly mentally disabled children had been pushed out of the school system—sometimes this meant being moved into residential institutions, where they became at risk for deportation and murder—thus leaving only those perceived to be capable of becoming "useful" for the state.[21] The Lebenshilfe parents and their expert allies urgently argued that their children, diagnosed as "ineducable," should be redescribed as at least "practically educable" (*praktisch bildbar*), a renaming intended to lend substance to the simultaneously legal and moral case that these children deserved access to state-funded public schooling.[22]

Lebenshilfe parents directly designed—and initially often themselves staffed—specialized day programs for their children, proving in practice that they could achieve therapeutic gains. In a remarkably short period of time, they created a national network of alternate kindergartens and schools, and subsequently—as their children aged—small dormitories and sheltered workshops. Already by 1965, the first school for the "practically educable" had received state support in Hessen, and more state-supported schools followed. In addition, the Lebenshilfe ran public awareness campaigns in newspapers as well as through fundraising events, seeking greater compassion among fellow citizens for the circumstances of the intellectually disabled. As schools for the "practically educable" were founded in towns across the nation, engaged parent activism to convince recalcitrant local school authorities remained constantly necessary, and recurrently it took locally and / or politically prominent families to keep pressing the case that such schools were needed, and still more parent effort to create spaces for all the children who were eligible. An especially moving and impressive example involved the odyssey of CDU parliamentarian Franz-Lorenz von Thadden in forcing Saarbrücken municipal authorities to open and maintain a school for children with physical and mental disabilities; initially the city had claimed there were only four children with special needs in the city. Once the school was opened, it became evident that there were more than 130.[23] (Von Thadden would later be among those Christian Democratic and Christian Social Union representatives, working closely with reform-minded psychiatrists, who were responsible for petitioning the Bundestag in 1970–1971 to launch the inquiry on the catastrophic state of psychiatry in West Germany—and make recommendations for remedies—that was to conclude with the publication of the *Psychiatrie-Enquête* in 1975.)[24]

The Association of German Special Schools (*Verband deutscher Sonderschulen*, VdS), the powerful guild of special pedagogues, thousands of members strong and extremely well-organized, did not stand in the way of the Lebenshilfe's or other parent-activists' goals—even as only very few of its members took an interest in developing expertise in pedagogical intervention for the "practically educable." During the 1960s, the association presided over a dramatic expansion of state-funded special schools segregated from the regular school system, by far the largest group of which were the schools for the (considered to be only mildly or moderately) "learning-disabled." These special schools were precisely the ones that in prior decades had pushed out the children whose abilities were considered too low to merit school participation. (By 1970, 1,890 of 2,600 special schools in all served more than 250,000 "learning-disabled" pupils, even as experts were estimating that the actual target population was well over 300,000.)[25]

The Lebenshilfe and related schools for the "practically educable" thus became just another one of a total of nine types of segregated special schools. In addition to the large majority which served the "learning-disabled," there were separate schools for pupils who were: physically disabled; blind; deaf; sight-impaired; hearing-impaired; speech-impaired; "behaviorally disturbed" (a rebranding of the former "difficult-to-educate" or "psychopathically inferior"); and now also the (deemed to be more significantly) "mentally disabled," renamed as the "practically educable." Once more, then, the long-standing self-evidence of hierarchized categories of cognitive impairment remained confirmed.

Some regions continued to be woefully underserved. A 1971 report found that in the state of Schleswig-Holstein, for example, there were 2,000 children who carried a "mentally disabled" diagnosis, but there was not a single school for the "practically educable" available to them—and jurists in the state capital of Kiel, ignoring the arguments put forward successfully by Lebenshilfe parents at the federal level, had defined these children as in any event "ineducable" and hence not requiring school attendance.[26] Everywhere, schools for the "practically educable" remained understaffed and underfunded.[27]

Meanwhile, albeit only gradually and unevenly, a shift began to take place in expert discourse away from the biologistic language of genetic transmission of mental defect and toward a language that acknowledged economic factors and the potential impact of sociocultural deprivation on children's performance in school. Even this incipient willingness to discuss class inequities, however, would retain elements both of parent-blaming and of the perceived irreparability of inherent deficiency. As of 1965, von Bracken himself was helpfully explaining that the "more severe" forms of intellectual disability were often a haphazardly occurring, not hereditarily transmitted condition (as indeed the typical middle-class Lebenshilfe family stories kept demonstrating, since the causes of their children's disabilities often lay in chromosomal abnormality, cerebral palsy or other forms of perinatal brain damage, or subsequently developed epilepsy). But he nonetheless continued to maintain that the larger group of more moderate forms of "learning disability" were likely to be the outcome of "heredity" (*Vererbung*).[28] So too, as late as 1967, seeking to explain the apparent "continuing increase of children in special schools"—figured expressly as a worrisome, "very considerable, and growing, burden on society"—a government report still alluded, as though it was an uncontestable fact, to the notion that there was "apparently increasingly more frequently occurring damage to the hereditary substance [*erblichen Substanzschäden*]" of the citizenry as a whole.[29] Long-standing convictions about the poor as inherently, biologically damaged proved extremely difficult to shake.

Yet by 1970, the undeniable evidence of the impact of economic inequities on learning outcomes was increasingly being thematized across the full gamut of ideological positions. Numerous studies found that a striking percentage of children tracked into "learning-disabled" schools had IQs equivalent to those who had been tracked into the lowest tier of the regular system, thereby calling into clear question, no matter what one thought of IQ as a metric, the justice of and rationale for their placement.[30] Historically, children in Germany were tracked after four grades of elementary school into one of three tiers. The top tier, Gymnasium, was for the elite, those likely to go on to university, the second was the Realschule, preparing pupils for a broad range of white-collar professions, while the third, the Hauptschule, typically served those who would go on to blue-collar work. Class mobility was possible, and promising pupils from the working classes did on occasion find opportunities to attend Gymnasium, but the tendency to transgenerational class stratification was unmistakable. By the late 1960s, a few West German states were trying out the possibility of having children from all classes share up to nine or ten grades in a more democratic and unified school, called Gesamtschule, but the model was highly contested. In this broader situation of rising tensions over the relationship between class background and educational outcome, it was well known that the function of the segregated "learning-disabled" schools was to be a "fourth tier" below the tripartite regular school system, de-burdening the third-tier Hauptschule of children assessed as unable to keep up even there.[31] But the numbers of children being shuffled out were rising to 5–8 percent of every age cohort (in some locales as high as 11 percent or more), and in the course of the 1960s alone, the numbers designated as "learning-disabled" nationwide had tripled.[32] Precisely the enormous regional variability in tracking practices, moreover, signaled significant confusion about the grounds on which students were directed into either the third or the fourth tier, and highlighted the subjectivity of experts' diagnoses. But the most scrutiny was directed to newly compiled evidence that tracking was not based on intellectual capacity but rather on class status. As one oft-cited essay of 1970 summarized, while in the past, "The essential causes of a lack of giftedness were seen in the child's constitution, in his hereditary disposition, or in later organic impairments"—primarily in some "hereditary factor" (*Erbfaktor*)—in truth at most 10–20 percent of all "learning disability" had a biological source and the plain fact was that those who ended up in the "learning-disabled" schools "originate above all from socially marginalized families of the lower class."[33] Meanwhile, and although the "fifth tier" of the "practically educable" continued to exist in a very different relationship to both the "learning-disabled" schools and the third-tier Hauptschule, it too was expanding its remit beyond the largely middle-class offspring of the activist founders. By the early 1970s, researchers were documenting that a disproportionate percentage of "mentally-disabled" pupils attending the "practically educable" schools also came from conditions of poverty and social marginalization.[34]

Why did the incidence of intellectual disability of some kind appear to be rising? Could it really be, one commentator fretted in 1974, as educators and politicians rushed to review the statistics and propose explanations, that the Federal Republic was becoming a "Volk of special education pupils?"[35] Or, as two other observers asked the year before: "Are working-class children dumber [*dümmer*]—or, in the final instance, just 'the dummies' ['*die Dummen,*' i.e., the 'losers']?"[36] What exactly was the causal mechanism within the evident correlation of poverty and disability, and what were the responsibilities of and possibilities for educators and policymakers to remediate the situation?

The convergence in time of this increasingly widespread recognition of the class dimension in tracking with a burgeoning perception that prejudicial attitudes toward disability in the wider public would need to be combated preemptively in early childhood if there was to be any hope of mitigating their virulence, prompted what was for most observers a dramatic and wholly unanticipated development. The *Recommendation of the Educational Commission for the Pedagogical Development of Children and Youth with Disabilities and at Risk of Becoming Disabled,* announced in the fall of 1973, altered virtually overnight the terms of the national conversation on how best to meet the needs of children with (diverse types of) disabilities—even as it was by no means universally welcomed (and indeed its vision has remained disputed to this day).[37] Written by University of Bochum pedagogy professor Jakob Muth, a liberal expert in regular, not special, education, the *Recommendation* insisted on "as much shared instruction of disabled and nondisabled as possible," and suggested that for that (assumed to be small) minority of more severely disabled children "for whom a shared instruction with the nondisabled does not appear sensible," it was imperative at least to "proliferate contacts with nondisabled children."[38] After a century in which segregated special schools were assumed to be the sole workable pedagogical framework, the *Recommendation* endorsed the idea that children with disabilities would be best nurtured by being integrated into the regular school system.

Yet an additional goal of the *Recommendation* was to change the attitudes of the nondisabled. It was not just, as the *Recommendation* emphasized, that in truth all children could benefit from "individualization of learning expectations," and that competitiveness and obsession with "the achievement-principle" (*Leistungsprinzip*), as inescapable as these might be in adult society, were damaging for children. It was also—and here sensitive attunement to the just-then-being documented problem of ongoing societal prejudice was palpable—that this represented a unique chance to advance "the humane acceptance of the disabled by the nondisabled." Further: "Humane acceptance means that the difference of the disabled person from societal expectations and assumptions is not seen as an inferiority, but as an individual distinctiveness. This insight must lead to the recognition of the disabled as an equally valuable partner in all areas of life."[39] Indicatively, the field of special education expressed vociferous disinterest.

The negative response was rapid—and lasting. Caught off guard both literally and conceptually, remaining themselves fervently attached to a hierarchizing perspective, and intent on preserving the prerogative on their own terrain, leading special education spokespersons rejected out of hand the idea of shared instruction of disabled and nondisabled pupils. Immediately in 1973, special pedagogue Ulrich Bleidick, professor at the University of Hamburg, took the occasion of his keynote at the seventy-fifth anniversary of the VdS to declare his displeasure, announcing his opposition to what he described frankly as "uncritical illusionism." While admittedly there were inadequacies in the extant school system, Bleidick asserted, it was "even more dangerous to indulge in social utopian dreams of integrating the disabled into mainstream schools."[40] Several years later, as resistance on the part of teachers across the nation to the implementation of the Commission's *Recommendation* had proliferated, Bleidick repeatedly returned to the topic, mocking Muth's call for "humane acceptance" of the disabled by the nondisabled, labeling it a naively "harmonized" vision not grounded in any "critical sociological assessment" of reality. As of 1977, Bleidick was pleased to report his findings that the handful of then-emerging experimental integrated classrooms revealed "unmistakable disadvantages for achievement-weak pupils" and, not least, to sum up that with regard to those who were "socially and economically disadvantaged," efforts at compensatory education displayed "up to now still disappointing results."[41] Other defenders of segregated schooling advanced their own objections to integration, among them the blatantly stated argument (put forward by Karl-Heinz Berg, professor at the University of Mainz) that segregated settings were necessary because it would be unacceptable for the "learning-disabled" to be exposed to potential antiauthoritarian behavior on the part of regular school pupils; given their "mental weaknesses," such a sight would only "confuse" the disabled and "endanger [their] development," robbing them of the "relative placidity . . . honesty and loyalty" that was the main, if not only, basis of their desirability as future workers. On these grounds—that the main purpose of special education for individuals with "learning-disability" was to prepare them to be docile laborers—Berg remained adamant in his "demand for authority-bound education." He specifically endorsed corporal punishment of special education pupils as well.[42]

Between Marx and Martin Buber

Such attitudes from the leadership of the special education guild were met by increasingly vocal and imaginative resistance from an insurgent movement *within* the guild, and it was precisely in the ensuing wrenching conflict—the pressing need to find persuasive counter-arguments and demonstrate the validity of radically integrationist counter-practices—that the most innovative new perspectives on intellectual disability in German history would be formulated. The conflict over integrated schooling, in short, was not just about integration per se; it provided the context for a more wide-ranging revolution in thinking about disability.

As it turns out, then, the most important advocates on behalf of people with cognitive impairments in 1970s–1980s West Germany were two dissident special education teachers. Wolfgang Jantzen (1941–2020) and Georg Feuser (1941–) would come to articulate, in a morally ardent blend of leftist secular-political and theological-philosophical concepts, a wholly new understanding of intellectual disability. Already by the late 1960s, Jantzen and Feuser were developing a comprehensive refusal of any and all hierarchization of people with mental disabilities and advancing practical ideas for a pedagogy and therapy that understood the other as a subject, not an object. By the turn from the 1970s to the 1980s, they not only added a rejection of all segregation into special schools or institutions, but called for a renovation of the entirety of the regular school system—and indeed of the society as a whole.[43] At every point, they defended the full equality of those human beings with the most severe impairments; they took the view that no one was unreachable or unteachable. There could be no exclusions, no compromises. There would be no "leftover group" (*Restgruppe*) that should be isolated from the rest of humanity; on the contrary, as Feuser would repeatedly underline, precisely those to whom the damage had been greatest were the most needful of social embeddedness and of highly qualified pedagogical engagement.[44]

Both men's activism grew out of concrete and personally transformative encounters with children with significant intellectual impairments.

In Jantzen's case—he himself had once been forced to repeat a grade, and had been constantly reprimanded for behavioral insubordination—the key experience was a vacation camp he ran on behalf of the Lebenshilfe in 1970. Here he adapted the Scottish reform educator A. S. Neill's experiential-learning-based approach expounded in *Summerhill* (in German: *Theorie und Praxis der antiautoritären Erziehung* [1969]) to the needs of children with intellectual disabilities.[45] This meant: playing in the landscape, including building dams of mud and canals at the local creek; daily intensive music-making, dancing, and other exercise; and demonstrative, unapologetic making-visible of disability to the public. Jantzen invited reporters from local newspapers on-site, and the whole group took excursions into the community: traveling on public transportation, to a swimming pool, and to the cinema. Two photos remain from 1970 that offer a glimpse of what was accomplished: Marion, endowed with Down syndrome, whoops with delight as she "sleds" down a grassy hillock in a plastic bucket, a game she—Jantzen stresses—invented herself. Horst, meanwhile, falls asleep trustingly in Jantzen's lap during the afternoon guitar-playing (figure 4.2). The camp was a great success in terms of both measurably reducing symptoms and inducing general joy. Over the course of the nearly three weeks, all the children made gains in capacities and independence, and Jantzen's confidence that youngsters with even more severe and multiple disabilities, including physical impairments, could be assisted just as well was firmly solidified.[46]

It was the obtuse reactions from experts on disability, however, that most determined Jantzen's future trajectory. Jantzen was livid at the Lebenshilfe's frank disinterest in having him report back individualized information about each child's history, wishes, and needs and what types of prior training for the accompanying caregiver volunteers would make future camps even more productively beneficial. But he directed his sharpest irritation at the sorts of reflexive responses he received when he first spoke about the camp in 1970 at a conference of pedagogues. His professional peers' main preoccupation appeared to be with the importance of "cleanliness" in camp facilities, rather than with any actual details of therapeutic work with the children.[47]

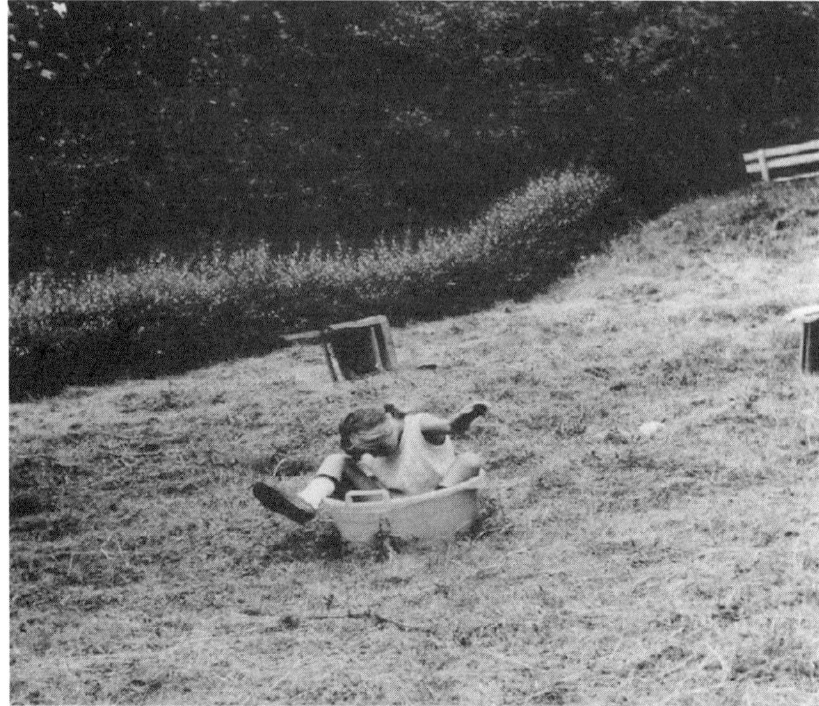

FIGURE 4.2. Photos taken during a joyous vacation camp organized by disability pedagogue Wolfgang Jantzen—at the invitation of the Lebenshilfe—in the summer of 1970. The wonderful encounters with the children—but also the subsequent confrontation with aggressive disinterest from his professional peers in learning about new and creative therapeutic possibilities—were life-changing for Jantzen. Writing about the experiences in 1972, Jantzen paraphrased Martin Buber, noting that a main task for pedagogic engagement with children with mental disabilities involved "recognizing, acknowledging, and valuing" every individual child "in communicative relation as *an equally valid* thou-partner." Reprinted from Wolfgang Jantzen, "Nein zur Macht: Ein Exkurs zu Freiheit und Befreiung," in Willehad Lanwer and Wolfgang Jantzen, eds., *Jahrbuch der Luria-Gesellschaft 2020* (Berlin 2020), 28–38, here 30 and 31. © Archiv Wolfgang Jantzen.

Also in his day job at a school in Lich, near Gießen, for the (moderately) "learning-disabled," Jantzen had gained the reputation of being a communist. His Protestant and female principal, a pastor's wife—known in local parlance by the redolent name *Frau "Kinderklau"* (Mrs. "Steal-the-Children") for her remarkable talent at tracking pupils

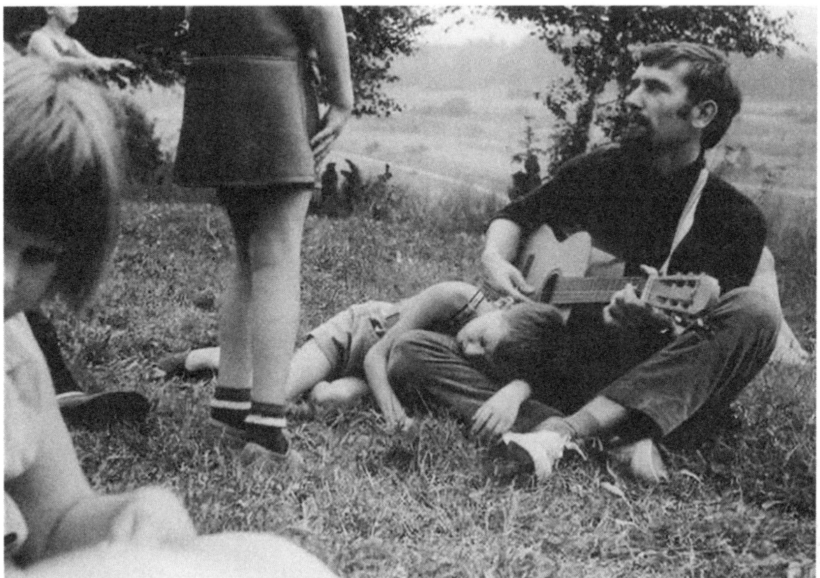

FIGURE 4.2. (*continued*)

out of the regular system and into her segregated school—advised her teachers to feel free to use corporal punishment to keep the children in line. After one day slapping a boy who fell asleep in class (because the boy had to rise at 5:00 to help his farm-laborer parents clean rabbit stalls before taking the long bus ride to school), Jantzen made a commitment that he would never hit another pupil again. He kept his promise. (His fellow teachers were furious that he set this precedent, as they said it gave their own pupils encouragement to noncompliance.) From von Bracken's works on prejudice, Jantzen gleaned that "learning-disabled" pupils had absorbed low self-esteem due to the constant biases they confronted; as antidote, he read to them from Bertolt Brecht.[48]

In Feuser's case, an uncompromising conviction about human worth and an ease of interaction with people with diverse impairments reached deep into his childhood. This included the remarkable experience that two women he dearly loved, coincidentally both diagnosed with schizophrenia (his own aunt, and the daughter of a neighbor), were successfully hidden in a small attic space during police raids as well as during aerial bombings when everyone else ran to the cellars – and protected collectively from the prying eyes of the Nazi apartment-building warden – by the entirety of the building's denizens through the duration of the Third Reich. In the immediate postwar, as his parents had moved to a rural village, among his close friends was an adolescent named Karl, known to others only as "the idiot" (*der Depp*). Karl miraculously survived the Third Reich (presumably because he was not institutionalized), living off handouts and petty thievery and sleeping in a barn. But as farming in the countryside was mechanized and his barn was needed to store tractors, Karl was—to Feuser's great horror—abruptly criminalized and dispatched by the villagers to an institution 60 kilometers away, never to be seen (or even mentioned) by the villagers again, as if he had never existed. This was Feuser's first lesson in the ugliness of postfascist mentalities.[49]

In contrast to Jantzen, Feuser was a superb pupil, and was already supplementing his schooling as a teenager with extensive independent reading at the state library (comprising early immersion in a wealth of classic literature, including the complete works of Fyodor Dostoevsky). When he acquired his first teaching post in 1963 at a remedial school in his home town of Rastatt, he was assigned the "C-class": those deemed (more severely) "mentally disabled" or "difficult." A substantial proportion were Yenish (persecuted under Nazism together with Roma and Sinti); many others came from families in which parents were un- or underemployed, or engaged in petty illegality. Feuser regularly extracted the children from police custody and from punitive parents alike; within six months the children had improved to the point that they could be taken as a group to the opera and the theater. In 1965, the state of Baden-Württemberg decided to turn the remedial school into an "achievement-oriented" school and ejected the "C-class" children diagnosed as mentally disabled while sending the behaviorally disturbed to a special school just for that newly designated category. This was precisely the "structural transformation" of the segregated school system to meet only the needs of the less severely disabled that the majority of special education teachers so self-congratulatorily applauded. Feuser chose instead to quit.[50]

By 1967, Feuser had moved to Hessen and prepared to open his own school in Gießen—the second one in all of West Germany for "practically educable" children—and determined that it should be named the Martin-Buber-Schule. Hessian state- and county-level authorities resisted, urging Feuser to choose a name of someone who had been involved with education for the disabled, thereby implicitly suggesting that Buber's dialogic "I-Thou" principle could not apply to people with cognitive impairments. In solidarity with Feuser and each other, parents of his pupils—from the most respectable professional to the very poorest—mobilized jointly to conduct an impromptu sit-in at the state administration building in Wiesbaden until the name was approved by the Minister of Culture. When the doors of the Martin-Buber-Schule formally opened in 1969, Feuser expanded its reach with yet another contingent—personally rescuing every one of the occupants from two psychiatric wards in the Gießen regional hospital where they had been warehoused in appalling conditions and most of whom carried marks of significant trauma. Feuser negotiated guardianships as needed and organized dormitory housing replete with support staff for these former "patients"-now-pupils.

The emphatic insistence on naming his school after an eminent Jewish philosopher of religion and education was no minor coincidence. From the start and consistently thereafter, for both Jantzen and Feuser—in their efforts as instructors at the University of Marburg in the early 1970s and in their decades (from 1974 and 1978 on, respectively) as professors in disability pedagogy at the University of Bremen—their two most significant intellectual orientation points were, in fact, Karl Marx and Martin Buber. However unlikely these thinkers may have seemed as resources—neither had ever had anything directly to say about disability—both proved indispensable. In time, ideas drawn from Marx and Buber would be supplemented by key concepts derived from numerous other thinkers. Most durably compelling for Jantzen and Feuser would be the "usable past" they found in the Russian cultural-historical school of psychology of the 1920s–1930s around the troika of Lev Vygotsky, Alexei Leontiev, and Alexander Luria, and the powerfully inspirational "elsewhere present" they found in the Italian "Democratic Psychiatry" movement around Franco Basaglia.[51] But over the years, numerous other thinkers would find citation—among them Theodor

Adorno, Hannah Arendt, Walter Benjamin, Pierre Bourdieu, Frantz Fanon, Michel Foucault, Paulo Freire, Antonio Gramsci, the Prophet Isaiah, Martin Luther King, Jr., Louise Michel, Jean-Paul Sartre, Baruch Spinoza, and René Spitz—as each particular occasion seemed to demand.[52] It was as though the message of Jantzen and Feuser was: We are insisting that people with intellectual impairments deserve the dignity of having their situations thought through with the most ambitious and rigorous philosophy; nothing less will do.

Marx was relevant for the understanding Jantzen gained, already in the early 1970s, for how the "moderately" disabled, who so consistently came from the ranks of the poor, were treated as "labor-power of inferior quality" (*Arbeitskraft minderer Güte*)—whether in factories and farms or in sheltered workshops run by the Lebenshilfe.[53] Marx was no less pertinent for explaining the blatancy of ongoing systematic disinvestment in education and life supports for those more "severely" disabled, who would never be able to work, as well as for making sense of the way, under Nazism, as Jantzen expressed the formula: "disability = incapacity-to-work = extermination."[54]

Yet a Marxist framework served two further purposes. One was as a moral language. By 1982, Jantzen had located a phrase—from Marx's "Critique of Hegel's Philosophy of Right" (1843)—that best expressed his overall sense of what mattered most: "the categorical imperative to overthrow all relations in which man is a debased, enslaved, forsaken, despicable being."[55] The second—and perhaps greatest—relevance of Marx was the way he supplied, for Jantzen and Feuser both, the language for a new notion of disability not just as socially constructed (in the sense that what counts as "normal" and what counts as "pathological" has changed historically), but also for coming to understand disability as socially co-produced. What manifested as "intellectual disability" became consolidated in the interaction between the environment (all too often terribly isolating) and the individual (in their extreme vulnerability), and only by starting from an understanding of that continual interaction between self and surroundings, and the purposefulness and logic of what appeared to outsiders as aberrant behaviors, could appropriate assistance be provided.

Marx supplied Jantzen and Feuser with a means to express not just an epistemological but an ontological challenge to their peers' tendencies toward condescending pathologization. When they were attacked and red-baited in 1973—by some of their peers in Hessen and, very publicly, by the nationally prominent professor Bleidick—for "openly professing neo-Marxism," "foreshortening special education . . . into political economy," and thereby (or so the accusation went) turning the disabled child "into the mere *object* of actions . . . misused as an instrument for the enforcement of society-transforming ideologies," Jantzen was provoked into clarifying that it was the accusers who had things backwards.[56] They were the ones who objectified their pupils: "A disability pedagogy that does not reflect on societal circumstances can solely see its clients as objects and thus is hardly capable of meeting their needs." In his book of 1974 on "Socialization and Disability" (*Sozialisation und Behinderung*), Jantzen demanded an end to the ways in which the disabled were continually conceived of as an "other" form of being, somehow incommensurate with the rest of humanity. If one did not understand "to what extent [a person's] disability is socially constituted" (*inwieweit gesellschaftliche Verhältnisse seine Behinderung konstituieren*)—and citing Marx's "Theses on Feuerbach," in which Marx had argued that "the essence of man is no abstraction inherent in each individual," but rather "in its reality it is the ensemble of social relations," Jantzen contended that disability, too, existed within that "ensemble of social relations"—then disability could only be understood as it had always been: "a fateful limitation of human life that is either biological or God-willed." But the result of believing either of the latter was that the person with disability became thereby "of a different sort" (*andersartig*), "of a different human quality" (*von anderer menschlicher Qualität*). This was the stance that needed to be overcome; the goal was a disability pedagogy that was unapologetically "partisan, that takes the standpoint of the disabled subject."[57] In a separate essay the same year, Jantzen went further, as he simply refused to see the nondisabled self as in any way qualitatively superior.[58] More generally, the point was to grasp that any symptom that seemed peculiar or problematic was actually "highly-purposeful"; every individual's behavior made sense within each one's unique history.[59]

This was how Buber came to matter just as much as Marx, and not least because in his book *I and Thou* and in his lectures on education, Buber offered a dialogic conception of pedagogy in which the moral imperative was one of mutual reciprocity in which the other was experienced as an absolute equal. As Feuser noted in 1970—in his first publication, describing his ultimately successful efforts to develop a connection with a severely traumatized, nearly catatonic twelve-year-old girl—in the more than a century since Guggenbühl had given some "early suggestions," no one had made any effort to build a pedagogy for those with the most significant impairments. Whatever had been recommended or done had been of more help to the parents, teachers, or caregivers than to the persons concerned. What a child needed, however, most fundamentally, was "the satisfaction of its specific needs for human contact" and to be "recognized and valued in communicative relation as *an equally valid* thou-partner" (emphasis in the original).[60]

Here were the beginnings of Feuser's later insistence on the absolute singularity of individuals with disabilities—each, in his view, far more distinctive and unique than people without disabilities.[61] Here too, there was the imperative that *the pedagogue*, not the pupil, needed to adjust and adapt to the other's needs. On these and related points, the Russian cultural-historical school of psychology, especially Vygotsky and Leontiev, were to become vital references as well. But Buber meant yet more to Feuser. This was both because in his theories of education Buber had emphasized a holistic approach, considering all dimensions of the human being before him, but additionally—and this was more difficult to articulate, but essential for Feuser—because Buber had found the language to express human *possibility*: the potential futurity that was already there within the present, no matter how damaged a person appeared. A Buber quote that would remain especially important for Feuser summed this up: "For the true educator does not keep merely the individual functions of his pupil in mind, as one would who intends to teach the pupil only certain knowledges or skills, but rather is always concerned with the whole person, and indeed with the whole person both according to his present actuality, in which he is living before you, and according to his possibility, as what may become of him."[62]

In *I and Thou*, Buber had famously declared: "It is through the Thou that the human being becomes I." To which Feuser added (here again the crucial idea was that the onus rests always on the teacher): "The human being becomes that I whose Thou we are to him."[63]

Far from considering these as matters merely of ethereal philosophizing, Feuser dedicated himself to teaching his university students to work practically, with children who had the most significant impairments—among other projects, he supervised the integration of Bremen's entire kindergarten system—and with those adults who had been for so long institutionalized or otherwise neglected that they were considered, in the conventional shorthand, "the hard core" (*der harte Kern*).[64] These were the people so "severely compromised in their psychosocial competencies" that they had been labeled as "incapable . . . of learning," subjected as they often had been to years of both emotional and social deprivation and isolation and who frequently demonstrated "severely self-injurious but also aggressive and destructive behaviors."[65] To these diverse ends, Feuser developed integrationist curricula in which children with and without disabilities could join together in small-group learning around a shared project, with the learning goals differentially tailored to each individual's needs (*zieldifferentes Lernen am gemeinsamen Gegenstand*), as well as comprehensive teacher training in which all students of pedagogy would work from the start with children with and without disabilities.[66] For the so-called hard core, Feuser developed an at once theoretically ambitious and inventive hands-on practicum program, a center for "crisis intervention," that brought to Bremen—into a set of repurposed rooms on the university campus—individuals deemed "beyond therapy." University students who had prepared themselves thoroughly for an entire semester for each individual case worked intensively and daily with that individual for up to a month. In almost all instances they would effectively recover contact and restore capacity for greater independence, and then accompany the person into either an old or new residence for several months to maintain the gains they had made.[67]

In all that he did, Feuser was always aware that his and his students' pupils and later their clients in the center for "crisis intervention" were precisely those who a few decades earlier would have been murdered.

Jantzen, for his part, extensively researched both Nazi and pre-Nazi developments in remedial education and psychiatry. He pointed especially to the insidious impact of Nazi teachings that taught all children to scorn and despise those who were weak (and that exaggerated the divide among those with intellectual disabilities, between—as one Nazi textbook had it—"idiots as adults still sitting senselessly in a sandbox" and those who, "despite limited mental powers," were "work-willing" and "good-natured").[68] And he reflected as well, in multiple settings, on the enduringly lingering effects, even after Nazism's military defeat, of what he came to call "the fascism in the heads."[69] It was this fascism, or more precisely this distinctive *post*fascism, that both men insisted had so urgently to be dislodged.

Against the Division of the Disabled

A baseline, foundational certainty about the full and equal personhood for individuals with intellectual impairments and psychiatric diagnoses would be, by the early 1980s, articulated by an ever-wider array of ardent advocates. Jantzen and Feuser—although remaining lightning rods for the animus of the special education field, whose leading figures continued for decades to attack them, reductively, as politically dangerous extremists—were no longer alone. Hundreds of new actors entered the conversation about mental disability. These included a younger generation of parents—first in Berlin, later scattered across the nation—passionately disinterested in segregated schooling options and intent on achieving integration for their children into regular kindergartens.[70] The majority of the new advocates of comprehensive equality for individuals with disability, however, were not personally affected by disability, but rather young professionals in healthcare or education or adjacent fields: nurses, doctors, occupational and physical therapists, psychologists, pedagogues, social workers. In their rebellion against business-as-usual in the various components of the disability care sector, they were convinced that new forms of interaction between disabled and nondisabled people were not only possible but urgently necessary. And they soon made connections with each other and organized collectively.

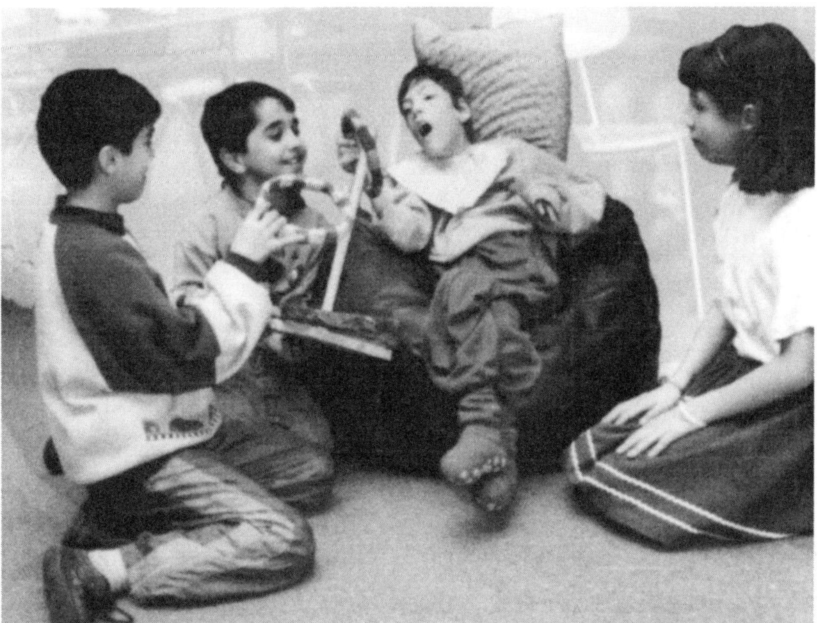

FIGURE 4.3. The picture of children with and without disabilities happily learning together was taken in a classroom at the Uckermark-Grundschule in the Schöneberg district of what was then West Berlin. Launched in 1982, it was modelled on the nearby Fläming-Grundschule founded in 1975, the very first example in German history of a successful experiment in school integration beyond the kindergarten years. The image served as the cover photo for Peter Heyer et al., eds., *Zehn Jahre wohnortnahe Integration: Behinderte und nichtbehinderte Kinder gemeinsam in der Grundschule* (Ten Years of Neighborhood Integration: Disabled and Nondisabled Children Together in Elementary School, 1994). Photo © Gisela Lau.

Two sites of discussion—and, most crucially, of practice—were especially important. One movement sought to integrate children with all types of disabilities, including mental disability, into the regular school system, beginning in kindergarten (with the ambition to continue integration into elementary school and even beyond; see figure 4.3). The other aimed to "dehospitalize" those individuals who had either been living indefinitely within large residential institutions for the mentally disabled, whether charity- or state-run (there were more than ninety of these across the nation, and many of them had multiple hundreds

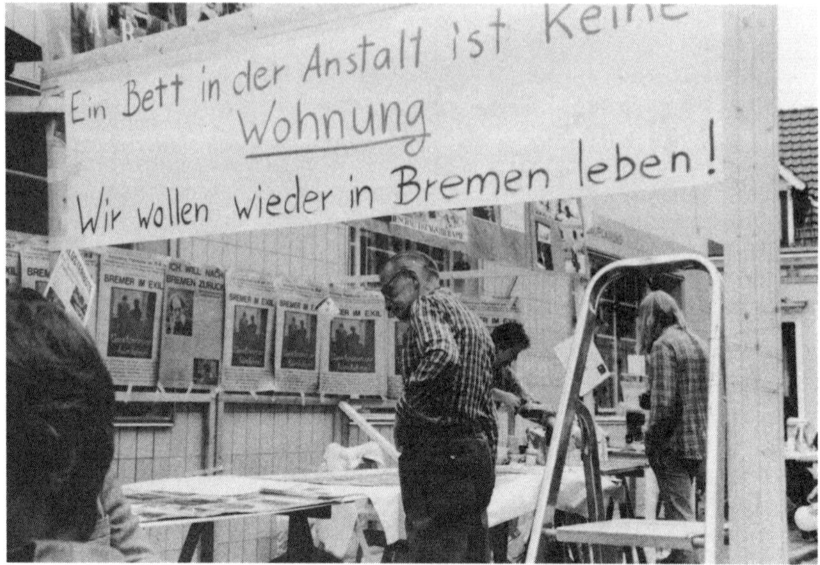

FIGURE 4.4. "A bed in an institution is not a *home*. We want to live in Bremen again!" Protest demonstration at a street festival in the district of Bremen-Walle in the context of deinstitutionalization activists' at long last successful campaign, in 1980–1982, to repatriate to Bremen, into group homes and supported independent living arrangements, 300 individuals who had been "mis-located," sometimes for decades, in the Kloster Blankenburg psychiatric clinic a half-hour's drive from the city. © Initiative zur sozialen Rehabilitation.

of beds), or had been for decades "mis-located" (*fehlplaciert*) within psychiatric hospitals, even though their diagnoses were for some form of mental disability, not mental illness. The idea was to move these long-term institutionalized individuals—with both on-site and mobile supports—into decentralized family-scale living arrangements integrated within ordinary neighborhoods[71] (figure 4.4).

Although on first glance, the two movements of progressive professionals were concerned with distinct constituencies, it is noteworthy that these were precisely the two groups with regard to whom disability-hostile death wishes had been most provocatively expressed already in the 1890s: young children with significant impairments and those who were long-term institutionalized. These were, additionally, exactly the two main groups of individuals with disabilities who had been targeted for murder by the National Socialists from 1939 to 1945. Recognizing the diffuse but pervasive disability-hostile attitude that Jantzen had termed the persisting "fascism in the heads" as having both deep prefascist roots and fascism-intensified manifestations, the most fervently pressed argument was that integration was not just an eventual goal, but already *the method itself* for reaching that goal.

In short, after one hundred years of segregation of people with intellectual disabilities from the wider society, the two activist movements of young professionals advocating for rights for those with intellectual disabilities in 1980s West Germany grew to challenge this segregation as both immoral in itself and intrinsically counterproductive. Indeed, and significantly, both the movement for integrated schooling and the movement for integrated living argued that the segregation caused, or at least exacerbated, the very symptoms that then were identified as signs of the disability and treated as indications of the person's ontological "otherness." Notably, too, as members of each movement aimed to refine their vision, they found themselves drawing on the works of Jantzen and Feuser.

Both movements, moreover, must be understood as *antipostfascist* movements.[72] In other words, they formulated their campaigns quite deliberately as counter-projects not just to prefascist segregation and fascist annihilation, but also to the profound inadequacies of the earlier postfascist settlement with regard to intellectual disabilities. This would bring them into constant conflict with the guild of special educators, on the one hand, and the directors of residential institutions as well as state-level welfare administrators, on the other. But it also brought them into direct conflict with the Lebenshilfe. As the first postfascist advocacy association, the Lebenshilfe remained—and, after all, not without justification—exceedingly proud and protective of the segregated kindergartens and schools for the "practically educable" and the latticework of hundreds of (medium-size) dormitories connected with sheltered workshops that it had succeeded in establishing throughout the country in the postwar decades, as well as of its good reputation and working relationship with politicians at municipal, regional, and national levels. The Lebenshilfe's leadership remained strongly invested in an image of West German society as becoming ever less prejudiced. For the integrationists, however, the Lebenshilfe was an obstacle, not an ally. Deinstitutionalization advocates, for instance, were outraged that the Lebenshilfe tied the right to live in its dormitories to the capacity to participate "productively" in sheltered workshop labor, and that it maintained a categorical distinction between "most severely" and "severely" disabled individuals.[73]

As a result of their antipostfascist convictions, the two new integrationist movements shared the radical and adamant refusal to exclude anyone from the project of integration, no matter how severely impaired. There could and should be no hierarchization of people with disabilities, no bottom below which inclusion was impossible. Taking this position was not a minor matter, and it had daunting practical consequences. Although there was, already from the mid- to late 1970s on, proving to be openness among politicians and school authorities in various locales to including learning-disabled children in the regular school system, at least experimentally, strong opposition persisted to including the more significantly mentally disabled or the multiply (both physically and mentally disabled) children.[74] Similarly, while regional welfare authorities and charity institutions had as of the mid- to late 1970s demonstrated openness to gradual devolution of their resident populations into decentralized, smaller-scale living settings, they were only willing to allow those perceived to be more capable of independence to make the move out into the world.[75] Precisely as a result of this partial liberalization, however, the old mega-institutions were becoming, as deinstitutionalization activists argued in dismay, "collection basins" for a tripartite "leftover group": the aged, the "severely and multiply" disabled, and those deemed to be most challenging because they were either self- or other-injurious.[76]

Meanwhile, at the turn from the 1970s to 1980s, there was a great deal of cross-borders traffic of young West German professionals in health-care and education to see firsthand and be inspired by the Italian deinstitutionalization and school integration model. Italy was a significant inspiration not solely (though also) due to the notoriety of the dissident "Democratic Psychiatry" movement around Basaglia, who by 1978 had succeeded—with the passage of Law 180—in shutting down entirely the antediluvian Italian asylum system and replacing it with community mental health centers.[77] In fact, the far greater impact within West Germany of the broader Italian "anti-marginalization" crusade of which Basaglia's initiatives were only a part was the transformation of the Italian school system: Law 517, going into effect in 1977, had dismantled all the segregated special schools and required integration of children with disabilities into their neighborhood-near [*wohnortnahe*] regular schools, and the Italians had also opted to abolish grading for everyone in the first eight years of schooling (replacing decimal grades with individualized descriptive progress reports). West German activists were enormously impressed by how Italy showed that, "without great fuss," one could simply implement integration—and then work out the finer details subsequently.[78] (This was in glaring contrast to many West German authorities' and experts' stubborn refusals even to countenance the transformation of the tripartite regular school system into the unified, more socially egalitarian Gesamtschule, which only a few states had tried and which remained a focus of perpetual contestation.)[79] Especially influential on the West German discussion was the German-Italian psychologist and prominent advocate for integration Ludwig Otto Roser (based in Florence, where he worked closely with the legendary specialist for children with cerebral palsy Adriano Milani-Comparetti, but a frequent visitor to West Germany). Roser's confident assurances that, in Italy, integration was no longer meeting any opposition and that the only complaints from the public concerned the desire to improve integration's efficacy, were orienting and motivating.[80] His observation that the social contact with nondisabled children was proving incalculably more therapeutic for children with disabilities than any corrective or remedial techniques that the most expert adults might be able to offer was received as revolutionary.[81]

No less significant for West German discussion was the steady stream of reports on the dozens of "islands" of experimental integration within West Germany itself. These reports included guidelines for reconceiving education more generally, for all children (for example: making all learning more emotionally engaging and "experience-near"; replacing "frontal" classroom instruction with small-group work; encouraging self-determined choice in learning foci; and emphasizing cooperative problem-solving). They incorporated concrete examples of cooperative learning assignments that could engage students of markedly different skill levels: from kindergarten projects in shared cooking or care of pet animals to elementary and middle school research projects on, for instance, the living conditions of the Berlin working class during the industrial revolution or the challenge of measuring and estimating spatial relations in a mathematical exercise.[82] Others in turn insisted on the myriad possibilities for further cognitive development that simply emerged in the daily-life environs of the pupils, from the architecture of the school building to the weather outside to the animals and plants in the nearest woods. And, perhaps most compellingly, these reports included not only the required documentation of gains made by both disabled and nondisabled children to assure readers that both were benefiting not just emotionally but also intellectually from shared instruction, but additionally anecdotes that revealed the children often to be far ahead of the adults in their ease of interaction across the boundaries of ability and disability.[83] Muth's wager that nondisabled children would grow up with less prejudiced, more socially inclined attitudes was being proven correct. So too was Roser's contention that daily contact with nondisabled children was therapeutically indispensable for children with severe disabilities. Significant debates unfolded around the advantages of mixed-age, mixed-grade classes and their special suitability for enhanced individualized learning, as well as around the desirable ratios between children with and without disabilities. One of the recommendations that emerged at this time was that there should be no more than two children with disabilities in an inclusive class, as the aim was to promote their comprehensive integration rather than grouping them together again. However, this proposal was already at the time competing with other models and is now again rightly controversial. In some inclusive schools today, ideal ratios of 3 to 20, 5 to 15, or 5 to 10 are aimed for; in others, no one is turned away from the local inclusive school and the corresponding communal structures of solidarity, simply on principle.[84]

Meanwhile, for those activists striving to make the case that the so-called hard core of long-term institutionalized residents would benefit from and be able not just to tolerate but actually to thrive in decentralized settings required still more comprehensively reconceived notions of "disability" and resourceful reconceptualization of pedagogic and therapeutic techniques in the face of often difficult behaviors that had seemingly become inextricable parts of the persons. As had been revealed in the *Psychiatrie-Enquête* of 1975, the commissioned report on the state of psychiatry in West Germany, not only were a staggering 36,000 "mentally disabled and chronically psychically ill" West Germans living in mega-residences under "wholly inadequate" conditions (nothing further than this had been said, in delicate discretion driven by the incentive not to insult the mammoth Protestant- and Catholic church-affiliated charity institutions). More unexpectedly, an additional 17,500 whose primary diagnosis was "mental disability" had already, and evidently for a long time, been "mis-located" within psychiatric hospitals.[85] Arguably, this overabundance of inappropriate placement was one long-term consequence—and this despite the intervening murder years and the significant entanglement of the psychiatric profession in them— of the power grab engaged in by psychiatrists back in the 1890s. At that time they had succeeded, after decades of manifest disinterest in "idiocy" and notwithstanding the near-complete inapplicability of a psychiatric skillset to the task of in any way remediating it, in wresting control of intake and treatment decisions at all the large residential institutions.

Yet this too went undiscussed in the media reception of the *Psychiatrie-Enquête* even as it surely counts as one of the glaring open secrets of postfascist psychiatry: Hospital administrators in the postwar decades had known full well that the mentally disabled did not belong in their wards, but had kept them around anyway as an (unpaid) labor force.[86] It was in doubly horrified response to this now incontestable evidence of the scope of the crisis—more than 50,000 human beings in "closed" institutions—and their own everyday experiences working in these large-scale and generally antiquated residences or psychiatric wards that an activist group of young professionals dedicating themselves to the needs specifically of the institutionalized mentally disabled was founded in 1979. It emerged as a subgroup from within the reform-oriented "German Association for Social Psychiatry" (*Deutsche Gesellschaft für Soziale Psychiatrie*) that had been established in 1970 by a group of progressive professionals that included in its leadership Gütersloh psychiatrist Klaus Dörner.[87]

Calling themselves the Fachausschuß geistig Behinderte (Committee on the Mentally Disabled), sustaining their clarity of mission not least through meeting every two to four months across the length and breadth of West Germany at different prominent residential institutions or as-yet-undevolved psychiatric hospitals, the Fachausschuß followed a twofold activist path. On the one hand, its members developed detailed analyses of the harms of institutional care—drawing not least on Canadian sociologist Erving Goffman's theories of the "total institution" elaborated in *Asylums*—but also, and for them most important, formulated implementable proposals for alternative, decentralized, family-scale housing constellations, promoting these ideas to the media, in publications in professional journals, and at a sequence of national conferences (figure 4.5). The titles of the conferences give a good indication of the Fachausschuß's commitments: "Living with the mentally disabled—out of the institution into the community" (1981); "The myth of the hard core—breaking the vicious cycle of exclusion" (1982); and "(Wrong) paths out of isolation—living spaces of mentally disabled people between institutional reform and integration into the community" (1986).[88] The central message was to be, as Fachausschuß member Christian Bradl put it in a summary that reviewed the results of all the conferences: "Against the Division of the Disabled."[89]

Fachausschuß members were strongly motivated by their acute awareness of what had happened in the Third Reich, but they also directed some of their most acerbic criticism at postfascist developments. This required finding frank language to pierce public and official complacency, to model that it was possible to identify with the most abject of fellow citizens, and to tackle what they saw as the rank hypocrisy of the Lebenshilfe's preferred focus on the moderately but not the severely impaired. As psychologist Rainer Nathow, one of the leading members of the Fachausschuß, observed bluntly and without any polite circumlocutions in a presentation in 1981, in a society obsessed with constant growth in "achievement" (*Leistung*) as well as profit and consumption, those perceived as "its weak and *unproductive* members" were seen as "a kind of *garbage*" (figure 4.6). It was all too telling that as the West German economy had recovered in the first post–World War II decades, the most severely disabled were kept *more* hidden than they had been

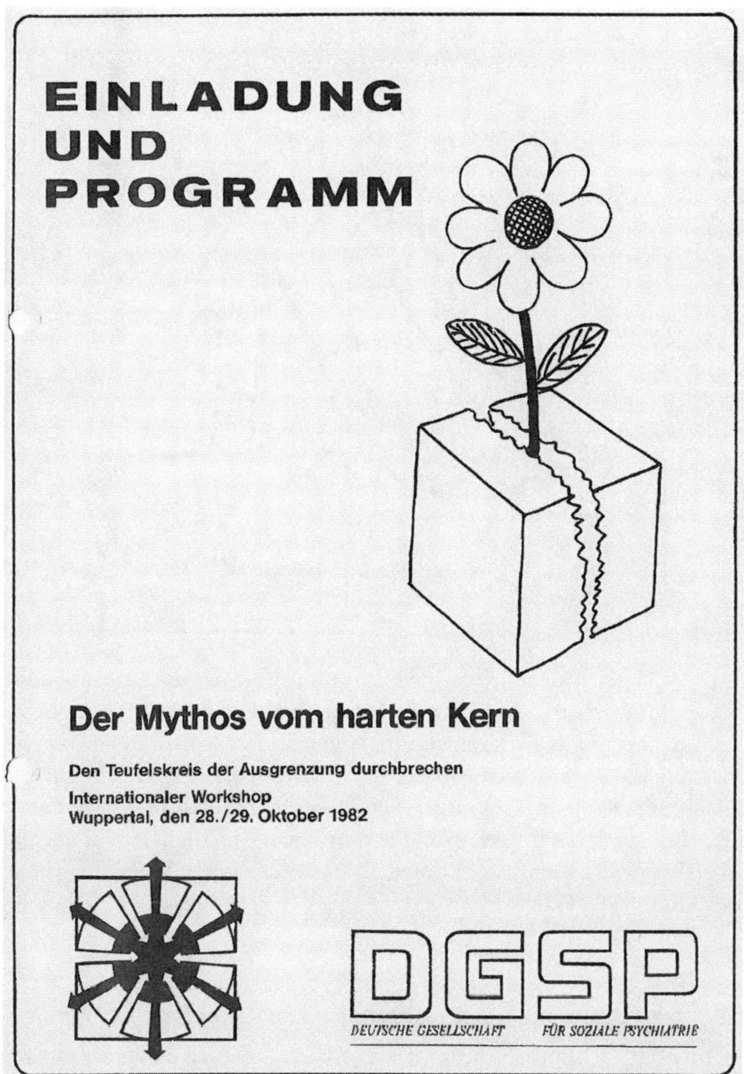

FIGURE 4.5. "The Myth of the Hard Core." Invitation and program flyer for the conference organized by the Fachausschuß geistig Behinderte (Committee on the Mentally Disabled) and held in Wuppertal in October 1982. Archiv Christian Bradl.

in the early twentieth century: "The euphoria of material prosperity should not be dampened with visible misery, especially of the sort that could have . . . unleashed distress, reflection, and shame."[90] Nathow, too, was influenced by Basaglia and his cohort of supporters, and was especially attuned to how easy it could be for even the most engaged

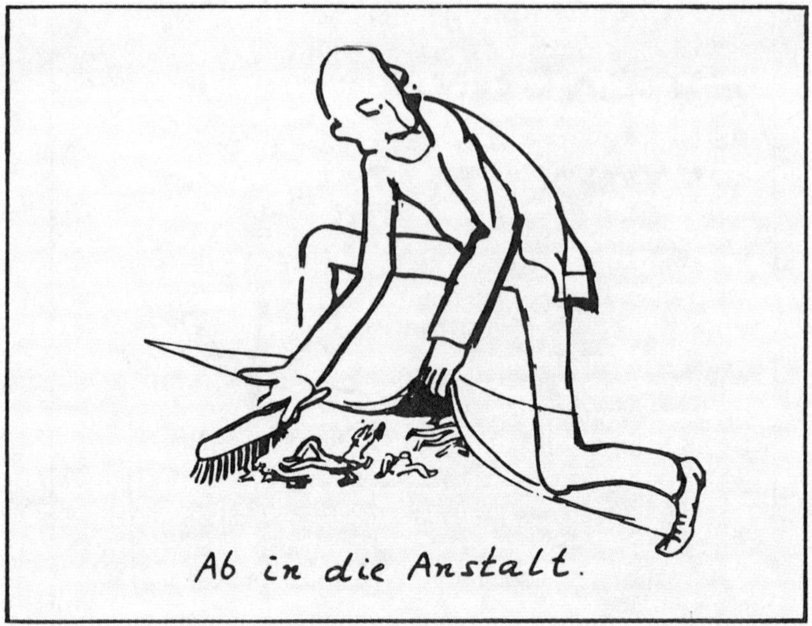

FIGURE 4.6. "Away with you, into the institution." The message is that people with disabilities were treated like trash and swept out of sight of the public. This critical cartoon by Fachausschuß member and deinstitutionalization activist Rainer Nathow accompanied the publication of the speech he gave at the Gesundheitstag in Hamburg in 1981. Reprinted from Rainer Nathow, "Die Entsorgung findet in den Anstalten statt" (1981), in Michael Wunder and Udo Sierck, eds., *Sie nennen es Fürsorge: Behinderte zwischen Vernichtung und Widerstand*, 2nd ed., Frankfurt / Main 1987), 129–132, here 129.

intellectuals to become unwittingly complicit, enjoying their newfound opportunities to explore integration with the not-so-severely-disabled and thereby once again leave behind those who had been most deformed by institutional warehousing.

On the other hand, the Fachausschuß's members agitated locally, each in their own municipal or regional settings, working to persuade politicians and welfare bureaucrats of the need for a fresh paradigm. This could mean devising mobile outpatient services to facilitate non-institutional living arrangements and enhanced integration also in other realms of life (as pioneered, for instance, in the city of Essen).[91] Or it could mean campaigning publicly, so as to prevent the construction of *new* mega-residences (this became a major issue especially in Bonn, where in the wake of the awkward revelation of the "mis-locations" on psychiatric wards, politicians had put pressure on welfare administrators to rectify the optics). Activists rallied to press the case that administrators were ignoring viable possibilities for deinstitutionalization and instead were moving forward—until exposed by Fachausschuß protest—with construction of a 200-bed facility (or, as activists phrased it in anger and dismay, the building of yet another "ghetto for the disabled").[92] Fachausschuß members offered instead an alternate proposal (inspired by Scandinavian and US models) for a combination of decentralized apartments with 4–5 residents each, a dozen one- or at most two-family-size houses, and a far smaller scale building for three dozen individuals with the very most significant disabilities also arranged in family-style groupings.[93] The protests and the proposed alternate plans failed in the short term, as new mega-facilities (albeit with a somewhat reduced number of beds) were built. But through their evolving campaigns, the protesters gathered experiences and refined their vision, developing a number of baseline principles that would subsequently become far more broadly propounded and implemented: As the maximum acceptable size of a group dwelling, they urged, "the measure has to be the dinner-table, around which one can sit and have a shared conversation." In all decision-making about group settings, priority (*Vorrang*) must go to consideration of the needs of the most severely disabled, rather than the least. Professionals should be shifted from a position of control to one of assistance, and clients treated as subjects rather than objects of intervention. And yes, the activists would be occasionally utopian in their aspirations. Sites of integrative praxis, they proposed, would have a double function: to help the individuals with special needs, but also to be "nuclei for a society with more solidarity."[94]

While the first half of the 1980s found special educators and residential directors alike caught off guard by the enthusiasm and moral righteousness being poured into both activist movements, by the second half of the decade the opposition to radicals' demands had grown more sophisticated. Integrationists' calls for complete abolition of the segregated special schools provoked powerful pushback (including the provocative contention made by Bleidick, in a comprehensive take-down of integration published in 1988, that the abolition would provide budget-conscious politicians an alibi for withdrawing funds for services and thus would directly harm the disabled).[95] And leading directors of charity institutions developed updated rationales that the large institutions provided a greater sense of "normalization" (*Normalisierung*) for individuals with mental disability than they could possibly experience outside of that safe and structured world; directors urged that activists should work together with them to bring better-trained staff into the institutions, rather than calling for their dismantling.[96] Peter Schlaich, the son of Ludwig Schlaich and his successor as pastor-director at the Stetten institution in Württemberg, pleaded angrily and earnestly in public controversy with Fachausschuß member Bradl that Stetten, far from being shuttered, should exist for another 130 years.[97]

The resistance from defenders of the segregated schools and the large institutions was strikingly effective, and radicals ultimately did not achieve the revolution they had sought. But, in spite of these defeats, they would in due time—although it took into the 1990s and in some cases the 2000s—achieve substantial reform of what went on *within* segregated settings.[98] As of the 1980s, they had already, and not least, succeeded in shifting what was speakable, teaching their most grudging and reluctant opponents to reconceive the "image of the human" (*Menschenbild*) to include also those individuals with the very most significant impairments.

Cripple-Movement and Benefactor-Perpetrators

In the early 1980s, the most noteworthy new participants in the debate about rights for the mentally disabled in West Germany would come from an unexpected quarter: members of the just-then emergent "cripple-movement" (*Krüppelbewegung*). This was a social movement, launched in the later 1970s, composed entirely of individuals with physical disabilities advocating on their own behalf and with verve and defiance challenging disability-hostile norms and practices in every aspect of social existence. Their visible impairments may have been caused by muscular dystrophy or polio, cerebral palsy or a car accident, or—if they were born in the early 1960s—thalidomide use by their mothers during pregnancy. But whatever the source, they shared the experience of being treated as a problem, and often as pariahs.[99]

The cripple-movement activists knew firsthand exactly how corrupt and poisonous the sociopolitical climate in the first decades after the Third Reich's end had been and in countless ways remained. For however ironic this might seem in decades-later hindsight, in the immediate postwar, Wehrmacht veterans with physical disabilities had had far higher moral status than civilians with physical impairments (whether congenital or incurred by accident). The former group, after all, had served the nation.[100] And although a law of 1961 aimed to regularize civilian status, many civilians with physical disabilities continued well into the 1980s to face a bevy of practical barriers in daily life, from difficulty finding jobs to high, uncut curbs, inaccessible staircases, and no wheelchair lifts on buses. They regularly faced contempt from physicians responsible for their healthcare and random passersby alike.[101] Patronizing opinions about the emotional maladjustment supposedly suffered by people with physical impairments prevailed not only in medical and pedagogical but also in charity and welfare circles.[102] Children with physical disabilities were all too often sent to segregated special schools far from home, and if adults could not live independently and were unable to organize their own care assistance, they were placed in residential institutions in which the climate was infantilizing, claustrophobic, and repressive.[103]

As of 1980, antidisability prejudice was still so routine, unquestioned, and pervasive that a Frankfurt / Main court had granted a West German tourist reimbursement from a travel agency for the fact that she had been impelled to endure the sight and sounds of individuals with physical disabilities—mostly cerebral palsy—enjoying their own beach vacation in Greece in the same hotel in which she had booked a room. Offensive, moreover, was not merely the decision, but the language in which the judges had legitimated it: "As desirable as the integration of severely disabled people into normal daily life is, it can certainly not be forced by a tour operator on its other customers. That there is suffering in the world cannot be changed; but a plaintiff cannot be denied if she does not want to see it, at least during her vacation."[104] In direct and outraged reaction, the first national demonstration of disability rights activism was held on May 8, 1980. Five thousand people descended on Frankfurt from all over the country. The banner held high above the crowd read: "Don't pity the disabled person. Pity the society that rejects him."[105]

Yet despite their intimate familiarity with antidisability prejudice, the difference for individuals with physical disabilities was that they could organize on their own behalf in a way that people with mental impairments could not. Moreover, the long unquestioned hierarchy in which those with mental disability were the most denigrated category of all remained in place. The significance of developments in the 1980s would be that an audacious and remarkable subset of cripple-movement activists would take it upon themselves passionately to defend the rights also of individuals with cognitive disabilities, thereby repudiating the pecking order by lived example.

The capacity imaginatively to identify across the border of types of disability was by no means a given, but rather a profound accomplishment.[106] The identification was substantially hampered not least by a very different idea of what the goal of disability rights activism might be. While the advocates for shared instruction of children with and without disabilities and for comprehensive deinstitutionalization organized under the watchword of "integration," the cripple-movement had expressed vehement disgust at that idea (figure 4.7). For them, "integration" implied the expectation that they as people with physical disabilities would strive to conform to the normative expectations of the nondisabled, and to seek acceptance from the nondisabled rather than defiantly going their own self-determined way. In addition, cripple-movement activists were highly critical of what they believed was a psychologically problematic "helper syndrome" prevailing also among those nondisabled individuals seeking to be allies and advocates, and an early, heatedly discussed topic involved the unacknowledged power dynamics between assistance-givers and assistance-recipients.[107]

Nonetheless, from the start there had been collaborative connections between cripple-activists and nondisabled allies. One of the most

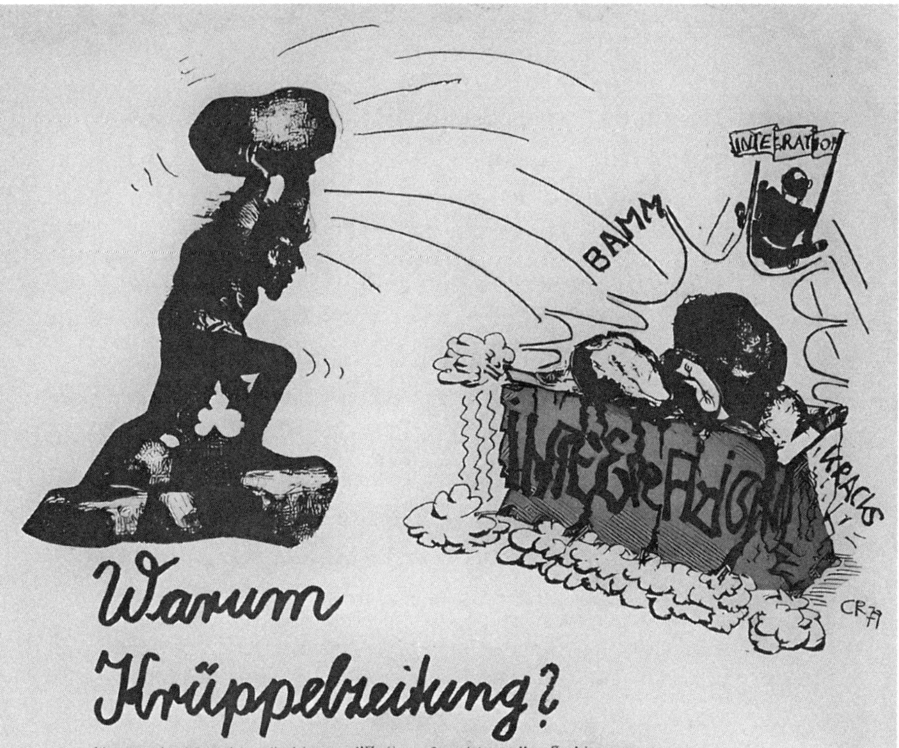

Warum Krüppelzeitung?

Warum heißt die Zeitung "Krüppelzeitung", Zeitung von
Krüppel für Krüppel - und nicht "Behindertenzeitung"?

Dies ist kein Streit um Namen, sondern es geht um
Inhalte. Der nichts sagende, etwas "sachlichere" Begriff
"Behinderte" wird heutzutage nicht ohne Grund verwendet.
Mit dieser Sprachregelung wollen die Gesellschaft und
auch die Nichtbehinderten Integration und Partnerschaft
vortäuschen.

Die Wirklichkeit ist: die Gesellschaft, die Institutionen,
die Nichtbehinderten beherrschen uns.
Der Begriff "Behinderte" soll uns vormachen, daß wir zwar
besondere Probleme haben, aber ansonsten sind wir Menschen
wie die anderen auch. Dies kommt auch zum Ausdruck, in
wievlel anderen Bereichen "Behindert" verwendet wird,
z.B. wird der Stürmer beim Fußballspiel auch sehr häufig
vom gegnerischen Verteidiger behindert.

Wir sind jedoch nicht mehr bereit, unsere Probleme mit
denen eines Stürmers auf eine Ebene stellen zu lassen;
denn wir werden beherrscht, sei es durch Institutionen
oder Nichtbehinderte, die uns vorschreiben, was wir zu
machen haben. Wir sind permanent von einer Persönlich-
keitszerstörung bedroht.

-3-

FIGURE 4.7. Drawing of Quasimodo (the sardonically chosen identificatory symbol regularly pictured in the *Krüppelzeitung*) heaving a boulder to smash the concept of "INTEGRATION" as idealized all too often naively—or so "cripple-movement" members contended—by nondisabled would-be "helpers" of people with disabilities. "Warum Krüppelzeitung?," *Krüppelzeitung* 1 (June 1979), 3.

acerbically vocal cripple-activists, who could be counted on to find fault with every other progressive constituency in the country, was movement co-founder Franz Christoph (who walked with two crutches due to polio he had contracted one year after birth). Christoph had published in 1979 in Georg Feuser's journal his sensationalist bid to be granted asylum in the Netherlands on grounds that in West Germany he faced political discrimination as a person with disabilities.[108] While he was writing what would become his first book, *Krüppelschläge* (Cripple-Strikes, 1983)—which analyzed critically not just conservatives' but also the New Left's discriminatory attitudes—he lived for months in Wolfgang Jantzen's family home. (Feuser and Jantzen certainly learned from Christoph as well, and cited his comprehensive challenges to "normality" in their own work.) And, together with dozens of fellow cripple-activists, though notably again with Feuser's and Jantzen's vigorous support, Christoph led the resistance to the paternalistic festivities organized in West Germany for the UN Year of the Disabled in 1981. Most sensationally, at the "REHA '81" convention in Düsseldorf, Christoph achieved widespread media attention when he deliberately struck Federal President Karl Carstens, a former Nazi, with one of his crutches twice (and then was not arrested, even though if he had been nondisabled he would have been), to highlight the situation of people with disabilities in West Germany and the cripple-activists' disgust at politicians' and welfare authorities' self-serving condescension. Still, none of this yet involved considered engagement on behalf of individuals with intellectual disabilities.

The tipping point came in 1984. Two other members of the cripple-movement, close associates of Christoph's and his successors as editors of the *Krüppel-zeitung* (Cripple-Paper), Nati Radtke and Udo Sierck, self-published what turned out to be an explosive book, as it ended up exposing as morally bankrupt members of several respected postwar professions. It had come to Radtke's and Sierck's attention that an apparent loophole in post-Nazi law was being quietly used—in 80 percent of cases without informed consent—to sterilize teenage girls diagnosed with mental disabilities. Although the Allies had dismantled the Nazi sterilization courts, and although it was illegal to sterilize anyone over the age of eighteen without their consent, physicians were skirting the restrictions by allowing parental or guardian permission to substitute for the individual's own knowledge or agreement. As the findings would soon be summarized in mass media, every year "hundreds, potentially thousands, of girls and women are being sterilized in the Federal Republic."[109] How was it possible that Nazi practices were being continued four decades after Nazism's demise? Radtke and Sierck's adroit title captured the answer with trenchant clarity: *Die WohlTÄTER-Mafia* (wordplay that merged the terms for "benefactor" (*Wohltäter*) and "perpetrator" (*Täter*), while highlighting with capital letters the "perpetrator" aspect).[110]

Precisely those three professions that had styled themselves as benefactors to the disabled—medicine, religious charity, and special pedagogy—were guilty of either implementing or abetting the sterilizations. Doctors who should have known that they were acting outside the law were performing the actual surgeries; other doctors were providing the expert opinions that served to legitimate them. But the strong encouragement to the parents or guardians to permit and pursue those surgeries was coming from the teachers in the special schools for the learning-disabled (as Radtke and Sierck had found, in these schools, often a third and sometimes even fully half of the females had been made infertile) or, in the case of girls and young women who lived in Protestant residential institutions, with the blessings of the charity institutions' own leadership. And then there was the fourth "benefactor-perpetrator" group: the Lebenshilfe. The very group that had begun as an initiative to reclaim dignity and rights for children with intellectual impairments would soon be revealed to be at the forefront of the only semi-legal sterilization project; for years already, the Lebenshilfe had been striving to convince the government to introduce a new sterilization law.[111]

Radtke and Sierck's self-published book was followed by a dramatic documentary episode of the popular television show *Panorama*. Among the most noteworthy elements of the episode was the revelation that the justifications for the sterilizations were being presented in the most liberal of postfascist terms: as facilitation of the rights of people with disabilities to engage in sexual encounters and romantic relationships. Yet the *Panorama* journalists were evidently unpersuaded of the innocence and empathy propounded by their interviewees—demonstratively juxtaposing the self-exculpatory statements of their interlocutors from the Lebenshilfe, the charity institution of Bethel, and special education teachers with clips from a Nazi propaganda film explaining the danger that Germany would be flooded with inferior people if those with mental disabilities were permitted to reproduce. The show further highlighted the implausibility of the virtuous elucidations precisely due to the secrecy as well as to the young ages at which the girls were being preemptively made infertile—well before their further development and potential ability to provide or refuse informed consent on their own—and included an interview with the progressive juvenile psychiatrist Charlotte Köttgen (a close associate of Dörner's), who explicitly compared the practices in the 1980s with Nazi decisions about what kind of life was "unworthy of living." Sierck, too, was interviewed on camera and made related points about disability-hostile assumptions in the wider public, and about how the secret sterilizations conveyed clear convictions about which kinds of lives were to be considered "worthy" or "unworthy."[112] Binding and Hoche's coinage of 1920 was continuing to haunt the 1980s present.

There had been a few precursor instances at which members of the cripple-movement had reflected briefly on whether they had much in common with people with mental disabilities. At the demonstration in Frankfurt in 1980 to protest the court decision about the beach vacation reimbursement, for instance (the court had added insult to injury by justifying its decision on the—as it happens untrue—grounds that the supposedly offending disabled tourists were not solely physically but also significantly mentally impaired), cripple-activist Gusti Steiner, in his speech to the crowd, had declared: "We are all affected. Those who discriminate against the mentally disabled today will discriminate against the physically disabled tomorrow."[113] And Sierck and fellow cripple-activists involved in the Green Party's disability policy division had in 1983 negotiated thoughtfully both with parents of children with mental disabilities and with activist professionals involved in the care work for those with mental disabilities about how to consult with each other before speaking on behalf of a different constituency.[114]

The publication of *Die WohlTÄTER-Mafia* in 1984, however, marked the first major moment in German history when individuals with physical disabilities put themselves on the line for individuals with mental disabilities. Moreover, the fact that they did so had a whole sequence of noteworthy consequences. The Lebenshilfe was greatly distressed to find its own actions being compared so directly, as the *Panorama* episode had, to Nazi propaganda and practices.[115] The Lebenshilfe additionally found itself having to submit to a great deal more public scrutiny about its previously discreet efforts to encourage policy-makers to introduce a new sterilization law.[116] In the meantime, prosecutors had begun looking into the cases of doctors who had conducted the only ambiguously legal if not illegal surgeries, and the national medical association had found it necessary to issue a warning memorandum to doctors to alert them about the actual state of the law. Most important, after the topic had blown up across the entirety of the welfare sector and the national media alike, new laws were ultimately passed that forbade anyone ever to be sterilized before the age of eighteen, and—in the context of a reconfiguration of the guardianship law—would only permit sterilizations for those unable to consent under the very most restrictive conditions. In the course of the extensive debates that the scandal had triggered—about how best to balance sexual rights with rights to bodily integrity—wholly unprecedented concepts of the rights of people diagnosed with mental disabilities to reproduction and to family creation were articulated.[117]

Radtke's and Sierck's commitment to advocating on behalf of individuals with mental disabilities proved durable.[118] In 1987, in the wake of the Chernobyl nuclear reactor disaster the prior year, an article was published in *Der Spiegel* reporting on a study that had identified unexpectedly higher rates of babies being born with Down syndrome in West Germany several months after the reactor meltdown, specifically in Berlin and in parts of Bavaria (where radioactive wind had blown). The essay was not neutral in tone, but rather was dripping with disability-hostile and demeaning language.[119] The three individuals who had the immediate perspicaciousness and nerve to conduct an impromptu sit-in in *Der Spiegel*'s foyer to protest the essay's representation of Down syndrome as (in *Der Spiegel*'s noxious phrasing) "the most common, just barely still compatible with life, malformation" (*die häufigste, gerade noch mit dem Leben zu vereinbarende Mißbildung*) were none other than three

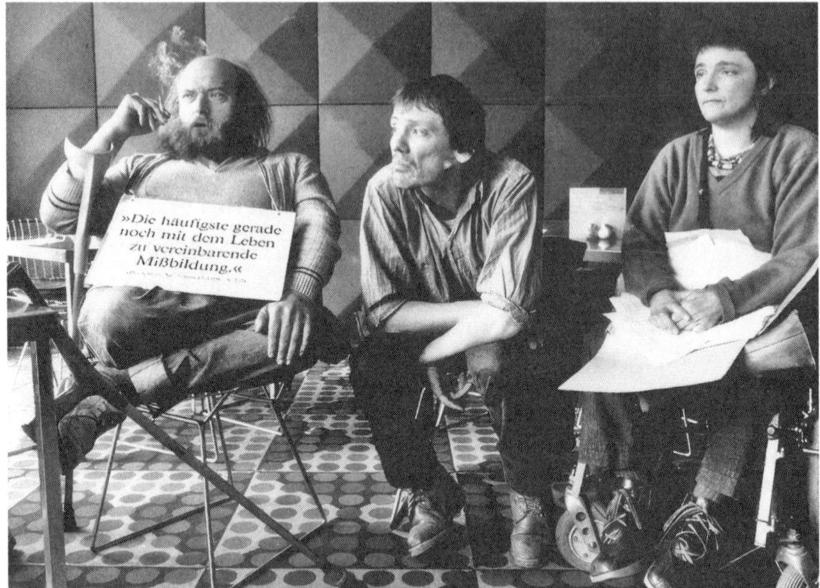

FIGURE 4.8. "Cripple-movement" activists Franz Christoph, Udo Sierck, and Nati Radtke occupied the foyer of *Der Spiegel* in 1987 in protest against the magazine's overtly disability-hostile language as it reported on a (putative) rise in cases of West German babies born with Down syndrome in the wake of the Chernobyl nuclear disaster of 1986. Photo © Gesche-M. Cordes, Hamburg.

members of the cripple-movement: Franz Christoph, Udo Sierck, and Nati Radtke[120] (figure 4.8). The sit-in blocked public access to *Der Spiegel*'s building for the remainder of day, although *Der Spiegel*'s management proved unwilling to concede that the essay had been offensive.

Yet two years later, when the Australian philosopher Peter Singer was scheduled to come to West Germany to explain why he believed that, from his utilitarian perspective, active infanticide of newborns with severe disabilities should be morally acceptable, *Der Spiegel* turned to none other than Franz Christoph to write the key rebuttal essay.[121] The cripple-movement had therewith arrived on the national scene as a voice to be taken seriously indeed. The terms of debate around all forms of disability in Germany would henceforth be set by the antipostfascist radicals and their allies.

5

Socialist Humanism Confronts Disabled Life

In state- and church-run homes we encountered living conditions that stand in crass contradiction to the humanistic character of our socialist social order. In some cases, important principles of human dignity and respect for the personality and the welfare of institutional residents are being grossly violated.

—REPORT OF THE EXECUTIVE BOARD OF THE FREE GERMAN TRADE UNION FEDERATION TO THE CENTRAL COMMITTEE OF THE SOCIALIST UNITY PARTY, CONCERNING CONDITIONS IN OLD-AGE AND NURSING HOMES IN THE GERMAN DEMOCRATIC REPUBLIC, 1973[1]

From the perspective of a Marxist-Leninist understanding of humanism, it is therefore indisputable that the severely disabled have a moral claim to respect for their personhood and the right to social care even in the extreme case of total inability actively to participate in social life and only minimal capacity to shape their life independently.

—REMARKS BY PHYSICIAN WOLFGANG PRESBER AND PHILOSOPHER OF SCIENCE ROLF LÖTHER, APPRECIATIVELY RE-PUBLISHED BY EAST GERMAN PROTESTANT DISABILITY CARE ACTIVISTS IN REFLECTIONS ON THE INTRINSIC CONNECTIONS BETWEEN MEMORIALIZATION OF NAZI "EUTHANASIA" AND THE ONGOING IMPERATIVE TO DEFEND DISABLED LIFE, 1986[2]

WHO WOULD count as fully human in a nation dedicated to the ideals of socialist humanism? The official answer to this question, so existential for the self-conception and self-presentation of the German Democratic Republic (GDR) as a model land, was: Everyone. The truth, however, was more ambiguous, for actually there was one group whose inclusion was consistently thwarted: those individuals who were so significantly disabled that they could not contribute, at least in some small way, "socially useful labor."[3] These were the human beings who, already since the 1890s and ever after, had been derogatorily labeled as "care-cases" (*Pflegefälle*). Yet this constitutive contradiction at the heart of the nation's organizing fiction would never be admitted by the communist Socialist United Party (*Sozialistische Einheitspartei Deutschlands*, SED), preoccupied as it was with projecting the image of itself as a morally superior nation, but above all with maintaining its tight grip on power.

This chapter shifts to the other side of the Wall, bringing into focus arguments put forward with regard to the value of disabled life under the auspices of the East German dictatorship. Would it be possible, in this society, to formulate a freshly conceived, explicitly secular—even expressly atheist—ethics in vigorous, affirmative defense of the value also of the most profoundly disabled life? Or, alternatively, could a dissident version of Christianity be articulated, one that shed the old paternalistic, ambivalently masochistic rhetoric that had for so long privileged the caregiver's dutiful service over the equal humanity of the person being cared for? What would be the relationship between post-Nazi memory politics in the East and the efforts to envision a transformed politics of education and care? How could one offer a convincing socialist humanist refutation to Karl Binding and Alfred Hoche's so durably influential and seductive viewpoint that murder was the most reasonable response to severe intellectual impairment?

The chapter considers the manifold consequences of the SED regime's conception of the GDR as above all a "workers' state" (*Arbeiterstaat*) intent on mobilizing the labor power of every single citizen—notably, also that of all women, including those who were mothers (and mothers of disabled children)—and its insistent antagonism toward anyone unwilling or unable to contribute.[4] And it details how the Nazi "eutha-nasia" murders, after an extended hiatus in which they were deemed pertinent by the regime only when their memory could be effectively mobilized for its incessant rivalrous competition with the democratic-capitalist, purportedly "neofascist" West, did eventually come to be commemorated both informally and formally in the GDR's final decade.[5] At the chapter's heart are explorations of three especially im-pressive concrete instances, as expressed in texts and in lived practice, of East Germans who strove to make a compelling case for the cherish-able value of the lives of precisely those humans who were most signifi-cantly impaired—and this despite the triply constraining context of insidious political repression, a highly constricted public sphere, and extreme material scarcity. These three instances deserve extended ex-amination not least because there simply are not many sources available that contain passionately expressed counter-testimonies to the menda-cious mystifications propounded by the SED. For genuinely humane care and education for people with disabilities was not just impeded by the perpetual lack of resources and the abysmally shabby physical plant in the institutions (whether run by church charities or by the state), the ever-inadequate ratio of staff to residents, and the government's sys-temic disinvestment and its vigorously pursued policy of concealing significant disability from public view. Another major impediment for any would-be advocate for expanded disability rights was the need to negotiate a space for critique amidst the welter of widely and repeti-tively propounded announcements that the government was deeply concerned for and committed to its disabled citizens, and was doing everything possible to assist them.

This deceptive fiction of a state that cared—a fiction that was upheld ingeniously and, as it turns out, with considerable success, as both insid-ers and surprised outsiders would discover after the fall of the Wall—posed distinctive problems for anyone trying to break through the cant and address fellow GDR citizens in a manner that enabled greater emo-tional identification with the disabled.[6] Yet to give away my argument up front: It was exactly in this social and political climate that in three very different instances the unexpected occurred. There were people in the GDR who succeeded—and who did so not least by inventively adapting many of the very same concepts, turns of phrase, and rhetorical framings propounded by the regime and its most dutifully genuflecting supporters—in rupturing, in quite innovative ways, the ugly ideas put into the world by Binding and Hoche.

Eastern Promises

It is not possible to make sense of how intellectual disability would be discussed in the forty years of the GDR's existence without recognizing how ideals of "socialist humanism" functioned as a shared moral framework—indeed a lingua franca—for an entire society.[7] The assumed meanings of a constantly referenced socialist humanism were formed out of a cluster of overlapping connotations. To adhere to "humanism" meant, among other things, to be inverting fascism's ruthless, blatant anti-humanism, but also, and simultaneously, to counter Christian or other religions' privileging of the divine over the human. Then again, it meant as well to position oneself as the latest bearer of the best of German cultural traditions, from the Renaissance through to the Enlightenment, especially as exemplified in the works of Johann Wolfgang Goethe and Friedrich Schiller, and it meant to trust more generally in the potentialities of human goodness, rationality, and progress. It implied, too, and even when the most programmatically stilted language was used, and when deferential nods to the correctness of a Marxist-Leninist understanding of history were strewn throughout a text, an affectively evocative gesture to Karl Marx's originally articulated dream of the liberation of all human beings from the bonds of unjust domination and exploitation by other humans.[8] To add the adjective "socialist," then, communicated the idea—endlessly repeated in official SED party propaganda but also in scholarship across many disciplines and in literature—that socialism was *the* at once economic, social, and political formation in which "true humanity" (*wahrer Humanität*), as the GDR's constitution of 1949 had put it, could be most fully realized.[9] "There was no other land on earth," an astute cultural critic noted in retrospect, where humanism was "discussed so much, so broadly and intensively, and in such a highly politicized way."[10]

In all instances when the topic of intellectual disability was permitted to be discussed in media directed at a general East German readership—whether in the rare moments when reference was made to the abuses of the Nazi era, or in the somewhat more frequent instances when the regime was eager to report on what provisions it was making to assist families with a disabled member—invocations of socialist humanism became predictably standard fare.[11] "In socialist humanism care for the human being, whether he is young or old, stands in the very center of a doctor's tasks," averred an author in the popular health magazine *Deine Gesundheit* (Your Health) in 1970.[12] Or as a professor of special education—in the GDR it was called "rehabilitation pedagogy" (*Rehabilitationspädagogik*)—declared in 1984, it was part and parcel for "socialist humanism" to prioritize the weakest and neediest of fellow citizens. For "in socialist society help and support for the physically-psychically impaired person does not derive from charitable thinking alone, but rather from the nature and character of socialism itself."[13]

Strikingly, and admirably, the SED's position on intellectual disability was expressly anti-eugenicist, interpreting the Nazi "efforts to purify the body of the Volk" as a tool to oppress and to harm mostly poorer members of the working classes—those who would be destined, as the author in *Deine Gesundheit* sarcastically put it, to serve as the compliant "coolies" (*Kulis*) for "the great nation" the Nazis were claiming to establish. This author educated readers not only to the facts of Nazi "euthanasia"—alluding to Binding and Hoche's coinages as he referenced, in distancing quotation marks, "the forcible elimination of 'ballast-existences'" and the "'annihilation of life unworthy of life'"—and noted how, despite an intricate system of camouflage, the Nazis' project of "mass murder could not remain hidden." He also explained the shaky evidence on which the 1933 coercive sterilization law had been based, its "misuse of the science of heredity" and the "violent crippling of human beings" that the law had permitted, pointedly observing the widespread complicity of the medical profession in the Third Reich.[14]

So too with respect to individuals with intellectual disability newly born into postwar East Germany, eugenic perspectives were emphatically sidelined. Experts relied on by the state went out of their way to underscore that cognitive impairments were by no means hereditary, nor a sign of parental moral failing, but rather a random stroke of unfortunate fate that could have many possible sources, yet none of which were transgenerationally transmissible. For example, when the mother of a young son with both physical and intellectual disabilities was empathically profiled in the major women's magazine *Für Dich* (For You) in 1977—the source of the disabilities in this case was cerebral palsy ensuing from difficulties in the birth process—and the mother asked not only "Why me?" but also "What is the cause?," the magazine segued immediately into quoting the prominent GDR physician Gerda Jun, director of a day clinic in East Berlin for children with neuropsychiatric disorders. Jun helpfully elucidated: "Approximately 0.5 percent of all children in our Republic are ineducable, but developable [*schulbildungsunfähig, aber förderungsfähig*]. The causes that lead to this severe brain damage are many and not in all cases fully explicable. The damage could happen during the pregnancy, during the birth, and could also be acquired after birth in the infant and toddler years." Jun then went on to list viral infections in pregnancy, metabolic disorders, perinatal oxygen deprivation, and household accidents—in short, every possible cause apart from heredity. She made a point of insisting that these children should not be thought of as "sick," but rather "healthy" although "disabled," that they could be "just as cheerful as other children are," and that most certainly the time was overdue for an end to "tactless comments" and "wrong attitudes, outdated prejudices." Touching photographs of several families attending with obvious devotion to their disabled children accompanied the article (figure 5.1). And—it could not be otherwise—acknowledgments of the beneficence of the SED state were included throughout. "In socialism, care for the impaired is the concern of the entire society," the *Für Dich* author asserted. And: "Our state knows the big problems these families face and does not leave them alone." Essential, too, were summaries of recent progress and anticipated further advances. Moreover: "More will be done."[15]

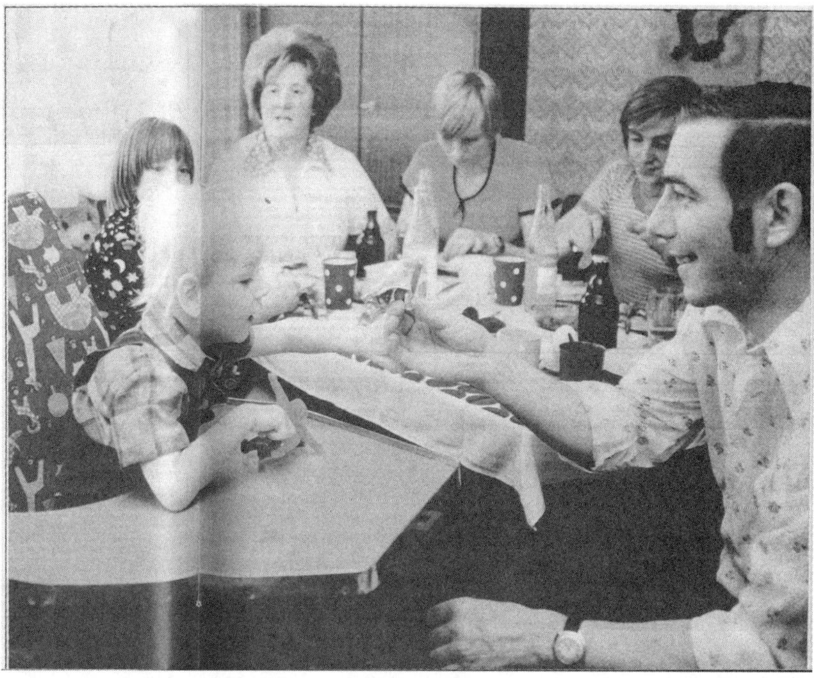

FIGURE 5.1. Two of the heartwarming, lovely photographs accompanying an article in *Für Dich*, the main women's magazine in the GDR, in 1977. The promotion of expanding services for children deemed "developable" helped to distract attention from abysmal conditions in many residential institutions. Courtesy of AddF—Archiv der deutschen Frauenbewegung, Kassel. Source: Karla Nitsch, "Damit sie nicht hilflos bleiben, *Für Dich*, April 1977, 24–27. © Wilfried Glienke.

No mass media representation of disability in the GDR could exist without the two key elements of praise and promises. On the one hand, every media item contained fulsome assertions that the state and its leaders cared for its citizens when they encountered challenging life situations, frequently followed by an enumeration of all the state had recently done to provide needed assistance. "Only in socialist society," an essay in *Deine Gesundheit* intoned in 1977, was "the impaired citizen recognized as a citizen with equal rights."[16] Another essay in the same issue dutifully referenced how the nation's leader, Erich Honecker, had declared at the Party Congress the year before that "Our concern is to improve the care of disabled people and to develop more rapidly the

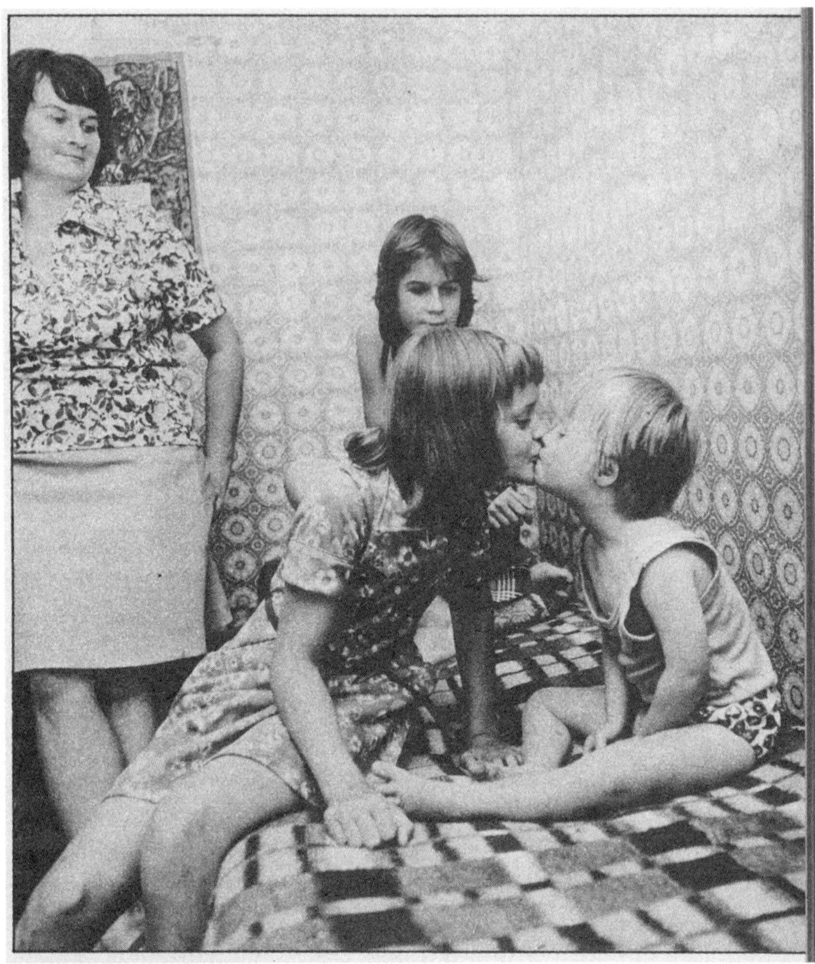

FIGURE 5.1. (*continued*)

material conditions for that purpose, from medical and social services to residential care homes, a protected workplace and recreational opportunities. These citizens have a right to be included in our social life as much as possible."[17] On the other hand, and although regularly conjoined with stock phrasing that conceded that the situation under discussion remained, alas, imperfect, there were reassurances that more help was definitely on the way soon and, above all, that everything was getting "ever better" (*immer besser*).[18] Thus the awkwardly named

"Ordinance on the Further Improvement of Social Support for the Most Severely and the Severely Impaired Citizen of July 29, 1976" opened with this assertion: "It is the concern of the socialist state through targeted social measures to enable the most severely and the severely impaired citizens as well as their families ever better to participate in societal life and to provide them with special care."[19] An orientation toward futurity so characteristic for the East had at least two dimensions. It enjoined all citizens to involve themselves in striving daily to build an improved society, helping to arrive at those "ever better" conditions.[20] *And* it consoled citizens in the face of the constantly frustrating (and worsening) realities of actual insufficient supports and constricted freedoms.[21]

However, there was still more going on with regard to children with disabilities and, not least, with regard to their (unmistakably overstrained) mothers. Dr. Jun's gesture to those who were "ineducable, but developable" alluded to a less pleasant aspect of SED disability politics: the regime's unapologetic maintenance of the age-old hierarchization of gradations of intellectual disability. All through the GDR's history, for those deemed intellectually impaired, the gradation of disability would persistently matter enormously. This was not just practice but policy as, by official ordinance from 1951 on, children labeled not only "ineducable" (*schulbildungsunfähige*) but purportedly even "undevelopable" (*förderungsunfähige*) were legally denied the right to any education. Both of the two lower-ranked groups—the "developable" and the "undevelopable"—were relegated to the auspices of the Ministry of Health, since the Ministry of Education rejected all interest in them and concerned itself strictly with those who were nondisabled and with the only moderately "learning-disabled" and those whose impairments were physical or sensory.[22] Those children Dr. Jun had described as at least "developable" had initially been neglected, but starting in the later 1960s and over the course of the 1970s–1980s, a far-flung network of therapeutic day program centers for these children were founded across the GDR, propelled forward by the efforts of Sigmar Eßbach, a professor of rehabilitation pedagogy at the prestigious Humboldt University in East Berlin.[23] This "in-between" group, in short, would ultimately fare rather well, and in the 1970s–1980s the day programs would be

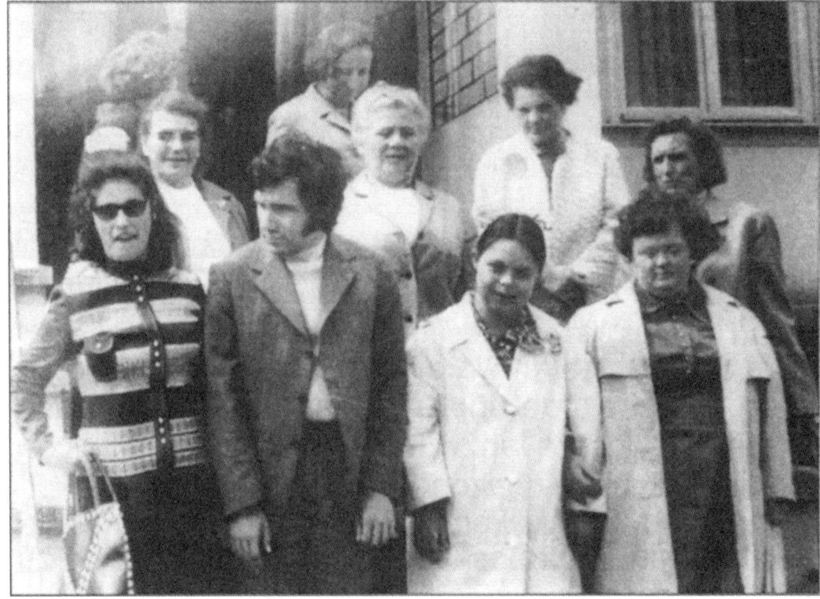

FIGURE 5.2. Hermine Fraas and her coworkers from the VEB Thermos factory in Langewiesen in the former GDR, where she worked from 1972 to 1988. Reprinted from Christine Fraas, *Leben mit Hermine*, Erfurt 1996, 78.

supplemented by a broad array of sheltered employment opportunities for their graduates—in conditions many believed were better than what was available in the West, not least as state-run businesses and industries were required to employ a quota of individuals with impairments and sometimes factories had entire subdivisions staffed by people with disabilities[24] (figure 5.2).

However, the situation was unquestionably worst for individuals with the most severe intellectual impairments. The regime gladly outsourced care for the most severely disabled to the otherwise strongly distrusted Christian churches while simultaneously systematically underfunding them. Generally, the best residential institutions were run by the Protestant Inner Mission, though church administration per se was no guarantee of excellent attention. Unless individuals with the most severe impairments could be cared for within their families of origin or had found a placement within one of those better-run large residential institutions, tens of thousands of these most defenseless human beings were warehoused, completely inappropriately, either in old-age nursing homes or in psychiatric hospital wards.[25] In short, much as the *Psychiatrie-Enquête* of 1975 had exposed for West Germany—although in the Eastern case including also minors and not just adults with mental impairments—thousands of children and adolescents with significant disabilities in the GDR were categorically "mis-located" and placed in the remit of utterly unqualified geriatric care staff or psychiatrists. In these settings, they were subjected to neglect and violence that has only begun to be systematically researched by scholars and formally acknowledged by political leaders. The conditions, to put it bluntly, were catastrophic. And yet all of this was studiously hidden from public view.[26]

This was where the often untenable position of mothers of children with disabilities intersected with a larger state narrative: The regime was intensely concerned that mothers should also be workers. Already in 1969, the Council of Ministers of the GDR—in their "Resolution on Measures to Develop, Educate, and Care for Impaired Children and Youth as well as Psychically Disabled Adults"—worried far less about the children and youth referenced in that typically unwieldy title, and rather more about their finding that at that point approximately 21,000 disabled children across the nation were still living at home with their parents, with the result that "above all mothers are being prevented from pursuing their careers, acquiring professional qualifications, and participating in political and cultural life."[27] (This was the finding that had prompted the genuinely beneficial spread of therapeutic day program facilities for "developable" children in the decades that followed, with more than 14,000 placement slots available by the GDR's end.) But, as the *Für Dich* piece was eager to underscore, at-home therapy could never be a permanent solution.

In this vein, *Für Dich* quoted the mother of the son with cerebral palsy as having anxiously worried—when his disabilities first became apparent and "our world collapsed"—not only "[H]ow will the boy develop, can he be helped [?]," but also "Will I have to give up my job forever?" The article further announced that an older daughter helped with the boy, dropping him off and picking him up from the day program—"so that the mother does not have to shorten her own workday." A different mother profiled affirmatively in the article had stayed home for three years after her son with Down syndrome had been born, "but now she derives self-affirmation and life-joy from her professional activity." Juxtaposed with these remarks and others, it suddenly becomes clear that a government promise that, soon, "fulltime employed mothers with a most severely disabled child . . . will only work 40 hours / week" could well have been experienced by many women as more of a threat than a graciously bestowed gift.[28] Yes, the GDR portrayed itself to its citizens and to the wider world as a society in which women's emancipation was at long last realized, the constitution guaranteed equality between men and women, and the organization of the society was one in which women could with aplomb and without any guilt combine career and motherhood. Yet lived reality existed at something of a slant to this stated ideal. It was not so much that women *could* combine employment with making babies; they were told, in no uncertain terms, that they *must*.[29] Economic considerations were paramount for the regime, as the chronic labor shortage meant all citizens of working age had to be drawn into the production process, but demographic worries were no less pertinent, because precipitously declining birth rates and the failure of various attempted incentives to reverse these had made state officials keen to make employment compatible with childbearing, and this in turn had prompted the provision of extensive childcare services. Nonetheless, children with disabilities massively disrupted this already imperfect calculus, and the regime's response did not include only the upbeat injunctions purveyed by popular magazines.

Mothers were often aggressively pressured to give up their children to the very residential facilities whose unsatisfactory conditions would make all but the most hardhearted recoil. One anguished mother wrote a letter to the Council of Ministers of the GDR in November 1989 (shortly before the fall of the Wall), reacting to a regulation passed in 1986 that required parents of disabled children to formally sign them up for residential placement if they wished to receive 200 Marks per month, until placement became available, to offset the cost of at-home care (she had declined to sign). Her letter was a reaction as well to the coercive maneuvers of local bureaucrats and doctors urging her to give up her ten-year-old daughter, who was blind and multiply impaired and for whom she lovingly cared; she found it deeply offensive to be told that her commitment to staying home was a sign of "laziness" or of wanting "vacation every day" (an example of the kind of accusations she faced as a professional—she was by training an economist—who had chosen to stay home): "What kind of a law is this, that compels a mother to commit her child to an institution?" She announced her intention to continue to refuse. Apparently knowing what the institutions were like, she reported simply that she could not reconcile giving up her daughter with her own conscience.[30]

As the example of the GDR demonstrates with particular clarity, then, rejecting a eugenicist framework alone would not be sufficient for ending endemic discrimination toward, and abuse of, individuals with the most significant cognitive impairments. The reasons for that insufficiency lay in the long-standing habit, formalized so explicitly in the late nineteenth century (though the roots of the impulse undoubtedly set centuries earlier), of hierarchizing human worth in accordance with the standards of "educability" and the capacity, or lack thereof, to contribute "useful" labor. This transhistorically pertinent preoccupation would remain continuously virulent, in ways both old and new, through the forty years of the GDR, not despite but because of the nation's foundational self-understanding as above all a "workers' state." The SED regime—notwithstanding, indeed in direct contradiction to, its numerous self-congratulatory pronouncements as a state that cared deeply about the well-being also of its weakest citizens—thus maintained the stigma that adhered to inability to work, with all that implied for those affected as therefore undeserving of either financial or emotional investment.

Importantly as well, organized group self-advocacy around disability issues was perceived by the regime with deep suspicion and officially prohibited – even if, as the newest scholarship is showing, individuals with physical impairments could at times at least individually, and occasionally also collectively, through petition letters to the authorities and other strategies achieve pertinent improvements in their living situations.[31] With regard to people with intellectual impairments, although here too individual initiatives, often by mothers, could sometimes achieve a great deal (for instance, within the Saxon regional Protestant church and under the auspices of the Inner Mission, family self-help groups were able to launch nine day-program centers and workshops between 1967 and 1975), an equivalent to the West German Lebenshilfe parent organization was forbidden in the GDR.[32] And there was no open public sphere in which conditions in the institutions could be—as they were, increasingly from the later 1970s on, in the West—productively scandalized.

Nonetheless, the most significant revelation provided by a look at the regime's propaganda is that censorship and suppression of all potentially politically embarrassing information was not the only strategy pursued; the regime's preemptive self-representation as motivated by great solicitude for its disabled citizens served as additional effective distraction and disguise. For, what the attention to those who were deemed (in the case of intellectual impairments) "developable" or (in the case of a physical disability acquired later in life) able to benefit from "rehabilitation" hid from scrutiny were the abysmal conditions available to those who were more significantly disabled. The evidence is by now extensive that this concealing was deliberate.[33] Foregrounding with satisfaction the growing network of therapeutic day programs and celebrating the expanding opportunities for sheltered work helped to assiduously hide from view those individuals incapable of work and the often ghastly conditions they were forced to endure.

Only after the Wall fell would dramatic media scandals occur. Two of the most significant were an article published in 1990 by the prominent Hamburg journalist Uta König in the magazine *Stern*, and a documentary film by Ernst Klee shown on reunified national television in 1993. Both uncovered atrocious conditions. König's piece, under the headline "Caged, Tormented, Forgotten" (replete with disturbing photographs), exposed the depth of depravity ongoing, quite flagrantly and unashamedly, at two East German state-run institutions: Children were systematically neglected, tied down to beds, in some cases literally caged (in dog cages), and with no professionally trained, therapeutically encouraging or engaging staff anywhere in sight.[34] In Klee's case, the filmmaking team documented the destitution and deplorable conditions continuing to structure daily life at an institution in Ueckermünde, on the Baltic near the Polish border, as well as at a psychiatric hospital near Dresden—even though at the point of filming at least two years had passed since the reunification of Germany.[35]

It is essential to note that similarly horrendous conditions had existed in the West just a dozen years earlier, including at facilities under the control of the Protestant Diakonie and Catholic Caritas (as the most recent scholarship is finally establishing beyond a doubt), and it is surely not irrelevant that it had taken the very same two singularly passionate individuals to expose to public outrage the disgraceful situation then also reigning in the West. König had found, at the Diakonie-sponsored Künausche Gründung in the Western city of Lüneburg in 1980, nearly identical conditions to those she would subsequently pillory in the East: children in metal cages, conditions "like in the Middle Ages."[36] And it had been Klee who delivered a stirringly sacrilegious speech as he gave, at a "cripple-movement" ceremony, the annual "Golden Crutch" award (given to the individual or organization that has done the most to offend the disability community) in November 1979 to the Alsterdorfer Anstalten in Hamburg: "Protestant therapeutic pedagogy, for many disabled people, has meant for all these many years: apathetic stupor, stinking rooms, beatings, subduing through overdosing of psycho-pills, straightjacketing and public collective shitting. . . . Jesus was crucified by the Romans. Now a few of his official church successors are crucifying mentally disabled people in charity-beds. They even collect for this kind of treatment 'care-fees.'"[37]

Nonetheless—and thus in its own way deeply revealing of just how effectively hidden conditions in the GDR institutions had been— Easterners were not prepared for the exposés brought by König and Klee, but rather reacted in furious indignation at being shown what had occurred in their very midst.[38] Legal charges were brought against Klee personally and the television station on suspicion of libel (although as of March 1994 these were dropped as the prosecutor found them groundless).[39] Klee received threatening correspondence and telephone messages from municipal and regional administrators and medical professionals condemning him for ignorant misrepresentations; media venues in the East accused him in histrionic tones of exploiting the disabled and representing them in outrageously undignified ways (including in their adult nakedness—even as one of his points had been to document that this mixed-gender nakedness during toileting and bathing was part of the scandalous abuse to which the residents were in fact subjected every single day, with the same washcloth used to wipe the bodies of an entire ward of individuals). And throughout, as Klee was dismayed to discover, there was quite evidently far greater distress at the public airing of the conditions than at the conditions themselves.[40] A few medical professionals, journalists, and ordinary citizens wrote poignant, thoughtful letters or published reviews of the film, expressing horror and shame.[41] Moreover, the film did prompt significant improvements, as the uproar around it led to a newly founded regional branch of the Lebenshilfe becoming formally involved, visiting Ueckermünde, confirming Klee's findings, and forcing excellent positive changes in the institution.[42] Only years later, as state security service and other archival records were scrutinized by scholars, did it become fully comprehensible that one of the tragedies of Ueckermünde was that it had been directed, in the 1980s, by an ambitious modernizer who had urgently wanted to improve conditions, especially on the psychiatric wards and in caregiver training, but who had been stymied repeatedly by corrupt local operatives of the SED.[43] In this sense again, then, the political constraints of life under supposed socialist humanism had contributed directly to the mistreatment of the most vulnerable and defenseless individuals. The entire situation had been rancid with hypocrisy and duplicity.

How, then, in the face of so much self-serving obstructionism, to pry open a space for an alternate vision? How to make a case, in this "workers' state," for the full humanity also of those who were incapable of work? Three pairs of protagonists, working from within the GDR during the years of its existence, deserve a closer look. In a society in which so much was unsayable, they had to find ways both to maneuver within and to stretch the boundaries of the rhetorical framework of socialist humanism; all modeled the capacity for identification with those who had for so long been demeaned as merely "care-cases." And, notably, they did so in both secular and dissident religious forms. For notwithstanding the distortions of socialist humanism as propounded by pro-SED propagandists, the ideal did also offer a vocabulary and a horizon of imagination in which an ethical and practical case for the full humanity of people with significant impairments could begin to be expressed.

The Responsibility of Socialist Society

How could one lobby for disability rights and make connections between care politics and memory politics when the mandated framework was the language of Marxist-Leninism? In 1975, Helmut F. Späte arrived as the new physician-director at the psychiatric center of Bernburg. Of the three former T4 centers on East German soil, Bernburg was the only one in the East (much like Hadamar in the West) that had served continuously through the postwar as a psychiatric clinic. Discovering in consternation that the former killing zone in the basement had been used, postwar, as a space for clinical work therapy—and would, due to severe shortage of space, have to continue to be used for that purpose—Späte resolved to confront the past: "In order to live with the weight of becoming director of an infirmary in which multiple thousands of ill people were slain, we began systematically in 1975 to preserve what was still to be found and to compile relevant material."[44] But Späte had to contend with strong popular disinterest. As in the postwar West, so too in the East, postwar prosecutions of "euthanasia" perpetrators had been met with a wave of petitions from ordinary citizens clamoring for the doctors to be set free (but in this case, under Soviet jurisdiction, the argument was that the doctors were in their hearts true "antifascists").[45]

From the perspective of the GDR government, memory of the "euthanasia" murders, where it existed, was allowed when it could be used to score moral points against the West. A prime example of this characteristic dynamic was the career of the brilliant lawyer Friedrich Karl Kaul. Kaul was a Jewish re-émigré to the East, deeply affected by his experiences as observer at the Eichmann trial in Jerusalem in 1961, and he went on to cooperate—with the SED regime's blessing—with Fritz Bauer's prosecutions both in the Frankfurt Auschwitz trial in 1963 and in Bauer's foiled attempt to bring T4 perpetrators to justice in 1964.[46] (So—legitimately—nervous had the West German authorities been about the potential damage Kaul might do in exposing, on international television, ex-Nazis in positions of political influence in West German society, they had stolen documents from his Jerusalem hotel room.) Kaul certainly saw his own work—in lectures, on the radio, in a 1963 television film about the Werner Heyde case, and a book, *Nazimordaktion T4* (Nazi Murder Program T4, 1973)—not only as shaming the West for its evidently lingering fascism but also as pertinent for educating and sensitizing the younger generation of doctors in the East.[47] And he put forward perceptive arguments about the links between the "euthanasia" murders and the Holocaust that in later years would be taken up far more widely in the West as well: "The 'euthanasia' action"—he had written in a private note in 1967—"was the beginning and the deliberate dress rehearsal for the millionfold gas murders in the concentration and extermination camps."[48] Appearing in court in Frankfurt / Main in a subsequent T4 trial in 1968—intent on showing that the perpetrators knew full well that they were committing crimes as they were doing so—he made the argument that "euthanasia" was the "prelude" (*Auftakt*) to that murder of "six million" whose violence "exceeds all human imagination": "The extermination of sick people and inmates of nursing homes selected as 'unworthy of life,'" he explained, "is in no way different in character, meaning and purpose from the 'Final Solution,' by which the 'racially unworthy' were killed in the same way."[49] (Notably, Kaul was here already mobilizing the sequentiality paradigm for connecting "euthanasia" with the Holocaust that would be adopted more broadly two decades later in the West.) Nonetheless, Kaul's concern with NS-"euthanasia" memory was about re-prosecuting the perpetrators, not primarily about humanizing the victims.

In the GDR, it would take until the 1980s before memorialization of "euthanasia" and advocacy for improved care were explicitly linked conceptually—and the SED's rivalry with the West could finally become strategically usable for beneficial ends. Here Späte in Bernburg, together with the medical historian Achim Thom of the Karl-Marx-University in Leipzig, would become an especially effective and impressive force. Thom, too, was a remarkable figure, at once a member of the SED in good standing and an East German university professor who was in regular conversation with disability rights activist-scholars like Klaus Dörner in the West, appreciated for his efforts on behalf of psychiatric reform within the GDR, and known for tolerating and supporting colleagues who hailed from dissident religious backgrounds—as well as a man who stood out among his East German peers for the numerous doctoral and medical students he mentored and encouraged as they researched critical aspects of the history of medicine under Nazism and of Nazi crimes against the disabled.[50] Yet no matter how well positioned Späte and Thom were both professionally and politically, even into the last decade of the GDR the regime would remain reflexively hostile to any effort to educate the public more broadly about "euthanasia," and the standard line, in response to those who wanted to honor Nazism's disabled victims, was that active "resistance fighters" needed to be honored first and foremost.

The effects of this enforced amnesia on levels of popular awareness of Nazi crimes—or rather, lack of awareness—were predictable. In the blunt assessment of East Berlin–based pastor Wolf-Dieter Talkenberger, who in the final year of the GDR had begun collecting testimonies from East Germans who had lost family members to the Nazi killing program: "[E]specially in the area of the former GDR there was among members of the congregation and in society generally as well a great ignorance of the euthanasia crimes."[51] Or, as one young memorialization activist who grew up near the T4 center of Pirna-Sonnenstein summarily recalled: "The 'euthanasia' victims could not be politically instrumentalized and were therefore not a topic for the official GDR historiography."[52]

In 1981, Späte and Thom together published arguably the single most important summary statement about conditions for individuals with severe cognitive impairments in the GDR, including as it did both urgent recommendations for improvement in therapeutic provisions—but also in cultural attitudes and government policy—and reflections on the inescapable shadow cast by the German past (figure 5.3). Appearing in the state-approved book series "Medicine and Society," the essay's title conveyed its moral message unequivocally: "The responsibility of socialist society for its intellectually severely disabled members." Späte

Die Verantwortung der sozialistischen Gesellschaft für ihre geistig schwer
behinderten Mitglieder

Von H. F. Späte und A. Thom

Die Sicherung angemessener humaner Lebensbedingungen für geistig schwer behinderte Bürger ist besonders in unserer Gesellschaft eine verpflichtende Aufgabe

Alljährlich ist – bezogen auf die Lebendgeborenen – mit einer Rate von etwa 7 %
Kindern zu rechnen, die für ihre Entwicklung und Betreuung besonders intensiver
medizinischer und sozialer Hilfe bedürfen. Etwa 4 % der Lebendgeborenen sind
geistig Behinderte, die zumeist auf Grund von Hirnschädigungen (infolge erblicher
Stoffwechsel- oder Chromosomenstörungen oder exogener Schädigungen vor und
während der Geburt) nur unterdurchschnittliche intellektuelle Leistungen zu er-
bringen vermögen. Während dabei etwa 75 % dieser Kinder mit leichter geistiger
Behinderung durch ein komplexes Angebot an medizinischer, pädagogischer und
sozialer Hilfe eine einigermaßen gute Integration in die Gesellschaft erreichen
können – wobei Hilfsschulen, eine spezielle Berufslenkung, Sonderberufsschulen
u. a. Bildungsformen genutzt werden – gestaltet sich das Schicksal der Gruppe der
schwerer geistig Behinderten schwieriger. Innerhalb dieser Gruppe sind die förderungsfähigen geistig Behinderten (in der traditionellen medizinischen Termino-
logie handelt es sich dabei um die Imbezillen mit einem IQ von etwa 55 – 20) nicht
mehr in den Hilfsschulen auszubilden, können jedoch durch gezielte Förderungs-
maßnahmen auf der Grundlage moderner rehabilitationspädagogischer Erkenntnis-
se zu relativer Selbständigkeit in der Umweltorientierung, zur sozialen Einordnung
und zu bestimmten Arbeitstätigkeiten geführt werden (Becker, R. u. a., 1978;
Eßbach, S., 1978; Franke, L., 1979). 1978 standen dafür in allen Bezirken spezielle Förderungseinrichtungen mit mehr als 11 000 Plätzen, ebenso ein organi-
siertes System der rehabilitationspädagogischen Qualifizierung der in diesen Einrichtungen tätigen Fachkräfte zur Verfügung. Die Restgruppe der geistig Behinderten bilden jene Personen, die wegen schwerster Schädigungen (oft auch psychischer und physischer Art) in den rehabilitationspädagogischen Einrichtungen nicht
mehr betreut werden können, sondern einer dauerhaften Befürsorgung bedürfen.
Da der für diese Formen der geistigen Behinderung oft verwendete Terminus der
"Förderungsunfähigkeit" eine allzu passive Haltung begünstigen könnte, sprechen
manche Autoren hier lieber von einer "Förderpflege" mit dem Ziel, Gefühle der
Sicherheit und Geborgenheit zu erwecken, relative Selbständigkeit in einfachen

FIGURE 5.3. First page of Helmut F. Späte and Achim Thom's pathbreaking essay,
"The responsibility of socialist society for its intellectually severely disabled
members." Reprinted from Uwe Körner, Karl Seidel, and Achim Thom, eds.,
Grenzsituationen ärztlichen Handelns, Jena 1981.

and Thom strategically embedded—all within dutifully effusive praise for the increasingly differentiated offerings in the GDR for individuals with "mild" to "moderate" disabilities—the delicately phrased but frank observation that conditions for those who had been categorized as "non-developable" were *not* satisfactory. And they used the (then recently published autobiographical) novel by Roswitha Geppert, *Die Last, die Du nicht trägst* (The Burden That You Don't Carry, 1978)—the story of a mother whose son was developmentally disabled due to phenylketonuria, a metabolic disorder (the novel was a bestseller in East Germany, and has since printed eleven editions)—to give voice to the fact that "occasionally even, with terrifying insouciance, the question is posed whether it is even 'worth it' to keep such life alive, given the high economic and personal expenditures required for its care and maintenance"[53] (figure 5.4).

Späte and Thom had three approaches to the question of how best to refute the assertion that there was human life that was "unworthy" of life: historically (reminding readers of the disability-hostile ideas advanced by Binding and Hoche and their introduction of cost-benefit financial calculations about the non-value of purportedly unproductive lives); practically (with regard to therapeutic approaches, as well as with regard to policy recommendations); and philosophically (as they worked to extend the ethical reach of the vocabulary of socialist humanism). Throughout, they tactically oscillated between reassuring readers that everything under socialism was for the best and getting better, including people's characters and reflexes, and a coaxing, reprimanding didacticism that reminded readers not to feel superior, and that disability could happen to anyone.[54] As they bluntly put it:

Whoever also in a socialist society is prepared, as an individual, to complain exceptionally that the establishment of old people's homes costs money, that chronically mentally ill people can only work to a limited extent or not at all and are nevertheless cared for by society, or that severely mentally handicapped people in institutions require a great deal of care and in the course of their lives may "cost" 100,000 or 200,000 or even more Marks, has not yet thought about the fact

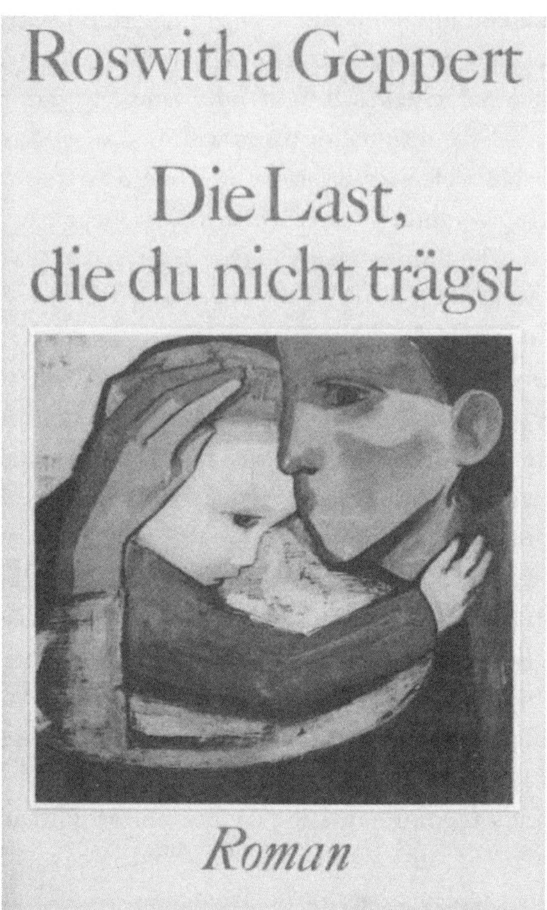

FIGURE 5.4. Original cover of the autobiographical novel by Roswitha Geppert, *Die Last, die du nicht trägst* (The burden, that you don't carry, Halle 1978). The title alludes to "an African saying" (probably from Zimbabwe) frequently quoted among Germans: "You don't know how heavy the burden is that you don't carry." Geppert's book was the first to convey to a wider East German readership the hardships confronted by parents of children with significant intellectual impairments; books by others on similar subjects followed. In the book, Geppert processes her sorrow that her son will never live independently, chronicles the breakdown of her marriage, describes her initial horror at and then growing affection for other severely disabled children she encountered in institutions, learns to give up her son, and ultimately returns to work. She became an addressee for hundreds of individuals confronting related challenges. The book was phenomenally popular, reaching eleven printings. It served as a touchstone reference also for Späte and Thom.

that he too will have to leave the labor-process one day, that he too could become schizophrenic, that his children or grandchildren could also be born with a serious chromosomal abnormality and that in all these cases the sustaining of his life is bound to the existence of this unrestricted system of life support and caring.

And they added: "We start from the premise that an individual born of a human and viable with social assistance, even if it is only capable of accomplishing modest cognitive achievements and due to its inadequate biological endowment for the entirety of its life will require social welfare-care, belongs to the human species and on the basis of this belonging must be regarded as a person [*Person*]." With regard to practicalities, Späte and Thom kept reiterating that what human beings most need in order not just to survive but to thrive were, most elementally, "feelings of safety." Above all it was vital to meet "social needs for security, recognition, love, and communication."[55] Finally, however, Späte and Thom persisted with a basic plea for decency: "The orientation toward satisfying social needs that we mentioned is something we consider so extraordinarily important because *it is in personal devotion to the intellectually disabled that our true degree of humanity is expressed*, and because precisely also for these people there exist only very few other possibilities for having those joyful experiences which effect satisfaction with life and a sense of secure human belonging in the first place."[56] Attitudes and actions toward the most vulnerable individuals with disabilities were no peripheral topic but rather were being placed at the very center of a theory of socialist ethics.

In sum: Späte and Thom's essay can be understood as a newly articulated rebuttal, sixty years later and in a language acceptable to the SED, to Binding and Hoche's call for "permission to annihilate life unworthy of life"—with reflections that are all the more noteworthy in view of the GDR's self-construction as a "workers' state," in which productivity was held up as such a high ideal. It is no less noteworthy that in 1981, Späte and Thom were anticipating by at least two years the conjunction of disability rights activism with "euthanasia" memory politics that would begin burgeoning in the West with Ernst Klee's and others' books from

1983 on. It is remarkable, too, that they not only alluded to the Nazi murders, but also demonstrated acute awareness of the *pre*-Nazi past, and the combination of economic and emotional arguments made by Binding and Hoche.

Nonetheless, the contempt of the SED state for the disabled remained, just as did the attachment of many of its functionaries to a particularly limited and self-congratulatory version of antifascism. Späte specifically had to negotiate with local party officials who held their own notions about which aspects of the Third Reich past should be publicly presented. From 1982 on, the municipal authorities were pressuring him to commemorate the murder, in the Bernburg gas chamber, of two Jewish female communist prisoners from Ravensbrück. Any Bernburg memorial center should emphasize "antifascist resistance" and not the victims of "euthanasia," he was firmly informed.[57]

Späte was of a different opinion. "Heritage preservation" must function as a "warning," he argued in 1983: "Overcoming the dark legacy of the fascist era is only possible if every citizen actively deals with it"—and such dealing, he contended, must also incorporate "the extermination-action against the psychically ill." Once more deftly adopting the tactic of, at one and the same time, acceding to the regime's terms and refusing them, Späte insisted that it was precisely the "euthanasia" murders that provided "an extraordinarily good opportunity to demonstrate, with a practical example, class struggle and fascist tyranny."[58]

Skillfully, too, Späte used the ongoing rivalry with the West to direct the regime's attention to the fact that at the comparable site in Hadamar, in the fall of 1983 there already had been an official exhibition, which had attracted positive international attention, and an accompanying public conference. This motivated Minister of Health Ludwig Mecklinger to get involved and, in 1986, to propose that Späte's concept for a memorial should in fact be realized. The contract for the design of the exhibition went to Achim Thom.

Not least due to the apparent sudden attention to "euthanasia" remembrance in the West, the government became increasingly comfortable with Späte's plans. On September 19, 1989—just weeks before the fall of the Berlin Wall—the Bernburg memorial was ceremonially inaugurated.[59] A final painful irony ensued: The financial upheavals and social vacuum of reunification plunged the memorial, which had just opened, into an existential crisis. It was not able to resume operations until 1991.

What Kind of Island in What Kind of Sea

The Samariteranstalten in Fürstenwalde, an hour's drive eastward from Berlin: For 450 individuals, ranging in age from toddler to elderly, it was home. *Was für eine Insel in was für einem Meer* (What kind of island in what kind of sea) was a photojournalistic account first published in the GDR in 1986, although the photos by Dietmar Riemann were taken in 1979–1981 and the texts were authored by the much-revered East German novelist and short story writer Franz Fühmann in 1981–1982, based on Fühmann's several visits to the institution. Fühmann's main text, in complement and counterpoint to Riemann's photographs, was a statement of what was imaginable and articulable with regard to severe disability within the language of socialist humanism at its best; it functioned as a tribute to and portrait of the remarkable goodness that could be achieved within the extant constraints. It was, in addition, a poetic testimony to Fühmann's own experience of being transformed by the encounter with individuals with disabilities and their caregivers.[60] As Riemann retrospectively recalled: "The encounter with the disabled and their caregivers overwhelmed him."[61]

On the occasion of his first visits—invited by a staff therapist who was well connected within the East German arts and culture scene—Fühmann already had developed authentic attachments to the residents and they to him. His (seven-part) main essay opened with the joy expressed by residents he had come to know who were delighted that he was returning and rushed up to embrace him. The types of disability represented at the Samariteranstalten included cerebral palsy, Down syndrome, epilepsy, autism, and organic brain damage; the references Fühmann brought to bear in his analyses ranged from Greek mythology to the Book of Exodus and the Gospels of Luke and John, and from Augustine to Shakespeare to Diane Arbus. And—not least—to Marx as, ultimately, the essay also became an exploration of the redemptive possibilities of non-exploitative, non-alienated labor. But no matter how erudite the references, the tone of the text was the furthest thing from inaccessible.

The text was, furthermore, attentive to all the anguishing difficulties that all too often attend to disability. On every topic—interacting with the disabled themselves (including his first experience of disabled individuals trying to touch him), observing their interactions with caregivers, their occasional violence toward themselves or others—Fühmann worked through the contradictions, dialectically as it were, acknowledging the complexity, the not-easy-ness, from multiple angles. He did not avoid the dark places, including his distress at witnessing the loneliness (and the evidence of a gross imperfection in the otherwise manifestly loving care provided at the Samariteranstalten) in the photo of one boy fixed in a straitjacket, in a crib with high bars, to prevent him from self-harming. He meditated at various points more generally on the fear and discomfort the disabled so often evoked in the abled, the brute reality that among the nondisabled, there inevitably arose a recurrent fantasy of the "merciful syringe" (*erlösende Spritze*), the "murder-thinking" that was presented with the excuse that it would be humane again to send the disabled "into the gas," as well as that other ugly reflex: to treat the disabled as "the pleasure-object of voyeurism, displaying those diminished physically or mentally or somehow different like animals before a public that, entertained by them, luxuriates in the bliss of its own normalcy." And—to set the tone for the reader—Fühmann foregrounded his concern with writing about people who could not themselves write; it pained him that the very act of describing them turned them into objects. He appreciated in Riemann's photographs the partnership with their subjects, the wooing of the subjects' participation that the images achieved, Riemann's success in avoiding the "tourist gaze" as well as any temptation to be "fascinatingly shocking."[62]

Several individuals emerged as central figures in the essay, beloved in their own right but also the bearers of an argumentative point Fühmann wished to make. One of them was Heike K., thirteen years old, who had cerebral palsy, was seated in a wheelchair, had very limited control over her arms and at best a dozen words and was, when Fühmann arrived for a visit, working with deep concentration on pushing little magnetic colored rhomboids into a design. The last time he was there had been more than half a year ago. But when she saw him again, she lit up, first with her eyes and then with her whole self. And far from finding it simply fleeting and of no particular relevance, Fühmann was so moved by the joy in this moment of mutual recognition he both suggested it was fully "an act of personhood" (*ein Akt der Person*) and—here summoning a famous phrase from Kierkegaard—that "the moment is not properly an atom of time but an atom of eternity." This notion of "an atom of eternity" recurred in the essay. But when it first appeared, it led into reflections on a sense of kinship with Heike and also his own struggles: "In a certain sense the labor of the spastic person resembles mine [as a writer]: extraordinary exertion, small successes, very long-persisting phases of unsatisfying effortfulness until there is any recognizable progress, constant doubt about the purpose of the daily work, profound crises to the point of despair. . . . No, the comparison is impermissible; subjectively, Heike's achievement is much greater."[63]

Another key character in Fühmann's account was Monika, a woman in her mid-thirties, with epilepsy and paralyzed from her knees down to her feet—and preferring to slide around on her knees on rubber sheaths, because that gave her far greater independent mobility than if she had been forced to sit in a wheelchair. In the midst of time spent in the work-therapy room—where products were made that were wildly popular with the public (leather bags, weavings, wooden puppets, change-purses, baskets, cuddly stuffed fabric snakes, and the "pieces made in the potter's workshop: jugs, crockery, the most fantastic animals"), therewith "augmenting the institutional budget considerably" (proceeds coming back to the residents in the form, for instance, of plants to decorate the space, or an improved weaving loom)—Fühmann experiences "a revelation" as he watched Monika push the heavy needle through the holes punched in the leather to make the bags (figure 5.5). Suddenly all around him in the workshop he saw "the human trinity" of heads and hands and objects worked on—by choice, he emphasized strongly, as no one was forced to participate and each resident was free

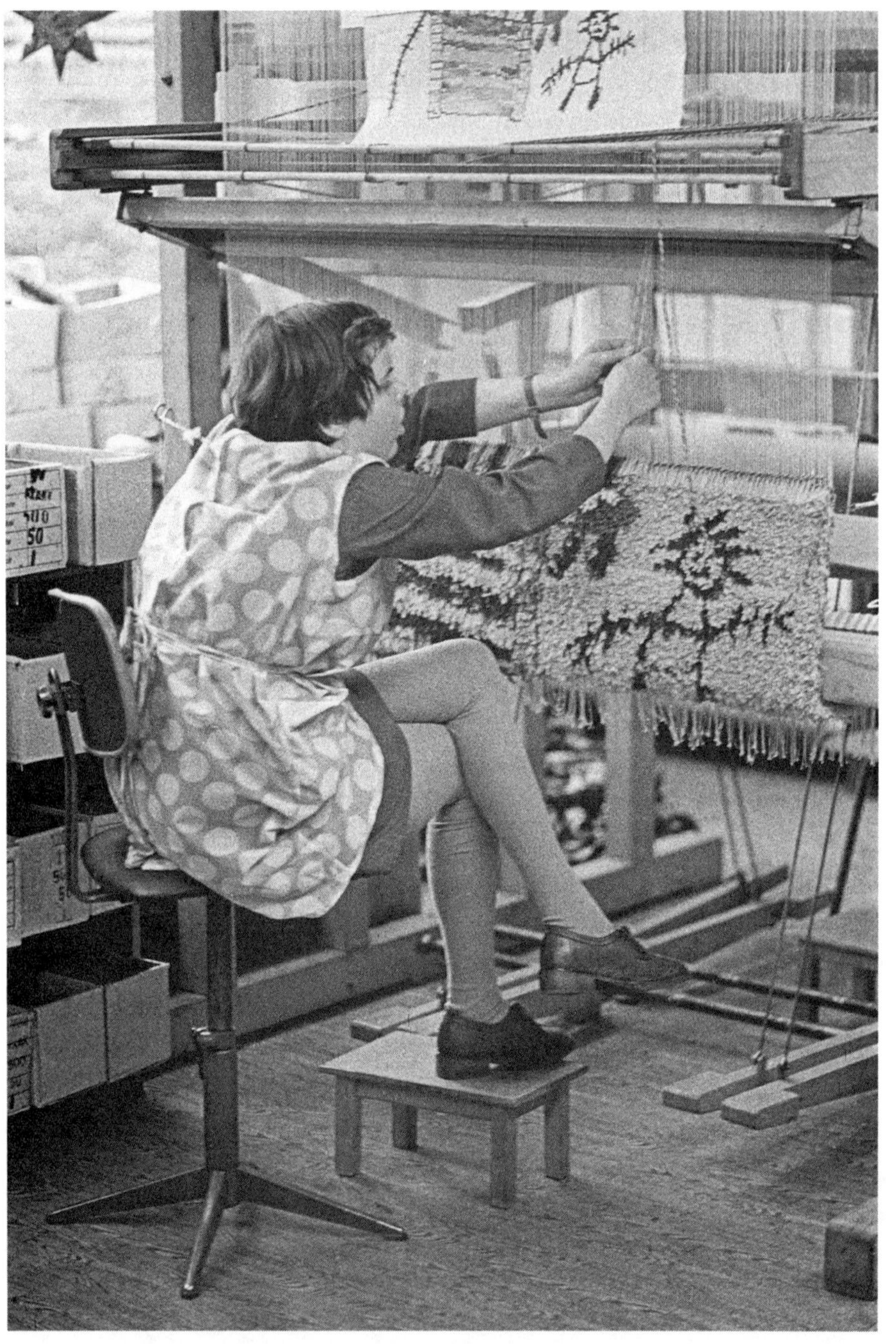

FIGURE 5.5. Photos from Franz Fühmann and Dietmar Riemann, *Was für eine Insel in was für einem Meer* (What Kind of Island in What Kind of Sea, 1985). These photos are from the section entitled "Work as Therapy." Photos © Dietmar Riemann.

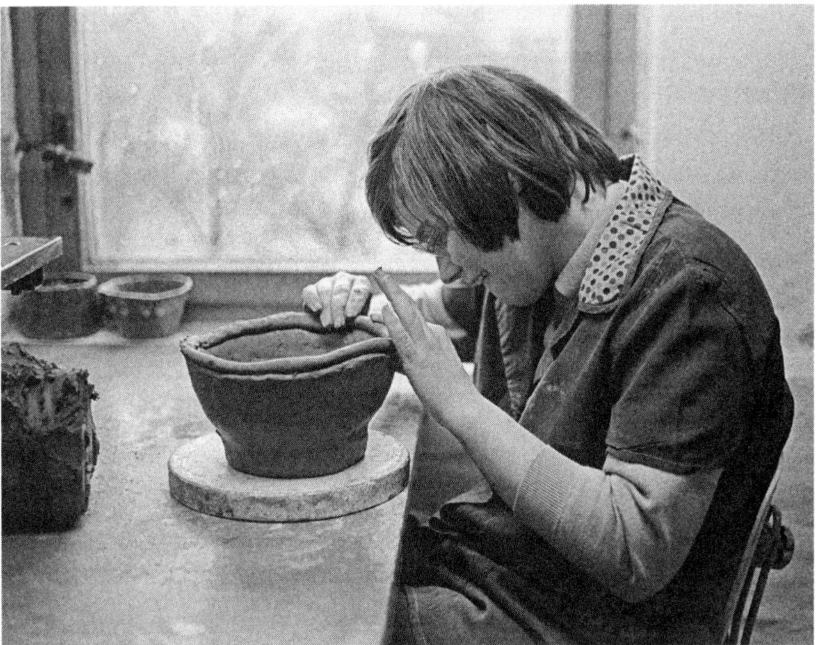

FIGURE 5.5. (*continued*)

to select which tasks to pursue or none at all, and as he recounted how Monika had, as the coworkers shared with him, first come to understand herself (via sanding wooden objects into palpable smoothness) as "the effecter of a transformation." He meditated on how he had always sought the experience of physical work, on the docks, at a construction site, in a mine. But it was only in the work-therapy space at the Samariteranstalten "that I suddenly grasp, what I for a long time already knew: that the human being through work enters into the object; he humanizes the piece of dead nature, and what flows into its materiality is human essence. . . . In his work, the human being is whole [*heil*]. . . . The result of this labor is more than its product: it produces not just a use-value, but a piece of humanness. In being play, too, and in providing immediate satisfaction to its completer, this work is profoundly human work, appropriate to the human, worthy of him, or let's just say it directly: unalienated labor."[64]

Unabashed about using religious language, Fühmann sacralized the labor of the residents and in so doing lifted the entire question of patient labor into a different frame. Here it was not a matter of unpaid, or underpaid, exploitation masquerading as (though perhaps also experienced as) therapy—as had been true for so many decades before the Third Reich and continued to be, in many places, for decades thereafter. And certainly here it was not the measure of a person's capacity to engage in labor as a reason for being permitted to live or be doomed to a cruel death, nor was it labor under duress facilitating the daily bustle and hum of mass homicide, as so much patient and resident labor between 1940 and 1945 turned out to be. Rather, the existential aspect of human work, its meaningfulness, was profiled, with abiding respect. And Fühmann went on expressly to contrast the aversion-inducing repetitiveness of monotonous factory conveyor-belt work ("the terrible price of our civilization") with what he called the "adventure" of each time anew re-finding—head and hands together—the movements that made the objects in this space. He knew he was elaborating an ideal. But he insisted that at the Samariteranstalten, "the quotidian comes close to this ideal."[65]

A third crucial character was Peter, a young adult with Down syndrome and "mental impairment of the third degree, the most extreme, most severe, that which in prior times one called 'idiocy.'" In the work-therapy space, he sometimes elected to sew purses, on other days he played with a ball or a doll, or drew, often a black dog with an overlarge head and two or three oddly splayed legs ("a creature of his own mythology")—and no one gave him a hard time. For Fühmann, the message of Peter's story was about human reciprocity. Upon his arrival at the Samariteranstalten, Peter had shown no reaction, could not hold urine or stool, could not lift himself up, had to be fed and put on the pot, and never gave so much as a smile as reward for those efforts. "A case for nothing but nursing care [*ein absoluter Pflegefall*]." That had been three years ago. Now he not only kept others company in the work space, but it was he who regularly pushed the wheelchair of his friend Ulli, who had cerebral palsy, when a group took walks (though he had to be watched not to direct Ulli into the passing traffic, as he treated cars as friendly beings).

"Also the Peter of today," Fühmann conceded, "would be sent by the Nazi doctor into the gas with a casual gesture. But for someone who knows Peter's development the meaning of therapeutic effort is radiantly evident." More precisely: "The person who integrally contributed to this quiet miracle of human unfurling is Gabriele D., in the photo [by Riemann] cheerfully giving him a goodnight kiss. She gave him this kiss also in the past, when he seemed like a hopeless case, every night, and this devotion of love and warmth, of hope and meaning, awakened the human dignity in Peter."[66]

Fühmann here referenced as well, and reworked, the passage in the Gospel of John often cited in the context of disability, in which the disciples asked Jesus, with regard to a man without sight, "'who sinned, this man or his parents, that he was born blind?'" and Jesus retorted: "'Neither this one nor his parents, but it was that the works of God shall become evident in him.'" Fühmann knew the centrality of this text for believing Christians, but wanted to stress that "it also does not lose its grip on many a one who has no faith, and he too needs to think it through to the end, to what this word might mean also for him. The notion of the meaning of a sickness as divine punishment, or as warning for others to steer clear of evil, or as stimulus to repentance, is ancient; from this the disciples' query arises." Fühmann took a brief detour into Sophocles, and Ajax's hubris in rejecting help from Athena—resulting in his death—only to return to the Bible: "Also Jesus' disciples still think wholly in the tradition of a causal connection, with sin as source and punishing sickness as consequence." But, Fühmann noted: "Rabbi Jesus breaks this chain: Neither the blind man nor his parents sinned, the sense of illness rather lies in God's power being made manifest." What could this mean, Fühmann asked, for an avowedly secular person? The point was not Jesus's miracle-making. "Rather it is in the very healing itself that the power of humanness unfolds, in the convalescent as in the one doing the mending." It was not just that Gabriele transformed Peter, Fühmann insisted further, for Peter also transformed the entire community of carers: "They are not only validated by him, they have been developed [*gefördert*] by him, by his meaning-filled existence." And this was the entire thrust of Fühmann's message: "That one doesn't just give to the impaired ones, but rather is also prepared to receive from them"[67] (figure 5.6).

There was far more to the essay, as it addressed discussions of the memory of Auschwitz and of the T4 centers alike, and declared with regard to people with disabilities that "we still owe them practically everything"—as they were "of all victims of the National Socialist murdering the ones who experienced the least empathy. . . . I know no memorial that reminds of them, no work of art has honored them, they have dropped out of literature, no one has reconstructed their life-journeys, as a group of persecutees they are not recognized, the names 'Hadamar' or 'Grafeneck' or 'Sonnenstein' or 'Eglfing-Haar' or 'Bernburg' or 'Hartheim' say almost nothing to anyone, even though there the first selections occurred." Throughout, Fühmann managed the tightrope balance of refusing all romanticization of impairment ("Just so nobody misunderstands me: I am by no means making a benefit of a bane") while simultaneously insisting on similitude in shared humanity ("But as long as they are among us, the carriers [of these disabilities] are of our kind and we of theirs: Whatsoever is done to them, is done to us as well." And—in his conclusion at last invoking Marx by name—Fühmann proposed that it was exactly with regard to individuals with disabilities that the rightness of the Marx phrase was best exemplified: "in which the free development of each is the condition for the free development of all."[68]

Yet his final words returned to one person in particular. Of all of Riemann's photographs, it was a portrait of Monika that Fühmann had chosen to hang—framed—on the wall of the room in which he worked, ate, and slept. "From her I learn, how I too can get on my knees and yet walk"[69] (figure 5.7).

The Invention of "Developmental Care"

Yet what did it mean, day after day, around the clock, year after year after year, to be not just an occasional visitor but rather the constructers and maintainers of such an island—and that in conditions of extreme paucity of resources and in a place quite far from the levers of power? In

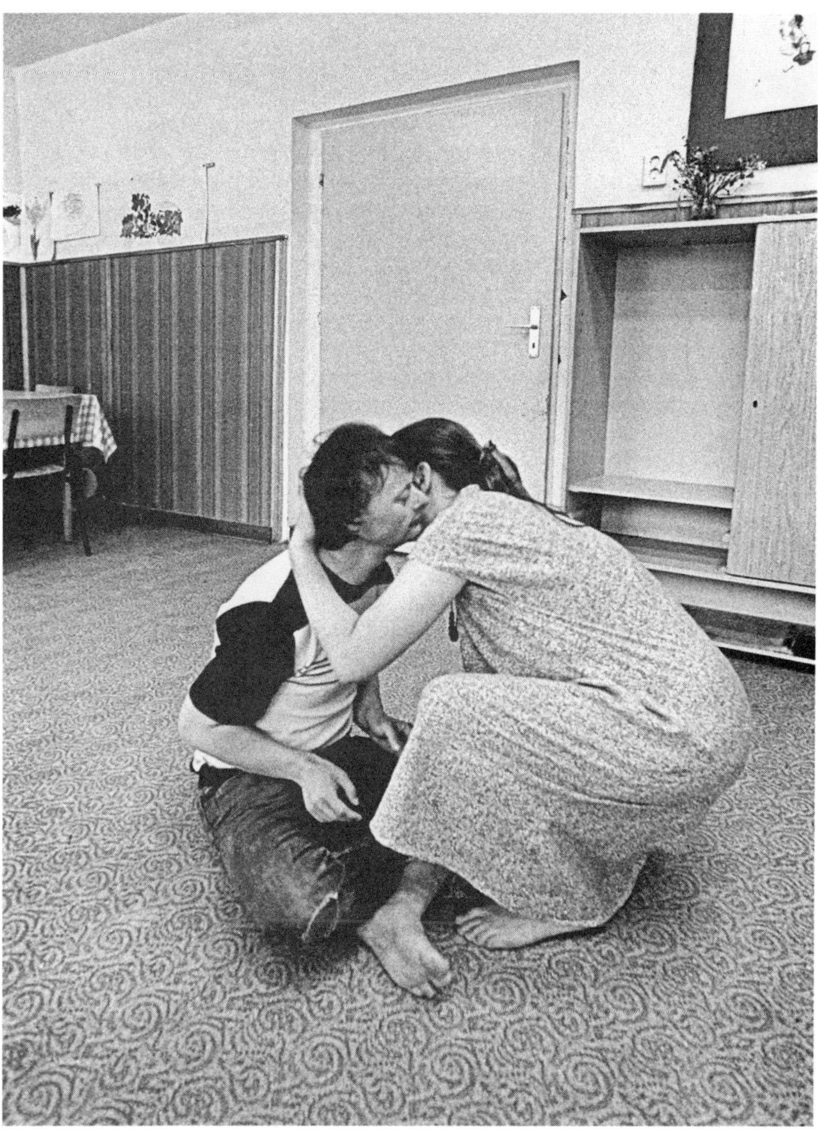

FIGURE 5.6. Photos of Gabriele, Peter, and Ulli, along with other residents. Photos © Dietmar Riemann.

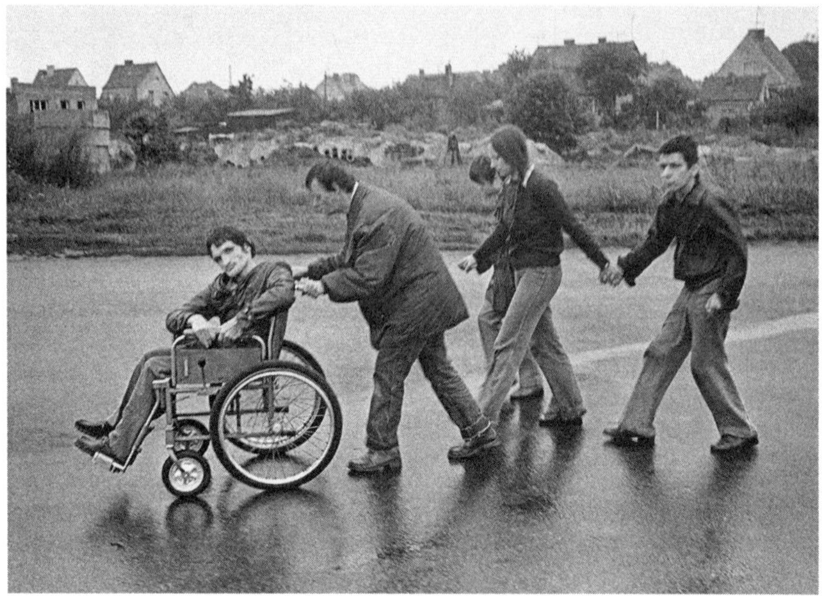

FIGURE 5.6. (*continued*)

1971, the young pediatrician couple Dr. Jürgen Trogisch and Dr. Uta Trogisch arrived to rebuild such a place: the Katharinenhof in Großhennersdorf in Saxony, an hour-and-a-half to the east of Dresden, near the Polish
and Czech borders. Founded in 1721 as an orphanage and school for the
poor, from 1911 to 1939 this was the institution that had been run by
Dr. Ewald Meltzer—the author, in 1925, of that most significant, albeit
complex and ambiguous, text attempting to rebut Binding and Hoche's
1920 call for "permission to annihilate life unworthy of life."[70] As of 1940,
224 children and 43 adults with intellectual disabilities had lived there;
more than 200 would be deported to their deaths—the majority, in
1941, at the T4 center Pirna-Sonnenstein, others to the Großschweidnitz
asylum.[71] By the mid-1960s, it was once again filled to capacity with purportedly "ineducable" (*bildungsunfähigen*) children.[72]

When the Trogischs arrived, to take over both the administration
and the medical and therapeutic care for 416 individuals, some of them
with evident long-term traumatization (indeed, six survivors of the deportations) and 185 of them categorized as severely disabled, and with
84 more names on a waiting list, the conditions on site were unfathom-
ably antiquated. ("Circumstances that are practically unspeakable now,"

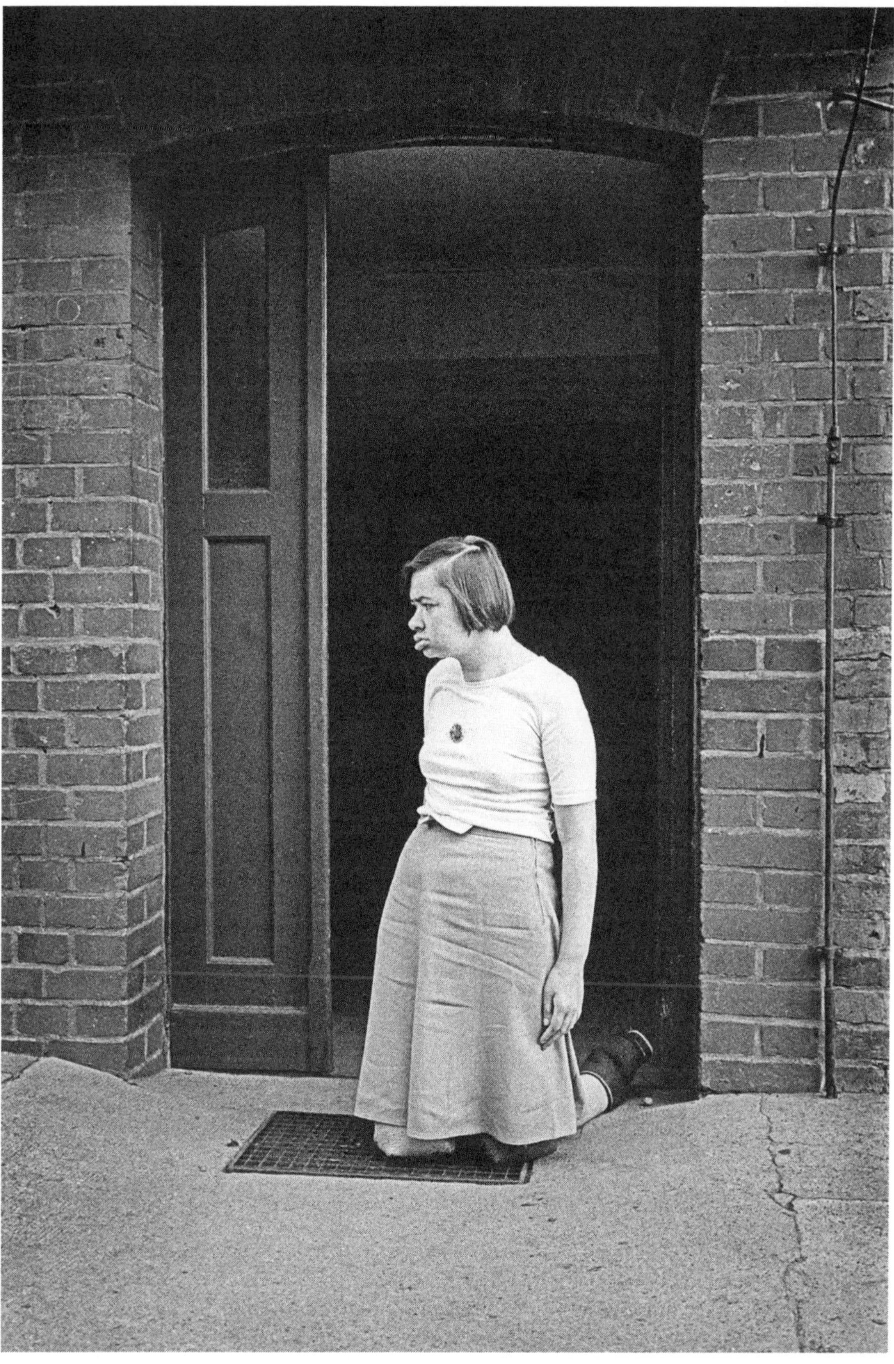

FIGURE 5.7. Monika. Not included in the published book, this was the photo that Fühmann hung on the wall in his bedroom. Substantial portions of Fühmann's essay that accompanied Riemann's photographs were a tribute to Monika and what he learned from her. He concluded the essay with the poignant statement: "From her I learn, how I too can get on my knees and yet walk." Photo © Dietmar Riemann.

Jürgen Trogisch said in 2021; and his wife described the rashes and bruises that come from scurvy, caused by deficiencies in vitamin C, and growth retardation and bone deformities, from insufficient vitamin D, that she had only ever seen before in textbooks.)[73] The residents were housed in thirty-bed dormitory wards (with one toilet, one sink, and one bathtub per ward), four dormitories to each level, with no private storage space anywhere; inadequate warm water; and inadequate living space for staff. The wards had uneven wooden floorboards throughout, covered in splinters, so that people whose main form of mobility consisted of sliding on their bottoms or on their knees constantly had boils and painfully infected abscesses, while bed-bound multiply disabled adults lay in low-to-the-ground cribs with wooden slats, over which staff had to bend to change and care for them. One hundred thirty-eight of the residents were in cloth diapers, which needed daily to be scrubbed, also of stool, and there was no dryer in the laundry. The place was bursting at the seams; meanwhile, the care subsidy granted by the state was less than 2.79 (East German) Marks per person per day. The extant, and numerically insufficient, staff were almost entirely lacking in professional training, and although in many cases conscientious and benevolent in their care provision, had no belief that the residents were capable of any growth. Meanwhile, especially for those most severely disabled, parents had often—"feeling guilty to have borne a disabled child, or ashamed to show themselves with their disabled child in public"—cut off contact.[74]

Over the years, the Trogischs instituted instrumental changes—inspired by houseparents at another, smaller institution they had met who took the view that "residents with disabilities should live the way our own children do."[75] At the Katharinenhof, the Trogischs insisted that the staff brainstorm and experiment with them to find ways to reach and to facilitate development in each and every individual. Unable to absorb people off the waiting list, they created a small respite ward, for ten individuals at a time, so that families with disabled kin at home could get a week or two of break; it was soon filled year-round. They created a guidance clinic for parents of children with disabilities, to give the mothers and fathers both strong positive affirmation and specific therapeutic skills to help them keep their children within the familial setting, despite the lack of state supports (and despite the state's pressures on women to give up disabled children to institutions so as to be able to participate in the labor force). The Trogischs felt fortunate, moreover, that they could receive not just monetary donations every year but also castoff items—a machine for lifting bedridden patients, for example, and adaptive vehicles for taking excursions—from sponsors in West Germany and Switzerland; staff from state-run institutions, Uta Trogisch noted in retrospect, no matter how personally dedicated, whenever visiting the Katharinenhof always looked a bit enviously at these recycled accoutrements to which they had no access.[76]

From the start in 1971, the Trogischs had coined a new term for provision of services for those with more profound intellectual impairments: "developmental care" (*Förderpflege*). The point was, strategically, simultaneously to respect and to defy the regime's distinctions between developability (*Förderfähigkeit*), on the one hand, and custodial care (*Pflege*), on the other. Publishing in the GDR's main continuing education journal for medical professionals, the Trogischs frontally challenged the idea that anyone could ever be deemed "undevelopable," and referenced with confidence the extensive therapeutic experience being gained by staff and residents in their own institution—no matter how "very unfavorable the external conditions."[77] The Trogischs emphasized that everyone had a right to learning, that all learning was socially mediated and involved interaction with the environment, and that even more than movement and sensory training, the targeted practicing of emotional connection was most imperative. As a baseline point, describing their "general goals," they observed that "*safety*" and "*security*" were in any event "essential, foundational needs of human beings"— adding "the concept of *well-being* from the World Health Organization's definition of health"[78]—but noted that this was all the *more* true for those who were "totally dependent on us" and that thus "the question: 'Have we done everything we can for the welfare, the safety and security of those entrusted to us?' is a very fine measure for the assessment of this work."[79] In 2021, Uta Trogisch would remark again that the idea of being "just a care-case" is "abominable." She noted that "still to this day I get goosebumps" when remembering how she herself came to conceive "utterly new benchmarks" for recognizing what an achievement in learning was (for example: "eye contact," or how it was when, upon the approach of a trusted caregiver, "a tetraspastically paralyzed child has a smile spread over his face and one arm starts to tremble with happiness").[80]

The Trogischs further pioneered the notions of "integration" and "inclusion" (the latter, the present-day watchword in disability rights), insisting on routinely making their residents visible on the streets of the neighboring towns, whether in wheelchairs or strolling independently, and attending local events. Regularly inviting visitors into the institution, they coordinated one-to-one sponsorships of individual residents, which often turned into lifelong attachments. And the Trogischs unabashedly ventured further afield, going on excursions and vacations with their residents, by bus and by boat, taking them to beautiful sites in the GDR, but also, in later years, as far as Poland and Czechoslovakia; frequently, they invited family members along—and for some parents, the experience provided a first-ever emancipation from "their dread and their shame."[81]

The past made itself felt indirectly. In September 1972, 66 children and young people, 20 staff members, and about 60 parents went on a boat trip by steamer on the Elbe from Dresden to Rathen to a friendly restaurant for coffee, and then back again (coincidentally—or not—passing the former T4 center Pirna-Sonnenstein twice). One of the fathers overheard in Rathen how an old man, looking at the children, had said: "'They should have been gassed too!'" One week later, in horrified rebuke, Jürgen Trogisch gave a lecture with the title "Life unworthy of life!?"[82]

In 1974, members of the Katharinenhof staff, with the Trogischs' support, creatively developed an inclusive worship service with candles, music, and simple blessings, designed to be meaningful for and appreciated by all (figure 5.8). More remarkably, in May 1981, in conjunction with events around the UN Year of the Disabled, the annual meeting of all the bishops of the Protestant Church from around the GDR was held at the Katharinenhof. Instead of providing a tour and presenting facts about the institution to the attendees, the emphasis was placed on "personal encounter." That was meant literally: Each bishop upon arrival was assigned a child with significant disabilities (and given a folder with information about that particular child), whom he then accompanied into town, helped the primary caregivers later to prepare for bed, and the next day joined at a worship service. The bishops returned home from

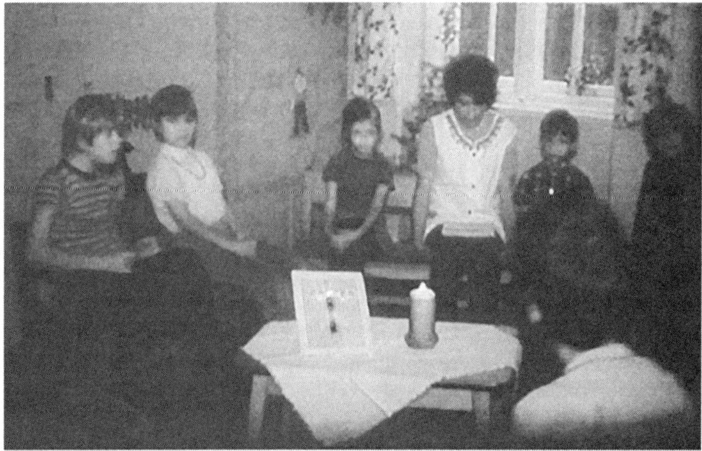

FIGURE 5.8. A simple worship service for children typical at the Katharinenhof in the later 1970s and early 1980s. Filmrolle © Archiv Katharinenhof Großhennersdorf.

the experience greatly affected. As one newspaper report summarized, this "direct encounter of church leaders with the disabled left an enduring impression that transcended all theoretical knowledge and experience."[83] (The worship services were in general a great success, and soon emulated at other institutions in the GDR. Nonetheless, specifically with regard to inclusive communion, it would take until 1985, after numerous arguments with their regional church authorities—who took the view that this category of persons "do not need [communion]," because they could not "understand" it—before services replete with shared communion also for the most seriously disabled residents, each paired with his or her own assisting companion and sharing with that person the wafer and grape juice, were able to take place.)[84] In another innovation, starting in 1974–1975, the Trogischs undertook a research project with the adolescents and adults to solicit the residents' knowledge base, views, and experiences with sexuality and partnerships—a further instance of taking the whole personhood of their residents seriously.[85]

Because the East German state, until the very end, refused to provide opportunities for formal acquisition of expertise in work with people with intellectual disabilities, church charities filled this lacuna and, from 1975 on, the Katharinenhof, in partnership with the Martinshof institution in Rothenburg / Oberlausitz, became a main destination for professional training in "curative educational care" (*Heilerziehungspflege*, HEP for short), bringing over the succeeding years dozens of committed young people into the field of disability services. Theologian Georg Kanig built the program, combining praxis-oriented rotations with theoretical-academic instruction and introducing from the outset Danish disability rights advocate Niels Erik Bank-Mikkelsen's model of "normalization" (the aim was not to adapt people with disabilities to any "norm," but rather to "normalize" their environment and daily lives in as many ways as possible); the emphasis lay on developing expertise in "individualized development and accompaniment" (*Einzelförderung und -begleitung*), and on the Trogischs' core concept of "developmental care."[86]

The Trogischs additionally took the view that the older children and the adults, too, deserved ongoing education and therapies. Thus defying the regime's categorical denial of education to those it deemed "undevelopable," in 1979, Uta Trogisch, together with Winfried Tippelt, a teacher from a nearby town specializing in pedagogy for the hearing-impaired, invented what was later called an "alphabetization program"—they referred to it simply as "the reading course" (*der Lesekurs*)—to assist individuals with cognitive impairments to learn how to read and write; the course was exceedingly popular.[87] There were no available guidebooks for teaching literacy to adults with learning challenges, so they simply adapted whatever materials they could find, such as picture cards (A for apple or auto) and special education textbooks for children.[88] Thirty years later, at the occasion of a reunion, it was apparent not only that some had learned to read and write, but many of those former young adult residents had become empowered enough to live independently.[89]

Despite all of these inventive advances, the situation was nothing to be idealized. Quotidian labor routines could be grueling; the ratio of residents to care staff could often be wide—in some instances as much as 12 to 1—making the commitment to individualized developmental attention something that could only be pursued intermittently, in focused but limited blocks of time.[90] No less pertinent to understand is the stark reality that, just as at other large institutions, East and West, so too at the Katharinenhof, the "fitter" residents were integrated of

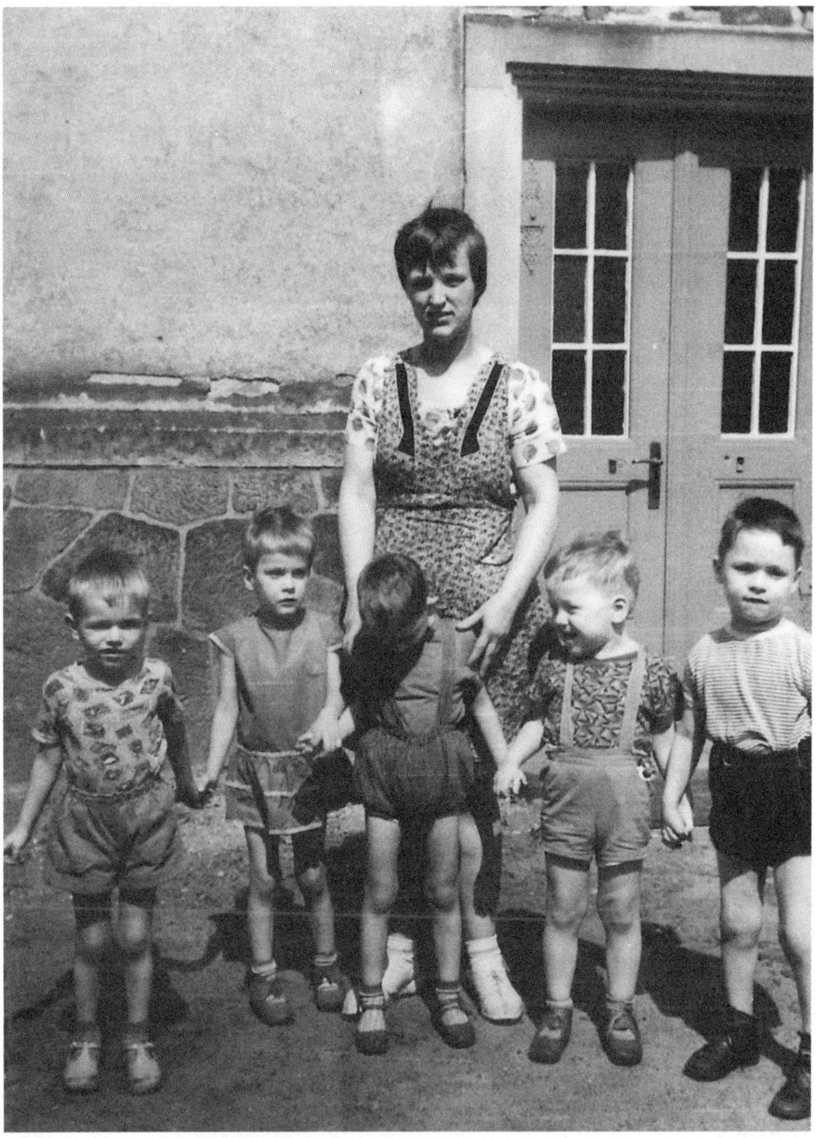

FIGURE 5.9. "Sieglinde Schloßbauer and 'her' children." Approximately fifty of the male and twenty-three of the female residents of the Katharinenhof provided labor on the premises; the institution could not have functioned without them. Sieglinde Schloßbauer was especially gifted at caring for the youngest children—she managed two dozen of them at once, almost every day. After the Trogischs took over the directorship of the institution, they paid salaries to these coworker-residents. © HERR, HÖRE MEINE STIMME. Stimmen aus dem Katharinenhof Großhennersdorf. With the permission of Sieglinde Schloßbauer.

necessity into the daily labor of institutional upkeep. This included not only work in and around the grounds, but also participation in care-labor for the "weaker" residents and especially for the children[91] (figure 5.9). The Trogischs regularized these work arrangements and also saw to it that residents were paid modest salaries for their labors.

Among the more unique features of life at the Katharinenhof was that its remote location on the easternmost edges of the GDR made it, by the 1980s, a destination for nonconforming and antiauthoritarian youth disenchanted by the SED regime; the area became a major center of environmental and peace activism.[92] A few were able to complete their alternative to military service on-site—conscientious objector status was far more difficult to achieve in the GDR than it was by the 1980s in West Germany—but the government quite evidently had the region under surveillance. Jürgen Trogisch, in 2021 writing a brief memoir for inclusion in a volume celebrating the now 300-year existence of the Katharinenhof, noted that it was only in retrospect, long after the GDR had ceased to exist, that it became clear to him and his wife just how many of his troubles negotiating with the authorities were due to the regime's double irritation: at their intense engagement with the residents and at the haven they provided for nonconforming youth. "[B]ehind the delay tactics, at the expense of the residents, lay the efforts of the state, to use the Katharinenhof as solely a place for custodial care and to block developmental work." But: "Also procuring living-space for new staff was difficult. Always again buildings we wanted were suddenly no longer available. Today we know from the files, that the Stasi [state security services] actively impeded the settling of staff in nearby communities because a few of them were involved in oppositional groups."[93] In short: What had for so long been mysterious and vexing became, after the Wall came down, fully, albeit dismayingly, explicable.

Meanwhile, many of these young people had been drawn into work at the Katharinenhof to alleviate the ever-pressing staff shortage even though disability care did not necessarily appeal to them. Jürgen Trogisch recalled trying urgently to explain: "People, this [work] *is* dangerous to the state!" (*Leute, dies* ist *staatsgefährdend!*).[94] Others, however, found the work deeply captivating. Quite a few stayed beyond the fall of the Wall. Some work there to this day.[95]

The Legacy of Antipostfascism

FOR THOSE morally engaged young professionals of the 1970s–1980s, West and East, that I have described as *antipostfascist* because of their dissatisfaction, if not horror, at the inhumane treatment of people with disabilities that had continued on both sides of the Wall into the first two or three—if not four—postwar decades, there was, despite their fervent searching, no adequately usable past to draw on.[1] As a result, these advocates had to invent, from scratch, a new "image of the human" (*Menschenbild*) and radically new ways of interpersonal encounter and interaction. The hierarchization of human value that had accompanied charitable efforts at education and care from their inception had to be jettisoned entirely, and revolutionary notions of equality, reciprocity, and human possibility had not only to be conceived but also put into practice. Moreover, the antipostfascists had to create new languages of moral persuasion. In order to convince their fellow citizens as well as the relevant local and national authorities of alternative approaches to pedagogy, therapy, and interaction in daily social life, the activists working on behalf of integration in schooling and deinstitutionalization in the West, or developing creative care practices or respectful memory politics in the East, freely repurposed and juxtaposed concepts drawn from a broad range of theological and philosophical traditions with wholly novel, previously untested ideas emerging out of their own direct encounters with people with disabilities. Depending on which side of the Wall they found themselves, the challenges of persuasion varied. For instance, because of the utterly different—generally denigrated and definitely disempowered—role of the churches within the GDR, Christianity could at times there provide a more subversive resource than it could in the FRG, where both the Protestant and Catholic churches along with their respective welfare divisions had long been more overtly complicitous in obfuscating their own entanglements, both ideational and practical, in the terrible events of the Third Reich.[2]

I am all too aware that the use of the term *fascism* to refer to Nazism—whether by the SED regime in the GDR or by New Left insurgents of the 1960s–1970s in the FRG—has been criticized, harshly and eloquently, as relativizing the distinctive qualities of Nazism and the centrality of the Holocaust to it, and as more generally diminishing our grasp of Nazism's extremity.[3] But I want to stress here that for the admirable individuals I discuss in this book, the word was by no means meant in either relativizing or diminishing terms. On the contrary, the word "fascism" captured for them the sheer ferocity and cynical hubris of Nazism, while "National Socialism" felt more generic and neutral. It was specifically *because* of their involvement with people with disabilities that they were attuned to dimensions of Nazism—particularly its trampling of all that was weak and vulnerable—that eluded other postwar interpreters, and it was this same attunement to the emotional dynamics of hostility to the defenseless that allowed them to have a finer grasp of the persistence of "the fascism in the heads" (as Wolfgang Jantzen phrased it) into the postwar decades.[4]

In communist East Germany, *antifascism* was of course the official state doctrine and constantly reduced to a shallow and hypocritical rhetorical or performative ritual. But—as the diverse contributions of Franz Fühmann and Dietmar Riemann, Jürgen and Uta Trogisch, and Helmut Späte and Achim Thom demonstrate—the conceptual framework offered by the SED's language of antifascism could also, strategically, be stretched to make room for honoring the needs and claims of people with significant intellectual impairments. Späte, in particular, was not only tactically ingenious—as he demanded of the SED government that it permit him to focus his memorial project at the former T4 killing center of Bernburg on the National Socialist "euthanasia" murders—but also intuitively correct in his insistence that doing so offered, as he put it in 1983, "an extraordinarily good opportunity to demonstrate, with a practical example, class struggle and fascist tyranny."[5] To emphasize the class warfare aspect of antidisability animus and policies, after all, was exceedingly perceptive. Historically, and even as contemporaries in every era argued over the exact mechanisms of causation or correlation, it was common knowledge that the vast majority of individuals carrying diagnoses of mental illness, intellectual defect, or behavioral disorder came from the poorest strata of society. Nor was it a mystery to anyone that the consistent patterns of disinvestment in their care were, at all times, rationalized with reference to the insufficiently exploitable labor power of those so diagnosed.

By contrast, activists and scholars in the West—confronted with the specific wording of West German reparations law granting official recognition as victims of Nazism only to those persecuted on grounds of "race, religion, or political worldview"—were faced with a quite distinct conceptual and political dilemma. Although she was indisputably part of a wider movement insisting that the mass coercive sterilization project was not a marginal but rather an absolutely central aspect of the Nazis' early agendas, the resourcefulness and brilliant acuity of historian Gisela Bock stands out. At the very same moment that Späte was making his case for remembering "euthanasia" as an instance of *class* politics, Bock was publishing her first analysis of the mass sterilizations and the intrinsic connections between Nazism's much-touted pronatalism and its brutal antinatalism as core parts of Nazism's *racial* politics. Bock was also well on her way to proving, as she would in book form in 1986 and in testimony to the Bundestag committee charged with considering all the "forgotten victims" in 1987, that Nazi racism had all along had a double dimension, and that these two dimensions were mutually inextricable. Nazi bureaucrats and propagandists—indeed, Adolf Hitler himself—had linked anti-Jewish and anti-disabled policy from the very start. Moreover, by reintegrating eugenics into Nazi racism (a connection that had, for decades after 1945, been strenuously denied), as she did, Bock called attention to the *aspirational* dynamics of Nazism in a way that explained so much about both its broad popular appeal and its viciously destructive effects. For the Nazi effort to eradicate perceived intellectual deficiency within the German Volk by mass sterilization and mass murder signaled both stunning conceit *and* profound unease about weaknesses and flaws *within* the would-be dominant group. Bock thereby offered an analysis that was more broadly relevant for understanding racisms of all kinds.[6] But it was most relevant for rethinking how we tell German history of the twentieth century.

Psychiatrist Gerhard Schmidt's long-suppressed masterpiece, *Selektion in der Heilanstalt* (Selection in the Asylum)—which finally saw the light of day in 1965 but which did not really become a touchstone text until the 1980s—had prefigured Bock's key insights into the phantasmatic quality of Nazi claims of racial superiority, and the insecurities animating those claims. Schmidt too had begun to adumbrate an analysis of the connections between anti-Jewish and antidisability hostility, which he expressed succinctly with the terms "racial hatred" and "racial anxiety" as the two, mutually mirroring, aspects of what he summarily designated as Hitler's "racial insanity."[7] Schmidt was, as it were, ahead of his time. It was Bock, in her antipostfascist context, who was able most comprehensively to explicate the point that the fury at flaws within the Volk functioned in *complementarity*, and not just parallelism, to anti-Jewish animus. This alternate modality she offered for theorizing the mutual imbrication of Nazi racism's two main forms has left a deep imprint on the historiography of Nazism overall.[8] It would be good if it were put to use more regularly in scholarship specifically on the "euthanasia" murders of 1939–1945 as well and their long pre- and post-histories, for this would give us a fresh vantage on how we can conceptualize the interconnections between the "euthanasia" killings and the Holocaust of European Jewry—beyond the compelling facts about overlap in perpetrators and chronological sequentiality with which I opened the introduction. The *complementarity thesis* can supplement the *sequentiality thesis* as we make the case for the broader implications of attending to the history of intellectual disability.[9]

This also means foregrounding, more than we have previously considered, the elements of Nazism that involved narcissism. More than half a century ago, Adorno made the point about the self-esteem bonus provided by all fascisms—the boost they give people who feel flattered at being thought superior. Adorno was primarily analyzing US extreme-right rhetoric of the late 1940s–early 1950s, but he unmistakably had the Nazis' and Hitler's popularity in mind as well. In Adorno's words: "The narcissistic *gain* provided by fascist propaganda is obvious. It suggests continuously and sometimes in rather devious ways, that the follower, simply through belonging to the in-group, is better, higher and purer than those who are excluded."[10] The important takeaway for our purposes might be that Nazism's eugenic and "euthanistic" projects were not furthered solely through malicious negative propaganda about how disgust-arousing people with intellectual disability were, and about how purportedly enormous was the expense of their care.[11] Instead, just as Nazism, in its libidinally inciting sexual politics, effectively inserted itself in people's most elemental desires for personal happiness—nurturing, in a Foucaultian sense, the positive and not just the negative workings of power—so too it bears constant emphasis how strongly and effectively Nazism played to many Germans' yearnings to become a Volk that was strong, healthy, beautiful—and smart.[12] But the extent and durability of the acceptance of vicious negativity has been, in the end, what has most required explanation.

Meanwhile, as the years of research and writing of this book have made vividly clear to me, centering the topic of intellectual disability raises questions about the craft of history more generally. This is so not just for the perpetual historians' puzzle of the relationship between evidence and interpretation: *Is* antidisability hostility a matter of class warfare or racial politics or personal self-aggrandizement or none-of-the-above or all of these at once? Relatedly, centering intellectual disability challenges us to reconceive questions of periodization and causation and the complex repercussions between multiple pasts and presents.[13] Here insights drawn from psychoanalysis can help greatly.

A few years ago, a US-based psychoanalyst glossed Freud's famous concept of *Nachträglichkeit* (in English, "deferred effects" or "afterwardsness" or, in French, *après-coup*), by summarizing its import thus: "The past may, under the influence of a later event, acquire not only new significance, but new force and consequence." He synopsized "deferred action" as the means "by which unassimilated, encrypted, past experience is reanimated, revised, and set to work in response to new circumstances." The crux of the matter was that "[i]n this scenario, the present may be understood in a certain way to 'cause' the past, or more precisely, to stand in a double temporal relation with the past in which the force of causality must be imagined to move in both directions."[14] These ruminations—especially the idea that the present may be "causing" the past, or that "the force of causality" can move in both directions—might on first impact sound mysterious or philosophically abstract, but they are, I submit, highly pertinent for understanding how pasts and presents have recurrently ricocheted in the history of intellectual disability.

Some examples: It is, on reflection, notable just how many of the empirical discoveries I made, in the years of research, involved time lags and postponements—especially with regard to the long battle, for people with disabilities, to be counted as fully human. But then again— perhaps because of the unresolvable trauma at the center of the twentieth century, or perhaps because of the many lies, rationalizations, and evasions that were promulgated in its wake—there were also numerous instances of recursive returns, of people being pulled back into various deeper layers of the past as they struggled to make sense of what it would take to shape a better present and future. It remains striking, for instance, that it was members of the several antipostfascist cohorts of the 1970s–1980s (most of them born either during the later years of the war or in the fifteen years after its end), disgusted as they were by the long shadow Nazism cast into the post-1945 years, who finally realized that the pre-Nazi 1920s were, specifically for people with disabilities, *not* the golden age of democratic experiment, sexual revolution, and inspirational legacies with which one might earnestly hope to reconnect, but rather an era when the pernicious pathologization that would legitimate the Third Reich's many cruelties against people with disabilities had already been incubating. In fact, these radicals came to realize, as they began to see through the haze of distortions propagated in the 1950s–1960s, that cruelly supercilious attitudes in regard to disability, precisely within the three supposedly responsible professions of psychiatric medicine, remedial pedagogy, and religious charity, were already becoming virulent in the 1890s–1910s.[15]

But there is more: One of the oddities of this book is that the "euthanasia" murders themselves are not discussed much in chapter 2, where one might think they fit chronologically—there they receive a mere two paragraphs—but rather show up in far greater detail in chapter 3, which concerns developments in the West in the post–World War II era. This was a deliberate decision. For it was only in 1983, with the publication of Ernst Klee's *"Euthanasie"* and its intense reception, that the prospect of widespread emotional identification with the victims (instead of with the perpetrators or with their prospective adversaries, the charity directors) even became feasible. With his idiosyncratic approach of retroactive re-creation, Klee made the past intelligible and palpable; he clarified the crass opportunism of the perpetrators; he made the gruesomeness of the killings something that could no longer be evaded; and in modeling for readers the possibility of imaginative affinity, he restored to the persecuted and tortured as much as he could of their human dignity.[16] However, not all the important perspectives I found entailed retrospection; there were other kinds of anachronism. For at every juncture, I was also intent on documenting the existence of people who were out of sync with the trends of their moment—and who, in whatever terms and framework was available to them, attested to a non-dehumanizing standpoint on people others considered deficient or impaired.

Further questions relevant for all historians present themselves when we revisit the riddle of the powerful consequentiality of phantasmatic notions. Scholars of antisemitism—most recently Jonathan Judaken—have given extended thought to what the medievalist Gavin Langmuir once dubbed "chimerical" hostility, that is, hostility based in delusions—as well as to Adorno's proposition that some forms of hostility are "functional" and manifest as projections onto a scapegoat not so much due to ignorance about the particular abjected minority, but rather because the stereotypes that have accrued (about Jews, Blacks, Mexicans—Adorno noted that hatreds were fairly interchangeable, and had exceedingly little to do with the nature of their objects) can provide orientation in an otherwise disconcerting and alienating world; they supply a canalization of anger for expressing displeasure at vaster social inequities whose actual sources are too complicated to be easily comprehensible.[17]

How might these theories require amending for the case of antidisability sentiments and actions? Far more remains to be understood about the seductive allure of eugenics.

As noted, especially in chapters 4 and 5, among the challenges the disability rights advocates of the 1970s–1980s faced was the difficulty of exposing as threadbare the eugenic assumptions that had acquired a kind of self-evidence over the prior half-century. Yet their problems remain our problems today. Nazi "racial hygiene" messaging was, like Nazi antisemitic propaganda, the "fake news" of its era. But it has been harder for historians to discern its falsity, if only because contempt for weakness and a feeling of superiority toward people with intellectual impairment can seem simply like a universally shared commonsense.[18] Here, more theoretically informed and especially transnationally comparativist research will surely be needed.[19] Yet the comparativist inquiry will, again and again, also lead us back to several particularities of Germany's twentieth century, and these will include at least three matters. One is the notable precociousness of Germany's establishment of massive networks of residential institutions and remedial schools already from the 1870s–1880s on.[20] A second is the wound to national pride—in contemporaries' terms, the "national humiliation"—that was incurred by the unforeseen and quite evidently disorienting defeat in World War I.[21] And third and not least is the exceptionally strong involvement of the Protestant church, not just in care provision but also in the elaboration of disparaging images of disability. What was in it, in the end, for the men of the Protestant Inner Mission in the 1920s, as they developed and lent their moral authority to a *theo-biopolitical* conceptual framework—a framework that was to assist greatly in smoothing the general German populace's acceptance of the Nazis' various antidisability projects? For we can recognize in the churchmen's words not solely a kind of "anticipatory obedience" (*vorauseilender Gehorsam*, to invoke the classic German expression). What is even more conspicuous is a sense that the rise of eugenics had given them a feeling of liberation from inhibition, a permission to be free to say derogatory things.

Nazi propaganda, which portrayed people with disabilities as an existential threat to the Volk both biologically and economically, was unquestionably artful and sophisticated.[22] Yet the enormous investment that the regime would make—financially, organizationally, and in terms of expenditure of psychic energy and effort—in designing thousands of lectures and seminars to "educate" teachers, pastors, physicians, party members, schoolchildren, and the general public and in developing propaganda that was cannily reflexive in taking up, and working through preemptively, potential concerns and counterarguments to the Nazi leadership's plans—itself should count as empirical evidence that antidisability hostility was *not* already a self-evidently shared baseline popular view (especially considering the substantial percentages of the Volk whose reproductive capacities the most avid eugenicists were intent on curtailing). The Nazis needed the Protestant Christians' help. And the churchmen gave it, indeed had given it already in advance.[23] Doing so apparently served multiple aims of their own. Developing a sumptuous blend of spiritual and quasi-scientific arguments as they overlapped the languages of sin, guilt, and redemption with the vocabulary of race, health, and strength, facilitated many things for leaders in Protestant welfare. Among these were: a justification for their own ambivalences about the people for whom they were responsible; an ability to self-position as modern, in contrast to Catholics; a strategy for defending against the accusation that in their provision of nurture for the unproductive, they were themselves contributing to the looming death of the Volk; and an updated paradigm for lending substance to their traditionalist conservatism around the themes of sex and gender amidst the so fiercely loathed loosening of mores in the Weimar years. If they could persuade citizens that sinful sex was the source of so much disability, perhaps they could reclaim the cultural hegemony that was slipping from their hands. Their eagerness, after the Nazis had come to power in 1933, to augment their already florid antidisability rhetoric with further anti-Jewish flourishes, speaks volumes about their self-interestedness.

In turn, the fact that in the initial postwar years in the West, both churches had striven to reclaim cultural authority by styling themselves as, on the topic of disability, the only moral alternative to Nazism, would make it yet more arduous for the cohorts of disability rights advocates who were coming of age in the 1970s–1980s—whether they were conscientious objectors providing their alternative service, or journalists, or professionals in medicine, education, or social work, or indeed young pastors- or deacons-in-training—to make sense of what exactly had happened in the past and to formulate fresh ideas about disability and a radically justice-oriented quality of care. The conjunction in time of being confronted with mendaciousness about the national past, on the one hand, and daily evidence of catastrophic insufficiencies in therapeutic approach especially to those vulnerable human beings who were institutionalized, on the other, would infuse with special urgency critical memory work and campaigns to professionalize care provision alike.[24] Enlightenment about the past and the demand for a revolutionized approach to praxis in the unfolding present became inseparable.

———

As Elisabeth Kunz, an East German woman who since the 1970s had been devotedly active in Protestant church–sponsored care and education for people with cognitive impairments, put the point in 2022, looking back in joyful affirmation: "[T]he real winners of reunification are the people with mental disabilities. For them, so very much has changed for the better."[25] Suddenly, those who in the GDR had been working in small niches, within extremely repressive political constraints, unable to be open about the fact they were providing schooling in addition to care, and amidst disinterest or even unkindness from fellow citizens, were liberated to develop new educational and therapeutic facilities— an infusion of funds facilitated the building of abundant new schools and residences—and to be openly present within the public sphere as well as to offer professional training in curative pedagogy and special pedagogy to thousands of new students.[26] Yet although numerous commentators, whether formerly Western or Eastern, have remarked on the transformative impact of reunification on the welfare infrastructure in the "new Bundesländer," the preponderance of historical evidence suggests that it was only after 1990 that things got increasingly better in the former West as well. Indeed, and although the causation may initially seem counterintuitive, the (not to Kunz but to many other Eastern Germans) initially irritating, patronizing attitude that felt disrespectful toward those who had spent decades developing practical strategies for improving the lives of people with intellectual impairments under obstinately difficult conditions, may actually have been most efficacious in stimulating the West to clean up *its* act and—at long last—to improve conditions on the ground in the "old Bundesländer" as well.[27] Spirited secular-ethical humanist and dissident-nonpaternalist Christian defenses of the precious value of disabled lives were also beginning to capture the popular imagination by the later 1980s, just at the historical juncture when apologetic and rationalizing interpretations of Nazi-era crimes could finally, in both halves of the German nation, begin to be more vigorously contested. In particular, uproar over the Lebenshilfe's ill-considered invitation to philosopher Peter Singer in 1989 to propound his views on the legitimacy of infanticide for disabled newborns provided an indispensable moment of reckoning for the profession of special educators.[28] And the "Singer-Affair" additionally marked the moment when the cripple-movement was catapulted into national attention and began to be able to set the terms of debate about numerous matters related to disability.[29]

But ultimately, it was to be over the course of the 1990s that the quadrilaterally conjoined efforts of self-representing "cripples" now newly allied across the former West-East divide, the ever-growing number of activist members of social service, healthcare, and pedagogic professions, members of the Green Party (strikingly often overlapping with the prior group), and morally and politically engaged independent and university-affiliated scholars finally bore fruit and succeeded in consolidating, culture-wide, a newly respectful attitude toward people with disabilities, past and then-present.[30] The very fact that the organization that had previously named itself Aktion Sorgenkind (Action Worry-Child), launched in the 1960s in response to the disastrous epidemic of birth defects induced by the morning sickness drug thalidomide, after careful consideration renamed itself in 2000 as Aktion Mensch (Action Human Being), testifies to the profundity of the implied shift.[31] At the latest since the turn of the millennium, then, what had once been a marginalized and embattled perspective finally conquered the political and cultural mainstream.[32]

Meanwhile, the importance of acknowledging and mourning the "euthanasia" murders and other Nazi-era crimes against the disabled has been firmly ensconced at the uppermost levels of the federal government.[33] The change has been as recent—in the first years of the twenty-first century, bureaucratic obstructionism was still routine—as it has been dramatic.[34] Learning about the past is being actively practiced every day at memorial sites across the country, especially at the six former T4 centers. "Stumbling-stones" honoring victims of Nazism murdered on grounds of their disabilities dot streets in towns across the nation.[35] A campaign to shed the shame surrounding disability and at long last to publicize the names of those killed on grounds of disability—carried by psychiatric patients' rights self-advocates as well as family members of victims—achieved a major victory in 2018.[36] As the Bundesarchiv's official press release acknowledged, the transformed cultural climate toward living people with disabilities meant that the fact of pervasive stigma could no longer be used as an excuse to withhold historical evidence of crimes and thereby also prevent proper honoring and mourning of the victims: "In the age of inclusion, the victims of Nazi 'euthanasia' must no longer be concealed and a more liberal handling of archival sources on Nazi 'euthanasia' is called for in the interest of scholarly and familial historical research."[37] Notably, moreover, individuals who themselves carry diagnoses of intellectual disabilities have begun to be more regularly included in official memorial festivities.[38] At the T4 memorial center in Brandenburg, people with cognitive impairments serve as the tour guides.[39]

Not least, as noted in chapter 5, also the *postwar* abuses in both West and East have begun to be recognized and addressed. In 2017, the Stiftung Anerkennung und Hilfe (Foundation for Recognition and Assistance) was launched, concluding its work in 2021. In the investigation process, hundreds of people with disabilities who were harmed in charitable or state institutions in the postwar decades could at long last be heard and receive some symbolic "reparation" (*Wiedergutmachung*), as belated and as paltry as the disbursed amounts are. And thus, with this date of 2021 in mind, we can say that it has indeed taken one hundred years for the stranglehold of Binding and Hoche and their coinage of "unworthy life" at long last to be broken. The Alsterdorf institution in Hamburg—to take just one concrete example—has made extraordinary efforts in recent years to come to terms with its multiple pasts, finally admitting openly, over the course of the 2010s, what brutalities were still common practice there until the 1970s and even into the 1980s—under expressly Christian auspices[40] (figures A.1–A.2.).

Attempts to reintroduce crass antidisability messaging—as for instance the far-right Alternative für Deutschland (AfD) party regularly does, in the Bundestag since 2017—are met with vigorous rebuke. Best known for its hostility to refugees and migrants especially when they are Muslim, and its complaints about a "culture of guilt" about the Holocaust, the AfD revels in a posture of taboo-breaking with regard to disability as well.[41] Yet in March 2018, when AfD party members presented a formal "inquiry" with regard to the (fantasized) issue of migrant families producing disproportionately more children with cognitive difficulties because of the (purported) prevalence of incestuous marriages between blood relatives among migrants, the rapidity of reaction was noteworthy.[42] Secular and religious spokespeople presented a united front. Eighteen advocacy organizations signed a protest declaration. Under the headline "This concerns all of us," it stated: "We are appalled by the AfD's inquiry in the German Bundestag about severe disability in Germany. . . . We say 'No' to any devaluation of people with disabilities and to any form of racism. Ideologies of inequality of human life have no place in this country."[43] A spokesperson for the Catholic bishops said the formal AfD query contained wording implying a difference between "life worthy and life unworthy of life, and as the Catholic church, we cannot accept this." Moreover, "For us, all disabled persons are equal, regardless of how the disability originated."[44] And Ilja Seifert (former East German, Linke party member, and paraplegic) of the Allgemeinen Behindertenverband in Deutschland (General Association of Disabled People in Germany) said at the time: "Why don't they ask about family policy among nobles? No, the AfD is about presenting disabled life as something avoidable. As something that causes harm. In

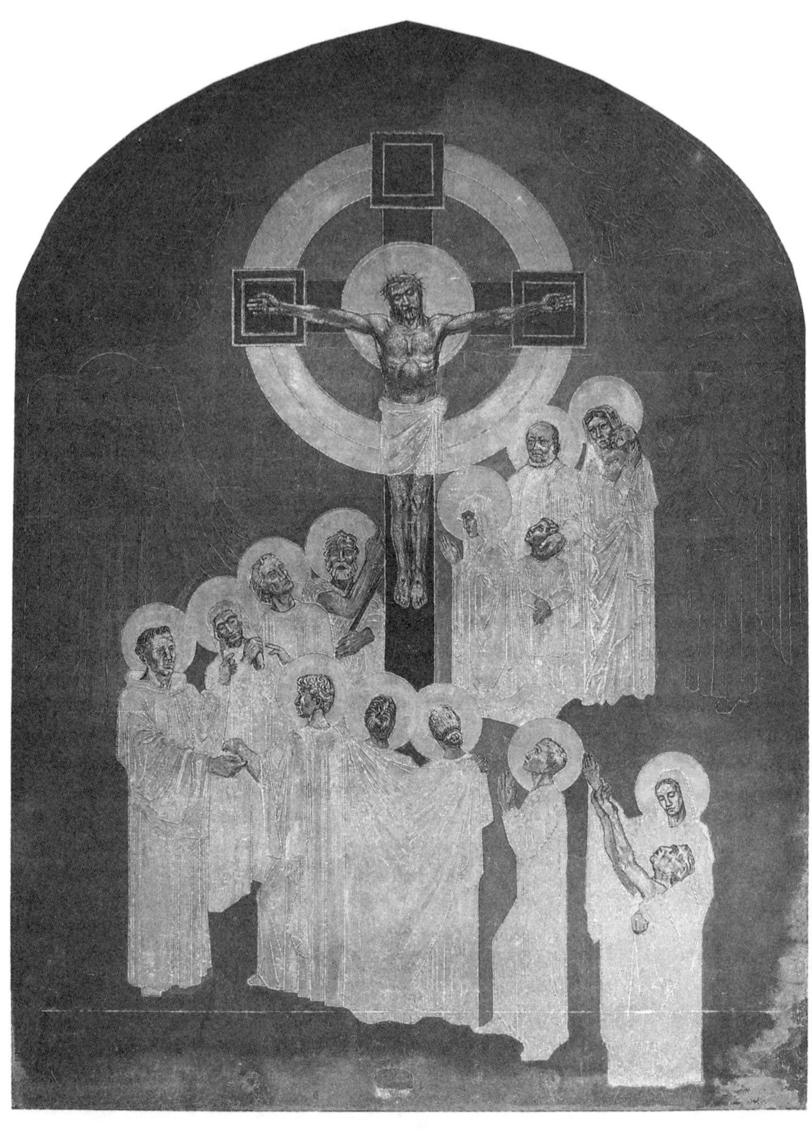

FIGURE A.1. Activist care staff long remarked on the offensiveness of the imagery in this example of Nazi sacred art designed by former pastor-director Friedrich Lensch and completed in 1938. Not only is Jesus strong and muscular, but it is solely the people with disabilities who lack halos. Archiv der evangelischen Stiftung Alsterdorf.

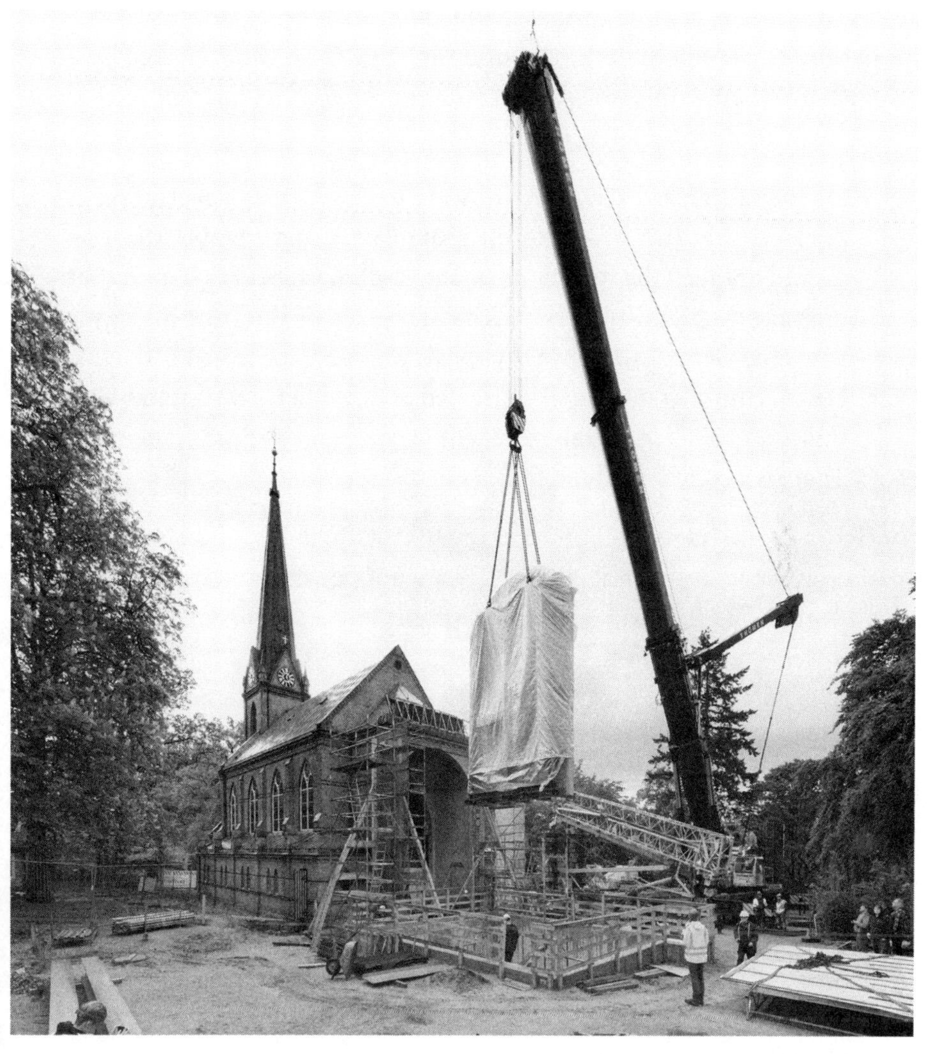

FIGURE A.2. In 2021–2022, the Alsterdorfer Anstalten (now Evangelische Stiftung Alsterdorf) removed the altar art from St. Nicolaus Kirche by lifting out the entirety of the church's 58-ton back wall, flipping it around and sinking it partially into the ground along a memorial path honoring the 511 residents deported to their deaths during the Third Reich. Archiv der Evangelischen Stiftung Alsterdorf.

the past, there was talk of 'useless eaters,' of 'eternal sufferers' who needed to be relieved of their suffering. That is not new." Asked by a reporter whether this wasn't just an attempt to goad liberals and leftists into consternation, Seifert noted:

> Of course, it is the usual provocation to stay in the conversation at the local pub. This falls on fertile ground with some people, that one should not feed the weaker ones, the "ballast existences," but rather promote the high achievers. . . . The AfD is always about the "us versus you." The Germans, the healthy, the Aryans on the one hand. The foreigners, the migrants and the disabled on the other. In my opinion . . . this is no coincidence, no oversight on the part of any staff member. There is a concept behind it.[45]

Here a comprehensive counter-vision to that of Binding and Hoche has simply become standard. Again, it bears noting what an extraordinary and precious historic accomplishment such a consensus stance represents.

In general: We are living, thankfully, in Germany as internationally, in the midst of an exponentialized growth in disability-positive messaging, much of it now carried by self-confident self-advocates—whether endowed with physical, sensory, psychic, or cognitive differences—and their families and allies.[46] Jürgen Dusel, the current (since 2018) Federal Commissioner for Disability Issues, also a lawyer and himself sight-impaired, launched his term with the upbeat and self-assured slogan "democracy demands inclusion." Moreover, the goal of inclusion, Dusel contended, is "not a question of humanitarianism, civilization or caring for people. Rather, my conviction is that democracy and inclusion are two sides of the same coin. Without inclusion there is no democracy."[47] Shrewdly and compellingly, in other words, Dusel moved disability thematically from the margins to the very center of what it takes to sustain a functioning and vital democracy. And the UN Convention on the Rights of Persons with Disabilities (UNCRPD)—cowritten, notably, by former cripple-movement member and feminist lawyer Theresia Degener and ratified by Germany in 2009—has most recently prompted significant improvements in German law, facilitating both increased possibility for self-determination and greater social integration in education, housing, work, cultural life, and political decision-making.[48] One important follow-up to the UNCRPD is the federal "Law for the Strengthening of Participation and Self-Determination of Persons with Disabilities" (*Gesetz zur Stärkung der Teilhabe und Selbstbestimmung von Menschen mit Behinderungen,* or *Bundesteilhabegesetz* for short). Passed in 2016 and going into effect in successive stages between 2017 and 2023, and notwithstanding whatever complaints can still be made about its insufficiencies, this law does signal the arrival of a thorough reorientation in social policy in numerous life-realms.[49] People with disabilities now have the recognized right to be treated as the authorities on their own lives.[50] Implementation of the principles of "assisted freedom" (*assistierte Freiheit*), "supported decision-making" (*unterstützte Entscheidungsfindung*), "advocatory assistance" (*advokatorische Assistenz*), and "accessibility" (*Barrierefreiheit*) are articulated as baseline expectations for all policy around disability.[51] It is also indicative that in the run-up to the Bundestag elections of 2021, all the political parties—with the telling exception of the AfD—provided detailed proposals for advancing disability rights.[52] Increasingly as well, disability rights organizations are taking on board the need to consider the intersectionality of disability with issues of ethnicity and migration and the importance of providing cross-culturally attuned and accessible support services. [53]

By no means is everything in order. In an all too painful irony, exactly those two groups that had served as *the* novel Archimedean points from the vantage of which the reigning "image of the human" needed so urgently to be revised, as the antipostfascist activists of the 1970s–1980s had insisted—children with significant impairments and those members of the so-called hard core that had been too long custodially warehoused in "closed institutions"—remain to this day vulnerable to the numerous exclusionary mechanisms that, alas, persist. Resistance to dissolving the segregated special schools and antipathy to comprehensive "inclusion" of children with impairments in regular school classrooms, while having many sources—not least of which is the neoliberal paradox by which disability-friendly vocabulary is coupled with austerity budgeting and therefore insures inevitable instructor overstrain, but also the long-standing disinclination to replace the tripartite hierarchically organized school system with a unified one—has recently intensified considerably.[54] Already in 2009, the minister for culture of Baden-Württemberg announced to reporters with confidence: "The UN can't tell us what to do."[55] More than a dozen years later, the pedagogic landscape across Germany remains thoroughly uneven, as German states that had committed, in the wake of the passage of the UNCRPD, to dissolving their special schools, are now backpedaling.[56] As Degener noted succinctly in an interview in 2019: "With regard to inclusion, Germany is far behind [other nations]."[57] That the retention of a segregated system is framed as giving parents choices and as allowing for each individual child's needs to be best met has continued to make it confusing for anyone not deeply versed in the issues to sort out what direction the nation—or even their own neighborhood—should take.[58] A handful of exemplary model inclusive schools are honored every year with the "Jakob Muth Prize," but their daily practical demonstration that inclusion can be enormously successful has not been broadly viewed as an ideal to be emulated.[59] In 2018, school integration pioneer Jutta Schöler, by then in retirement—in the 1980s she had brought many dozens of young West Germans to Italy to learn how integration could very well succeed—observed in a tone of acerbic resignation that something she had been told years ago was, apparently, true: "that the German school system" would "be harder to reform than the Catholic church."[60]

Along related lines, with regard to adults with disabilities, a reflexive desire to have more significantly impaired individuals be kept in institutions largely out of mind and out of sight of the general public is by no means an artefact only of the past.[61] Meanwhile, dedicated individuals working at those institutions frequently remark that there remains a drastic shortage of qualified care staff, that the working hours and conditions are undesirable, and that profit-conscious administrators increasingly seek to maximize efficiency by moving staff around, even if this means rupturing bonds of trusting relationship between residents and specific caregivers. The wider public typically only hears of these deficits when there are scandals—even as, obviously, better training and improved staff-to-resident ratios and regular unannounced monitoring visits would help prevent the scandals from happening at all.[62] But on the most fundamental level, as the German Institute for Human Rights observed summarily in 2021: "The goal has to be deinstitutionalization" (*Ziel muss die Deinstitutionalisierung sein*).[63] This, of course, had been *the* central demand of activists on behalf of the "hard core" since the 1980s. Yet the statistics for 2023 indicate that more than 190,000 people with disabilities in Germany continue to live in "a special living situation" (*einer besonderen Wohnform*—the new term of art for institutions of various sizes); 64 percent of these are individuals carrying a diagnosis of "intellectual disability."[64]

Nonetheless, without question, the standards for what is acceptable have changed, and profoundly so. As the firm rebuffs to the AfD demonstrate, openly derogatory and condescending language is no longer socially acceptable and can expect to meet critical retorts. The necessary monetary investment in improved pedagogical, living, and work settings continues to be substantial, at both federal and local levels; the arrival of a transformed paradigm—in theory and in praxis—is reasserted appreciatively and with regularity. And even as there are setbacks, new initiatives in favor of inclusion emerge almost every day.[65] The learning curve since the revolution in perspective propelled by a minority of militants in the 1970s–1980s has been steep and impressive. In sum, it is everywhere manifest that both the public messaging and the practical initiatives of such (meanwhile energetically self-reformed) prominent advocacy organizations as the Lebenshilfe and, just as significant, the animating concepts for the Protestant Diakonie and the Catholic Caritas, have become in large measure oriented to the radically egalitarian human rights paradigm that was initially most forcefully articulated by the antipostfascist cohorts of the 1970s–1980s. This is their legacy. It is up to all of us to complete the revolution in practice and in attitude of which the antipostfascists first dreamed.

ACKNOWLEDGMENTS

THE FOLLOWING individuals, living witnesses to and / or expert scholars of the intricately imbricated histories I tell here, have honored me with precious gifts of evocative reminiscences and acute interpretive insights: Esther Abel, Götz Aly, Meike Sophia Baader, Hans Becker, Heike Bernhardt, Erik Bittner, Gisela Bock, Christian Bradl, Nancy Bullard-Werner, Heike Bůžek, Dagmar Drovs, Heinz Duchscherer, Jürgen Dusel, Sieglind Ellger-Rüttgardt, Georg Feuser, Claudia Fraas, Conrad Frohn, Maresa von Fürstenberg, Uta George, Uwe Gerrens, Klaus Gubener, Michael Häusler, Harald Jenner, Roselore Jurjanz, Harald Kalteier, Uwe Kaminsky, Jürgen Kampmann, Elke Klee, Charlotte Köttgen, Dinah Kohan, Gerhard Kneuker, Elisabeth Kunz, Julia Latscha, Patrick Lau, Klaus von Lüpke, Hagen Markwardt, Hans-Georg Matthes, Ulrike Menzel, Marina Meyer, Barbara Michel, Jürgen Moltmann, Nati Radtke, Wolfgang Rose, Janine Runge, Tatjana Ruge, Jonathan Sarna, Kai-Uwe Schablon, Dietrich Schabow, Hans-Peter Schick, Christoph Schneider, Brigitte Schwan-Steglich, Michael Seidel, Udo Sierck, Wulf Steglich, Gabriele Sterzing, Rainer Stier, Kerstin Stockhecke, Kerrin Stumpf, Sonja Süß, Johannes von Thadden, Winfried Tippelt, Jürgen Trogisch, Uta Trogisch, Bettina Westfeld, Michael Wunder.

This project began thanks to a daunting but wonderful opportunity to deliver the 2021 Adorno Lectures in Frankfurt / Main provided by Eva Gilmer, Martin Saar, Almut Poppinga, and Ferdinand Sutterlüty; their input has been indispensable. Along the way, during the years of writing, Yanara Schmacks, Miranda Brethour, and Tamara Maatouk provided truly outstanding research assistance. Warm gratitude goes as well to Hanna Leitgeb, Andreas Huyssen, Gunter Schmidt, Joan Wallach Scott, Detlef Siegfried, Kurt Starke, Mischa Suter, and Anson

Rabinbach for their readings of drafts at crucial junctures and for their sustaining support. Priya Nelson and the entire team at Princeton University Press have been terrific to work with at every step, and I thank Karen Verde for stellar copyediting.

A handful of cherished human beings put their good energies to the task of making sure I would not fall through the cracks in the universe in the sorrow-drenched autumn of 2023. For their steadying care and companionship, I thank especially Lucy Staub, Brendan Hart, Anne Montgomery, Kevin Riley, Johanna Schoen, Lily Saint, Jim Henle, John Kucich, William Kelly, Stefanos Geroulanos, Gary Wilder, John Barnhill, Stuart Michaels, Todd Shepard, Omer Bartov, Ayelet Barkai, Chelli Riddiough, Jonathan Fine, and Caroline Arni.

Without Michael Staub, this book would not exist. Every thought in it was developed together with him. It is dedicated, in unending love, to his memory.

NOTES

Introduction

1. A note on terminology: T4 is a reference to Tiergartenstrasse 4, the address in Berlin from which the first main phase of the "euthanasia" murders was organized; 70,273 human beings were asphyxiated in one of six gas chambers: Grafeneck, Hadamar, Bernburg, Brandenburg, Pirna-Sonnenstein, Hartheim. Throughout this book, I put the word "euthanasia" in quotation marks, as most German scholars also do, to distance myself from what was a mendacious euphemism for a singular mass murder project. An excellent and accessible survey of the latest scholarly findings on all the dimensions of Nazi "euthanasia" is Gerrit Hohendorf, "The Extermination of Mentally Ill and Handicapped People under National Socialist Rule," SciencesPo Online Encyclopedia of Mass Violence (November 17, 2016), https://www.sciencespo.fr/mass -violence-war-massacre-resistance/en/document/extermination-mentally-ill-and-handicapped -people-under-national-socialist-rule.html.

2. The best study on the multiple interconnections is Sara Berger, *Experten der Vernichtung: Das T4-Reinhardt-Netzwerk in den Lagern Belzec, Sobibor und Treblinka* (Hamburg: Hamburger Edition, 2013).

3. The state of scholarly discussion by the early 1990s is well analyzed in Gisela Bock, "Krankenmord, Judenmord und nationalsozialistische Rassenpolitik: Überlegungen zu einigen neueren Forschungshypothesen," in Frank Bajohr, Werner Johe, and Uwe Lohalm, eds., *Zivilisation und Barbarei: Die widersprüchlichen Potentiale der Moderne—Detlev Peukert zum Gedenken* (Hamburg: Christians, 1991), 285–306. The most recent expert studies question the chronologically sequential (and thereby implicitly causal) paradigm of "euthanasia"-Holocaust interrelation, pointing out rightly that transfers of technology and personnel back and forth between the two mass crimes were not solely sequential but rather recurrently reciprocal, and that both genocides, as they developed in parallel, were, in any event, multi-sited, diversely motivated, driven by numerous actors and forces, and reliant on a broad variety of murder modes. In no way, however, do these findings and analyses undermine the extraordinary moral and political achievements of the 1980s–1990s in their success at forcing acknowledgment of the humanity of the "euthanasia" victims. See Jörg Osterloh and Jan Erik Schulte, eds., *"Euthanasie" und Holocaust: Kontinuitäten, Kausalitäten, Parallelitäten* (Paderborn: Schöningh, 2021). Formal legal-historical considerations regarding the applicability of the category of genocide were aired in a roundtable on "A Conceptual Exploration of Genocide: The Case of Nazi 'Euthanasia,'" Medicine, Holocaust and Genocide Studies Program, Cedars-Sinai Medical Center, Los Angeles, May 4, 2023.

4. Henry Friedlander comments at a conference in Heidelberg in 2006 (published in Maike Rotzoll et al., eds., *Die nationalsozialistischen "Euthanasie"-Morde* [Paderborn: Schöningh, 2010], 347–49, here 349); and at the Lessons and Legacies conference of the Holocaust Educational Foundation in Evanston, Illinois, 2008.

5. Henry Friedlander, *The Origins of the Nazi Genocide: From Euthanasia to the Final Solution* (Chapel Hill: University of North Carolina Press, 1995), xii–xiii. Cf. the exemplary new book by Ari Joskowicz, *Rain of Ash: Roma, Jews, and the Holocaust* (Princeton, NJ: Princeton University Press, 2023).

6. "Nazi Persecution of the Disabled: Murder of the 'Unfit,'" https://www.ushmm.org /information/exhibitions/online-exhibitions/special-focus/nazi-persecution-of-the-disabled (last accessed January 20, 2023).

7. Kenny Fries, "Before the 'Final Solution' There Was a 'Test Killing,'" *New York Times*, January 8, 2020, https://www.nytimes.com/2020/01/08/opinion/disability-nazi-eugenics .html. Diverse additional public-facing projects and scholarship in English that theorize in innovative ways aspects of the nexus between "euthanasia" and the Holocaust include: Susanne Knittel, *The Historical Uncanny: Disability, Ethnicity, and the Politics of Holocaust Memory* (New York: Fordham University Press, 2014); Frank Schneider et al., *Registered, Persecuted, Annihilated: The Sick and the Disabled under National Socialism* (Heidelberg: Springer Medizin, 2014); Edith Sheffer, *Asperger's Children: The Origins of Autism in Nazi Vienna* (New York: Norton, 2018); Cameron S. Mitchell and David Mitchell, *Disposable Humanity*, https://www.disposablehumanity.com/; Avril Alba, Jennifer Barrett, and A. Dirk Moses, "The Holocaust and Human Rights: An Inclusive Critical Field for Museums," *Museums Galleries Australia Magazine* 27.1 (Summer 2018), 42–45, https://issuu.com/museumsaustralia/docs/mam_vol27_1__summer _2018_-_web/s/46713.

8. Key early example: Klaus Dörner, *Der Krieg gegen die psychisch Kranken: Nach 'Holocaust' Erinnern, Trauern, Begegnen* (Rehburg-Loccum: Psychiatrie-Verlag, 1980).

9. Kathrin Braun and Svea Luise Herrmann, "Unrecht zweiter Ordnung: Die Weitergeltung des Gesetzes zur Verhütung erbkranken Nachwuchses in der Bundesrepublik," in Sonja Begalke, Claudia Fröhlich, and Stephan Alexander Glienke, eds., *Der halbierte Rechtsstaat: Demokratie und Recht in der frühen Bundesrepublik und die Integration von NS-Funktionseliten* (Baden-Baden: Nomos, 2015), 223–241.

10. "25 Jahre Bundestagsbeschluss zum Benachteiligungsverbot," *Netzwerk Artikel 3* (2019), http://www.netzwerk-artikel-3.de/index.php/134-25-jahre-bundestagsbeschluss-zum -benachteiligungsverbot.

11. In the 1990s, an especially disturbing—though eventually inspirational—case involved the extended struggle to remediate the catastrophic conditions at the Evangelisches Hospital Lilienthal (now Diakonische Behindertenhilfe). See Diemut Roether, "'Behinderte werden totgemacht,'" *taz*, March 8, 1993; Wolfgang Jantzen, *". . . die da dürstet nach der Gerechtigkeit": Deinstitutionalisierung in einer Großeinrichtung der Behindertenhilfe* (Berlin: Marhold, 2003); Undine Zeidler, "Hans Menckes Abschied auf Raten," *Weser-Kurier*, March 27, 2015.

12. Georg Feuser, "Advokatorische Assistenz," in Tobias Erzmann and Georg Feuser, eds., *"Ich fühle mich wie ein Vogel, der aus seinem Nest fliegt": Menschen mit Behinderungen in der Erwachsenenbildung* (Frankfurt / Main: Peter Lang, 2011), 203–218; Kirsten Ehrhardt, *Henri—Ein kleiner Junge verändert die Welt* (Munich: Heyne, 2015); Julia Latscha, *Lauthals Leben: Von Lotte, dem Anderssein und meiner Suche nach einer gemeinsamen Welt* (Munich: Knaur, 2017); Christian Bradl, "Systemische Risiken für Gewalt und mangelnden Gewaltschutz in Einrichtungen der Behindertenhilfe bei erheblich herausforderndem Verhalten," *Behindertenpädagogik* 61.4 (2022), 358–383.

13. Ernst Klee, "Der alltägliche Massenmord: Die 'Euthanasie'-Aktion war der Probelauf für den Judenmord," *Die Zeit*, March 23, 1990. On the long-standing resistance of academic historians to researching Nazi "euthanasia," see Dirk Blasius, "Der 'Historikerstreit' und die historische Erforschung des 'Euthanasie'-Geschehens," *Sozialpsychiatrische Informationen* 2 (1988), 1–6; Michael Burleigh and Wolfgang Wippermann, "Hilfloser Historismus: Warum die deutsche Geschichtswissenschaft bei der Erforschung der Euthanasie versagt hat," in Karl Ludwig Rost, Till Bastian, and Karl Bonhoeffer, eds., *Thema: Behinderte* (Stuttgart: Hirzel, 1991), 11–23.

14. The sense of ethical urgency felt by young scholars who were among the first to grapple with and name the cynical ruthlessness with which the project to "purify the 'body of the Volk' from all that was unhealthy, foreign and bothersome" was pursued amidst Nazism's distinctive "interlacing of annihilation and modernization," their intensely personal attunement to the enmeshment of their parents and grandparents ("with whose hopes, crimes and achievements in repression we are familiar") as well as their keen awareness that also for their own generation, "there can . . . be no prospect of closure, either emotionally or ideologically," is well conveyed in Götz Aly, Angelika Ebbinghaus, Matthias Hamann, Friedemann Pfäfflin, and Gerd Preissler, "Editorial," *Aussonderung und Tod: Die klinische Hinrichtung der Unbrauchbaren* (Berlin: Rotbuch, 1985), 7–8. The stubbornly hostile, concrete opposition this cohort faced over a long postwar period is captured powerfully in Götz Aly, "To Prevent Further Unfounded Aly Constructions!," in Sabine Hildebrandt et al., eds., *Recognizing the Past in the Present: New Studies on Medicine before, during, and after the Holocaust* (New York: Berghahn, 2021), 298–325.

15. As two British disability rights feminists once described succinctly: "Disability is not just one difference among many, but a difference that changes everything." Margrit Shildrick and Janet Price, "Deleuzian Connections and Queer Corporealities," *Rhizomes* (Fall 2005–Spring 2006), http://www.rhizomes.net/issue11/shildrickprice/index.html. See also Catherine J. Kudlick, "Disability History: Why We Need Another 'Other,'" *American Historical Review* 108.3 (June 2003), 763–793; Elsbeth Bösl, *Politiken der Normalisierung: Zur Geschichte der Behindertenpolitik in der Bundesrepublik* (Berlin: transcript, 2009); and Susan Burch and Michael Rembis, eds., *Disability Histories* (Urbana: University of Illinois Press, 2014). Bösl aptly notes—even as her book primarily concerns physical, not mental or emotional, disabilities—that in postwar West Germany, disability was treated as "the ultimate Otherness" (*das ultimativ Andere*) (337).

16. Of course, then and now, the "it" that is referred to as "disability" has never been any one obvious thing and that is not just, though most certainly also, because notions of "normality" and "pathology" are constantly changing. The term "disability" is inescapably a political one, both ascribed and self-chosen, and it continues to encompass a capacious and elastic category of being, including as it does physical, sensory, psychological, and mental variability and impairments, and increasingly also "invisible" disabilities like chronic illnesses.

17. Karl Binding and Alfred Hoche, *Die Freigabe der Vernichtung lebensunwerten Lebens: Ihr Maß und ihre Form* (Leipzig: Felix Meinen, 1920), 53.

18. For an excellent analysis of German eugenicists' and medical professionals' own acute awareness that they were unsure about the hereditary nature of intellectual disability—and that even an extensive mass sterilization program would not successfully reduce the prevalence of intellectual disability in the populace by very much at all—and the ways they compensated for their lack of proof with quasi-religious cosmic faith-claims about the Volk's future glory, see Uwe Gerrens, *Medizinisches Ethos und theologische Ethik* (Munich: Oldenburg, 1996), 42–48. For a helpful overview of the comparative state of debate in the United States and the UK in the 1930s, along with a critical explanation of the already-then-evident weaknesses in the scientific claims made, see David Barker, "The Biology of Stupidity: Genetics, Eugenics and Mental Deficiency in the Inter-War Years," *British Journal for the History of Science* 22.3 (September 1989), 347–375.

19. In fact, there was one individual already at the time who did so: the perspicacious (blind) jurist and disability rights activist Rudolf Kraemer. In 1933, Kraemer published an impressive countertext to Binding and Hoche and to the rising chorus of eugenicists (or, as they called themselves in Germany, "racial hygienists"): *Kritik der Eugenik: Vom Standpunkt des Betroffenen* (Criticism of Eugenics: From the Standpoint of One Affected). Here Kraemer did not mince words as he labeled those endorsing Binding and Hoche's proposals for killing as motivated by nothing more than "ugly hangman-lusts" (*häßliche Henkergelüste*). Eugenics, he further averred, was not just "mischief" (*Unfug*) but "nonsense" (*Unsinn*), based as it was in both erroneous

math and inaccurate science. The ambitious dreams of reducing the number of disabled people being born into the German nation by more than a single percentage point through a sterilization program had, he noted, almost no chance of succeeding in anything less than "300, 400, 500 years"—if then. Yet Kraemer's was a lone voice. Nonetheless, his very existence proves it was possible to imagine and understand otherwise. For more on Kraemer's breathtaking acerbic acuity, see the analysis in Carol Poore, *Disability in Twentieth-Century German Culture* (Ann Arbor: University of Michigan Press, 2007), 135–138.

20. Maike Rotzoll, "Krankheit schreiben in der Psychiatrie um 1900? Diagnosen, Kranken- und Patientengeschichten von Opfern der nationalsozialistischen 'Euthanasie'-Aktion 'T4,'" in Yvonne Wübben and Carsten Zelle, eds., *Krankheit schreiben: Aufzeichnungsverfahren in Medizin und Literatur* (Göttingen: Wallstein, 2013), 109–128; Petra Fuchs, "Zur Selektion von Kindern und Jugendlichen nach dem Kriterium der 'Bildungsunfähigkeit,'" in Rotzoll et al., *Die nationalsozialistischen "Euthanasie"-Morde*, 287–296; Herwig Czech, "Nazi Medical Crimes, Eugenics, and the Limits of the Racial State Paradigm," in Devin Pendas et al., *Beyond the Racial State: Rethinking Nazi Germany* (New York: Cambridge University Press, 2017), 213–239.

21. "Menschen mit Behinderung—Wohnen, leben, arbeiten," *Caritas Deutschland*, https://www.caritas.de/hilfeundberatung/ratgeber/behinderung/wohnenlebenarbeiten/wohnenlebenarbeiten.aspx.

22. "Hilfe bei Behinderung," *Diakonie Deutschland*, https://hilfe.diakonie.de/hilfe-bei-behinderung; Sarah Spitzer, Ulrike Pape, und Martina Menzel, "UN-Konvention über die Rechte von Menschen mit Behinderungen" (April 30, 2021), *Diakonie Deutschland*, https://www.diakonie.de/wissen-kompakt/un-konvention-ueber-die-rechte-von-menschen-mit-behinderungen.

23. "Schon viel erreicht," *Aktion Mensch*, https://www.aktion-mensch.de/ueber-uns/chronik/chronik-detail.

24. Strikingly, and in this way in strong contrast to how the law could serve as a resource, already by the late nineteenth and early twentieth centuries, for advancing some psychiatric patients' rights (for example in arguments over involuntary confinement), the law for a long time did not serve individuals with intellectual impairments very well at all. This was so both with regard to the gruelingly difficult post–World War II battles to bring perpetrators to justice and get crimes against the disabled recognized as crimes at all—a project which met a major setback in 1964 with the dissolution of the case brought against high-level "euthanasia" perpetrators due to the successful suicides of key defendants—and with regard to the broader struggles to improve education and care for the living. The ratification in 2009 of the UN Convention on the Rights of Persons with Disabilities at long last shifted the entire force field dramatically, and the law has become a vital resource for expanding the rights of individuals with all types of disabilities, but especially also intellectual disabilities, for the first time in German history.

25. Sebastian Barsch and Elsbeth Bösl, "Disability History," *Zeithistorische Forschungen* 2 (2022), https://zeithistorische-forschungen.de/2-2022/6039#footnote-035-backlink.

26. Raymond Williams, "Structures of Feeling," in *Marxism and Literature* (Oxford: Oxford University Press, 1977), 128–135, here 132.

27. Nicholas Manning, "'Intensity is a signal, not a truth': An interview with Lauren Berlant," *Revue française d'Études Américaines* 154.1 (2018), 113–120.

28. Theodor W. Adorno, "Education after Auschwitz," in *Critical Models: Interventions and Catchwords*, trans. Henry Pickford (New York: Columbia University Press, 1998), 191–204, here 201, 193, 195. German original: Theodor W. Adorno, "Erziehung nach Auschwitz," in *Erziehung zur Mündigkeit* (Frankfurt / Main: Suhrkamp, 1971), 88–104.

29. Adorno, "Education after Auschwitz," 203.

30. On the constellation of considerations prompting Hitler to react to von Galen's sermon by abruptly shutting down the gas chamber phase of the killings, not least the felt need to reduce

any potential foci for popular unrest since launching war on the Soviet Union in June 1941, see Götz Aly, "Die jähe Unterbrechung der Aktion T4," in *Die Belasteten: "Euthanasie" 1939–1945. Eine Gesellschaftsgeschichte* (Frankfurt / Main: Fischer, 2013), 174–192. On research with regard to contemporaneous public attitudes toward "euthanasia," see Petra Lutz, "Herz und Vernunft: Angehörige von 'Euthanasie'-Opfern im Schriftwechsel mit den Anstalten," in Heiner Fangerau and Karen Nolte, eds., *"Moderne" Anstaltspsychiatrie im 19. Und 20. Jahrhundert: Legitimation und Kritik* (Stuttgart: Steiner, 2006), 143–167; Thomas Stöckle, "Die Reaktionen der Angehören und der Bevölkerung auf die 'Aktion T4,'" in Rotzoll et al., *Die nationalsozialistischen "Euthanasie"- Morde*, 118–124. The scope and details of the second phase, in which killing was mostly done by medication overdose, poison, and starvation, and in which the perceived need continually to "re-locate" residents of institutions to make room for emergency hospital wards as Allied bombing increased on the German home front, were poorly understood by contemporaries and scholars alike until the 1980s–1990s. An outstanding analysis of the most important trends in scholarship on all the dimensions of "euthanasia" since the 1990s is provided by Uwe Kaminsky, "Die NS-Euthanasie: Ein Forschungsüberblick," in Klaus D. Henke, ed., *Tödliche Medizin im Nationalsozialismus: Von der Rassenhygiene zum Massenmord* (Köln: Böhlau, 2008), 269–290.

Chapter One: The Problem of Incurability

1. Remarks of Heinrich Matthias Sengelmann in "Die erste Hauptversammlung," in E. Reichelt, ed., *Bericht über die V. Konferenz für das Idiotenwesen. Frankfurt a. M., vom 14.-16. September 1886* (Dresden: Kgl. Hofbuchhandlung von Hermann Burdach, 1886), 9–24, here 9. Sengelmann (1821–1899) was not only director of the Alsterdorfer Anstalten in Hamburg, one of the largest residential institutions in all of Germany, but also the founder and president of the directors' conferences, held triannually since 1874.

2. For comparative perspectives on developments in the UK and the United States, see Mathew Thomson, *The Problem of Mental Deficiency: Eugenics, Democracy, and Social Policy in Britain c. 1870–1959* (Oxford: Clarendon Press, 1998); James Trent, *Inventing the Feeble Mind: A History of Intellectual Disability in the United States* (New York: Oxford University Press, 1995); Steven Noll and James W. Trent Jr., eds., *Mental Retardation in America: A Historical Reader* (New York: New York University Press, 2004).

3. Christian Bradl, *Anfänge der Anstaltsfürsorge für Menschen mit geistiger Behinderung ("Idiotenanstaltswesen"): Ein Beitrag zur Sozial- und Ideengeschichte des Behindertenbetreuungswesens am Beispiel des Rheinlands im 19. Jahrhundert* (Frankfurt / Main: AFRA, 1991); Uwe Kaminsky, *Zwangssterilisation und "Euthanasie" im Rheinland: Evangelische Erziehungsanstalten sowie Heil- und Pflegeanstalten 1933 bis 1945* (Köln: Rheinland-Verlag, 1995); Volker van der Locht, *Von der karitativen Fürsorge zum ärztlichen Selektionsblick: Zur Sozialgeschichte der Motivstruktur der Behindertenfürsorge am Beispiel des Essener Franz-Sales-Hauses* (Opladen: Leske & Budrich, 1997); Dagmar Drovs, *Heilpädagogik im deutschen Judentum: Eine Spurensicherung 1873–1942* (Münster: LIT, 2000); Hans-Walter Schmuhl and Ulrike Winkler, *"Der das Schreien der jungen Raben nicht überhört": Der Wittekindshof—eine Einrichtung für Menschen mit geistiger Behinderung, 1887 bis 2012* (Bielefeld: Verlag für Regionalgeschichte, 2012); Tatjana Ruge, *Die Israelitische Erziehungsanstalt für geistig zurückgebliebene Kinder in Beelitz: Eine Stätte des Segens und der Hoffnung* (Berlin: Hentrich & Hentrich, 2022).

4. Sieglind Ellger-Rüttgardt, *Verloren und Un-Vergessen. Jüdische Heilpädagogik in Deutschland* (Weinheim: Deutscher Studienverlag, 1996); Bettina Lindmeier and Christian Lindmeier, eds., *Geistigbehindertenpädagogik* ("Studientexte zur Geschichte der Behindertenpädagogik," vol. 3) (Weinheim: Beltz, 2002); Ingeborg Thümmel, *Sozial- und Geistesgeschichte der Schule für Geistigbehinderte im 20. Jahrhundert: Zentrale Entwicklungslinien zwischen Ausgrenzung und Partizipation* (Weinheim: Beltz, 2003); Alexandra Schotte, "Jena als Ort der Heilpädagogik," in Ralf

Koerrenz, ed., *Laboratorium Bildungsreform: Jena als Zentrum pädagogischer Innovationen* (München: Fink, 2009), 111–139; Vera Moser, "Kontroversen behindertenpädagogischer Geschichtsschreibung," in Oliver Musenberg, ed., *Kultur—Geschichte—Behinderung: Die kulturwissenschaftliche Historisierung von Behinderung* (Oberhausen: Athena, 2013), 83–99; Johannes Gstach, *Kretinismus und Blödsinn: Zur fachlich-wissenschaftlichen Entdeckung und Konstruktion von Phänomenen der geistig-mentalen Auffälligkeit zwischen 1780 und 1900 und deren Bedeutung für Fragen der Erziehung und Behandlung* (Bad Heilbrunn: Klinkhardt, 2015); Sieglind Ellger-Rüttgardt, *Geschichte der Sonderpädagogik: Eine Einführung* (Stuttgart: UTB, 2019); Jona Garz, Vera Moser, and Stefan Wünsch, "Die 'Kielhorn-Rede': Ursprungsmythos der deutschen Hilfsschule," in Sabine Reh et al., eds., *Schülerauslese, Schülerbeurteilung und Schülertests 1880–1980* (Bad Heibrunn: Klinkhardt, 2021), 29–45.

5. Hans-Walter Schmuhl, *Rassenhygiene, Nationalsozialismus, Euthanasie: Von der Verhütung zur Vernichtung "lebensunwerten Lebens," 1890–1945* (Göttingen: Vandenhoeck und Ruprecht, 1987); Paul Weindling, *Health, Race and German Politics between National Unification and Nazism, 1870–1945* (Cambridge: Cambridge University Press, 1989); Dirk Blasius, *"Einfache Seelenstörung": Geschichte der deutschen Psychiatrie 1800–1945* (Frankfurt / Main: Fischer, 1994); Klaus Dörner, *Bürger und Irre: Zur Sozialgeschichte und Wissenschaftssoziologie der Psychiatrie*, 3rd ed. (Hamburg: Europäische Verlagsanstalt, 1995); Michael Schwartz, "'Euthanasie'-Debatten in Deutschland (1895–1945)," *Vierteljahrshefte für Zeitgeschichte* 46 (1998), 617–665; Volker Roelcke, *Krankheit und Kulturkritik: Psychiatrische Gesellschaftsdeutungen im bürgerlichen Zeitalter (1790–1914)* (Frankfurt / Main: Campus, 1999); Eric J. Engstrom and Volker Roelcke, eds., *Psychiatrie im 19. Jahrhundert: Forschungen zur Geschichte von psychiatrischen Institutionen, Debatten und Praktiken im deutschen Sprachraum* (Basel: Schwabe, 2003); Heiner Fangerau and Karen Nolte, eds., *"Moderne" Anstaltspsychiatrie im 19. und 20. Jahrhundert: Legitimation und Kritik* (Stuttgart: Steiner, 2006); Anne Cottebrune, "Zwischen Theorie und Deutung der Vererbung psychischer Störungen: Zur Übertragung des Mendelismus auf die Psychiatrie in Deutschland und in den USA, 1911–1930," *Zeitschrift für Geschichte der Wissenschaften, Technik und Medizin* 17.1 (2009), 35–54.

6. Heinrich Damerow, "Zur Cretinen- und Idiotenfrage," *Allgemeine Zeitschrift für Psychiatrie und psychisch-gerichtliche Medizin* 15.4-5 (1858), 499–545, here 499.

7. Max Kirmsse, "Die deutschen Anstalten für Geistesschwache und Epileptische am 1. Januar 1911 nebst Rückblick," *Zeitschrift fur die Behandlung Schwachsinniger* 31.3 (1911), 62–66 and 31.4 (1911), 81–84, here 82–83.

8. Appreciative overviews of Guggenbühl's therapeutic approach and significance: Heinrich E. Stötzner, "Auf dem Abendberge," *Zeitschrift für die Behandlung Schwachsinniger und Epileptischer* 20.5-6 (May 1904), 83–88; Max Kirmsse, "Guggenbühl, Johann Jakob, Dr. med," in Adolf Dannemann et al., eds., *Enzyklopädisches Handbuch der Heilpädagogik*, 2nd ed., vol. 1 (Halle: Carl Marhold, 1934), 1036–1039; Leo Kanner, "Johann Jakob Guggenbühl and the Abendberg," *Bulletin of the History of Medicine* 33.6 (Nov.–Dec. 1959), 489–502. See also Johann Jakob Guggenbühl, *Briefe über den Abendberg und die Heilanstalt für Cretinismus* (Zurich, 1846), 3, 17–19, 57–67; Guggenbühl, *Sendschreiben an Lord Ashley, Mitglied des Englischen Parlaments* (Basel: Bahnmaier, 1851); Guggenbühl, *Die Heilung und Verhütung des Cretinismus* (Bern and St. Gallen: Huber & Comp., 1853). Translator and contemporary of Guggenbühl, William Twining, medical doctor at Balliol College at the University of Oxford, reported already in 1845 that the Abendberg was then home to 25 children and funds raised in England and Holland were helping to expand it further, that "in several cases" Guggenbühl, in his "devoted attention," had been "perfectly successful," that he had acquired "an assistant in the laborious task of teaching the Cretin children," and that he also had "two Sisters of Charity from the Protestant establishment at Lausanne to attend them." W. Twining, "Preface," in Dr. Guggenbühl, *Extracts from the First Report of the Institution on the Abendberg, near Interlachen, Switzerland, for the Cure of*

Cretins, trans. W. Twining (London, 1845), 3–4. In the United States, Samuel Gridley Howe, referring to the Abendberg as a "holy mount," founded the Massachusetts School for Idiotic and Feeble-Minded Youth in 1848 in Boston. Retrospectively, Leo Kanner observed: "Guggenbühl must be acknowledged as the indisputable originator of the idea and practice of the institutional care for feebleminded individuals. The hundreds of institutions now in existence derive in direct line from the Abendberg." Kanner, "Johann Jakob Guggenbühl," 499.

9. Guggenbühl, *Die Heilung*, 106.

10. Guggenbühl as translated by Kanner, "Johann Jakob Guggenbühl," 492; the original quote is in Guggenbühl, *Sendschreiben*, 9.

11. Guggenbühl, *Die Heilung*, 107; cf. Guggenbühl, *Briefe*, 26.

12. See Ferdinand Kern, "Gegenwart und Zukunft der Blödsinnigenbildung," *Allgemeine Zeitschrift für Psychiatrie und psychisch-gerichtliche Medizin* 12.4 (1855), 521–574, esp. 546–549; Damerow, "Zur Cretinen- und Idiotenfrage," 509–518. It bears emphasizing, however, that this theme of a special affinity or sensibility for the divine among individuals with cognitive disabilities would prove to be an exceedingly durable one among the directors of Protestant and Catholic residential institutions alike for decades thereafter.

13. The 1858 report is reprinted in F. Kölle, "Ueber Dr. Guggenbühl und seine 'Kretinen-Heilanstalt' auf dem Abendberg," *Zeitschrift für die Behandlung Schwachsinniger und Epileptischer* 15.5 (May 1899), 92–99 and 15.6 (June 1899), 113–117. In his opening remarks, Kölle commented on how "unfortunate" it was that a "religious cloak" had been cast over the whole enterprise; he also noted that perhaps there had been a "kernel of rot" all along and, like other retrospective evaluators, he reported that Guggenbühl had taken in not only children afflicted by cretinism, but also individuals with various other forms of "idiocy" (92–93). Within the report, a Professor Demme is cited as having been especially offended by the *"religious comedy"* of the Abendberg (95). In another indication of what would become a persistent need to self-distance, in an earlier issue of the same journal Kölle had already reprinted a mocking satire of Guggenbühl purportedly penned by a grateful cretin (who had risen to be a town councilman), ridiculing Guggenbühl's self-representation as the cretins' savior. F. Kölle, "Über Dr. Guggenbühl auf dem Abendberg," *Zeitschrift für die Behandlung Schwachsinniger und Epileptischer* 14.4-5 (June 1898), 89–91.

14. Carl Heinrich Rösch, *Über die Heilung und Erziehung unentwickelter oder kretinischer Kinder mit besonderer Rücksicht auf die Guggenbühl'sche Stiftung auf dem Abendberge bei Interlaken im Schweizerkanton Bern, und eine in Württemberg zu errichtende Anstalt dieser Art* (Stuttgart: F. H. Köhler, 1845); Carl M. Saegert, *Die Heilung des Blödsinns auf intellectuellem Wege* (Berlin: E. H. Schroeder, 1846); Adolf Albrecht Erlenmeyer, "Die Errichtung von Heil-Anstalten für Idioten," *Correspondenz-Blatt der Deutschen Gesellschaft für Psychiatrie und Gerichtliche Psychologie* 5.4 (February 28, 1858), 25–27, 5.6 (March 31, 1858), 42–44, and 5.12 (June 30, 1858), 92–93; Kern, "Gegenwart." Guggenbühl himself repeatedly emphasized that cretinism, because of its obvious somatic dimensions which (he believed) appeared to be at least partially remediable in childhood with improved nutrition and a healthful environment, was "curable" in a way that significant brain damage manifest in other forms of mental disability could never be. Only "very rarely" was there, for cretins, not at least some "improvement in their lamentable condition," he averred, and in the years of the Abendberg there were always instances, he asserted, of "complete cure of cretinous children." But "during this time an idiot has never been healed." Guggenbühl, *Sendschreiben*, 8–9; cf. Guggenbühl, *Briefe*, 10, 22.

15. Édouard Séguin, *Traitement moral, hygiène et éducation des idiots et des autres enfants arriérés* (Paris: Baillière, 1846).

16. Occasionally these valuable ideas would be picked up and further elaborated on by later practitioners, and some of the approaches became simply standard wisdom. Examples include: the remarks of Dr. Koehler about his time in Hubertusberg in Saxony, learning how to use passive gymnastics in order to help the most severely disabled children "first of all learn to feel," in

the directors' conference discussion of Direktor Rall (Mariaberg), "Das Turnen in den Idioten-anstalten," in E. Reichelt, ed., *Bericht über die III. Konferenz für Idioten-Heil-Pflege, Stuttgart, am 13.-15. September 1880* (Dresden: Johannes Pässler, 1880), 36–39, here 38; the impressive compre-hensive lesson plans developed by Großhennersdorf-based teacher Gustav Nitzsche, "Aus der Praxis der Vorschule," *Zeitschrift für die Behandlung Schwachsinniger und Epileptischer* 14.4-5 (June 1898), 52–66, 14.6 (August 1898), 81–88, 14.7 (October 1898), 108–127; and the myriad inge-nious uses of a footstool (*Hitsche*) for teaching practical concepts to and strengthening the "self-activity" of the most severely disabled children in Reinhold Gürtler, "Mein Anschauungsunterricht bei Geistesschwachen auf der untersten Stufe streng nach dem Prinzip des Selbsttuns," in Jacob Schwenk, ed., *Bericht über die XIII. Konferenz des Vereins für Erziehung, Unterricht und Pflege Geist-esschwacher vom 13. bis 16. September in Wiesbaden 1910* (Idstein: Grandpierre, 1910), 125–137.

17. An early summary of the consensus was articulated in 1862: "After centuries of the doc-trine that the idiocy of children was incurable, and as a consequence idiots were rejected by all who should have felt called to stand up for them, all at once the perfect cure of idiocy was envisaged, and physicians as well as teachers really lived in this delusion or, in spite of better insight, sought to spread the new doctrine of the curability of idiocy. Among the physicians, it was especially Guggenbühl who advocated for this doctrine, and enthusiastic tourists, sensitive ladies and philanthropic physicians echoed him in this new gospel. The religious nimbus, with which he surrounded his efforts and especially his person, prevented any sober examination of his activities for a long time." Gustav Brandes, *Der Idiotismus und die Idiotenanstalten mit beson-derer Rücksicht auf die Verhältnisse im Königreiche Hannover* (Hannover: Carl Rümpler, 1862), 94–95. Heinrich Matthias Sengelmann at the Alsterdorfer Anstalten, who had originally been enormously inspired by Guggenbühl and was perceptive about both the imaginative strengths and the self-indulgent weaknesses of Guggenbühl's efforts, became one of the loudest and most insistent self-distancers. See Heinrich Matthias Sengelmann, *Idiotophilus*, vol. 1 (Norden: Soltau, 1885), 69–78, esp. 76; Sengelmann's remarks in "Die erste Hauptversammlung" (1886), 9, as well as Karl Barthold's comments in "Zweite Hauptversammlung," in Reichelt, *Bericht . . . 1886*, 29; Heinrich Matthias Sengelmann, "Zur Orientierung über die bisherige Arbeit an den Idioten und ihren Leidensgenossen," in E. Reichelt, ed., *Bericht über die VI. Konferenz für das Idiotenwe-sen: Braunschweig, vom 10.-13. September 1889* (Dresden: Hermann Burdach, 1889), 3–15, here 4–5 and 14 (jabs against the—misinterpreted—efforts of Carl M. Saegert in Berlin and of the sig-nificant early French experimental educator Édouard Séguin were built into the comments as well). Further instances of self-distancing: Kölle, "Ueber Dr. Guggenbühl," 92–93; J. P. Gerhardt, "Hans Jakob Guggenbühl," *Zur Geschichte und Literatur des Idiotenwesens in Deutschland* (Ham-burg: Selbstverlag, 1904), 95–97.

18. To be clear: The goal of "usefulness" was well-intentioned and meant in the most empa-thetic, expansive way. Sengelmann, for instance, in 1889 defended "work-instruction" as just as valuable as "school instruction" for the determination of "educability": "That child appears to me as educable which, by one path or another, can be brought to prove himself useful to others and himself." Sengelmann, "Zur Orientierung," 9. At the same conference, teacher Heinrich Kielhorn (19, 28), teacher E. Reichelt (33), Director Schaarschmidt from Braunschweig (35), and Dr. Wulff of Langenhagen (43) all invoked the ideal of making pupils or residents "useful" as a self-evident goal. Six years later, at the 1895 directors' conference in Heidelberg, the consensus was expressed again (this time by "educational inspector" Piper) that "Our feeble-minded children are meant to be developed as fully as possible into useful members of human society." Piper, "Der grundlegende Sprachunterricht bei stammelnden, schwachsinnigen Kindern," *Zeitschrift für die Behandlung Schwachsinniger und Epileptischer* 12.1-2 (February 1896), 11–22, here 11. Also the most impressive and dedicated remedial education experts—whether focused on sensory disabilities like blind-ness or deafness or on cognitive impairments or behavioral challenges—felt the need to frame their commitments in related terms. For instance, when the editors for the new Vienna-based

German-language (and internationally exceedingly well networked) quarterly journal *Eos* (named for the Greek goddess of dawn) published their mission statement in the first issue in 1905, they made the typical move of stressing that "We know it well and will proclaim it loudly that *we do not achieve any successful cures* with the youthful abnormals, but rather our whole striving must go toward harnessing their diminished powers for the aims of ennoblement of character and usefulness in human life [*Veredlung des Charakters und der Brauchbarkeit im Menschenleben*]." Moritz Brunner, Salomon Krenberger, Alexander Mell, and Heinrich Schlöss, "Zur Einführung," *Eos: Vierteljahrsschrift für die Erkenntnis und Behandlung jugendlicher Abnormer* 1.1 (1905), 1. The journal, published continuously until 1920, was outstanding, providing critical assessments of all the latest pedagogical trends as it additionally strove to recover historically significant innovators. Krenberger in particular—initially the founding director of a school for "feebly-abled children," later the director of the Israelite Deaf-Mute Institute in Vienna—was especially remarkable and deserves far more study. He is to be credited particularly for bringing into German translation the pioneering work of the French American remedial pedagogue Édouard Séguin, *Die Idiotie und ihre Behandlung nach physiologischer Methode* (Vienna: Graeser, 1912).

19. A peculiar contrapuntal subplot that does not integrate easily into the overall trajectory of German attitudes about disability involves a debate between and among Jewish and non-Jewish medical professionals, from the early 1900s to the mid-1920s, over the statistical finding that Jews were disproportionately represented among those diagnosed with either mental disability or illness (whereas physical disabilities were proportionately more prevalent among Catholics and Protestants), even as Jews represented less than 1 percent of the German population. Might this phenomenon have its source in Jews' greater tendency to live in urban centers (as urban life was thought to exacerbate nervous illnesses)? in Jews' greater willingness to consult medical experts (and hence likelihood of being diagnosed at all)? or indeed, in Jews' tendencies toward endogamy (which might, particularly in the cases of marriage between individuals with kinship ties prevalent among *some* Orthodox groups, especially from Eastern Europe, increase the risk of instances of children born with intellectual disability)? A few suggested—while others vigorously refuted this—that Jews might have an inherent tendency to mental illness, a *psychosis Judaica* (usually understood as a predilection toward manic depression), and some speculated that processes of secularization could explain the apparently higher rates of suicidality among Jews, while others—for instance, the directors of the Jacoby'sche Anstalten in Sayn near Koblenz—suggested that it was the stubborn persistence of aggressive antisemitism among gentiles itself that made Jews more vulnerable to nervous strain. See for example (the anti-antisemitic) *Der Israelit*, March 24, 1902, in "Sayn (Stadt Bendorf, Kreis Mayen-Koblenz): Jüdische Geschichte/ Jacoby'sche Anstalten/ Synagoge in der Anstalt," https://www.alemannia-judaica.de/sayn_anstalt.htm; (tendentially antisemitic) Alexander Pilcz, *Beitrag zur vergleichenden Rassen-Psychiatrie* (Leipzig and Vienna: Franz Deuticke, 1906), esp. iii–iv, 1–24; (anxiously balanced) Max Sichel, *Die Geistesstörungen bei den Juden: Eine klinisch-historische Studie* (Leipzig: Kaufmann, 1909); (neutrally remarking) S. Behrendt and S. A. Rosenthal, "Israelit. Heil- und Pflegeanstalt für Nerven- und Gemütskranke Sayn bei Coblenz," in *Deutsche Heil- und Pflegeanstalten für psychisch Kranke in Wort und Bild* (Halle: Marhold, 1912), 426–433, here 431; and (conflictedly puzzling) Karl Jaspers, "Rasse," *Allgemeine Psychopathologie: Ein Leitfaden für Studierende, Ärzte und Psychologen* (Berlin: Springer, 2013), 307–309, here 308. Although the arguments ranged widely, the very existence of the debate conferred a sense of legitimacy to the question. Hence, some authors also emphasized data demonstrating Jewish mental health. Sichel, for instance, recurrently stressed that the prejudicial *perception* of "a special Jewish disposition to psychic illnesses" could be the result precisely of the "well-known solicitude" traditionally shown by Jews to their ill community members, and their readiness to seek out expert medical advice. Max Sichel, "Die psychischen Erkrankungen der Juden in Kriegs- und Friedenszeiten," *Monatsschrift für Psychiatrie und Neurologie* 55

(1924), 207–228, here 207, cf. 223. See also Joseph Walk, "Jüdische Sondererziehung im Dritten Reich," in Ellger-Rüttgardt, *Verloren und Un-Vergessen*, 45–70, here 45. Walk cites the so-called invalid count (*Gebrechlichenzählung*) of the year 1925 as finding that for every 10,000 inhabitants in Germany, 48.7 Jews were "mentally invalid" (*geistig Gebrechliche*) in comparison with 35.8 Protestants and 37.6 Catholics. Although his focus is more on psychiatric illness and not intellectual disability, see also the important and helpfully contextualizing discussion (for instance also on Pilcz's antisemitism) in Sander Gilman, "Zwetschkenbaum's Competence: Madness and the Discourse of the Jews," in *Love + Marriage = Death: And Other Essays on Representing Difference* (Stanford, CA: Stanford University Press, 1998), 91–112, here 105–109.

20. Julius Disselhoff, *Die gegenwärtige Lage der Cretinen, Blödsinnigen und Idioten in den christlichen Ländern: Ein Noth- und Hülferuf für die Verlassendsten unter den Elenden an die deutsche Nation* (Bonn: Adolph Marcus, 1857); Erlenmeyer, "Die Errichtung" (5.4), 25; [Heinrich Matthias Sengelmann], "Das Knabenhaus der Alsterdorfer Anstalten," *Briefe und Bilder aus Alsterdorf* 2 (February 1877), 5.

21. Johannes Miquel's words of welcome in "Die erste Hauptversammlung" (1886), 9.

22. Cruelty was pervasively and persistently thematized. Two typical examples, decades apart: Dr. Koehler from the Hubertusberg institution in Saxony remarked summarily in 1877, regarding the need for institutions, on the "lovelessness" and "pranks," the "injustice, torments, and abuses" to which individuals with intellectual disabilities were subjected within families and communities alike. In 1912, in a handsome, photo-laden volume profiling dozens of the established institutions, a boy is quoted telling the pastor who is his religion teacher, after hearing the statement of God in the Bible when the Ten Commandments are introduced, that "I am the Lord your God, who led you out of the land of Egypt, out of the house of bondage"—the statement that reminds Jews to keep God's commandments—that he had been pelted with stones as a child and now felt so grateful that "the good Lord has also led me away from evil Egyptland," and that he had been given a safe home in the institution. The stone-throwing was "just like it was for the Jews in Egypt. And now I am in Hephata, that is as though I had come to Canaan, now I will also gladly be obedient to the dear Lord." Koehler quote in Bradl, *Anfänge*, as epigraph; boy's response to Bible story in "Treysa (Bez. Kassel), Anstalten 'Hephata,'" in Paul Stritter and Ewald Meltzer, eds., *Deutsche Anstalten für Schwachsinnige, Epileptische und psychopathische Jugendliche* (Halle: Carl Marhold, 1912), 125–148, here 130.

23. Miquel's remarks in "Die erste Hauptversammlung" (1886), 9. The numbers were cited by Sengelmann in "Vorversammlung," in Reichelt, *Bericht . . . 1886*, 4–8, here 7.

24. Heinrich Matthias Sengelmann, "Das Kirchlein der Alsterdorfer Anstalten," *Briefe und Bilder aus Alsterdorf* 1 (January 1877), 1.

25. Pastor Karl Ulrich Kobelt, Neinstedt, in Reichelt, *Bericht . . . 1880*, 46; Probst Palmer, Neuerkerode, in Reichelt, *Bericht . . . 1889*, 48.

26. As of 1904, of the 93 "German institutions for idiots and epileptics," 19 had been founded by Catholics. By 1910, of the 226 institutions harboring 34,404 individuals with intellectual disabilities, only 46 were Catholic-run, but many of these were large, in total serving more than a third (14,750) of the residential clientele. The staff at these facilities was largely drawn from religious orders: 1,763 nuns and 353 male religious. See Hans Wollasch, *Ein Jahrhundert der Sorge um geistig behinderte Menschen*, vol. 2 (Freiburg: Verband katholischer Einrichtungen für Lern- und Geistigbehinderte e.V., 1980), 11; Michael Fischer, "Die Entwicklung der Schwachsinnigenfürsorge," *Krankendienst* 5 (1924), 73–78, here 78.

27. Quoted (and contextualized in the inadvertent effects of the *Kulturkampf*) in Bradl, *Anfänge*, 410.

28. And: "In the interest of the cause and of truthfulness I consider it necessary to say these things to the public, which keeps harboring the opinion that through the institutions the imbeciles and the weak could be cured." Pastor Kobelt in Reichelt, *Bericht . . . 1880*, 31.

29. Dr. Oswald Berkhan, director of an "idiot-institution" in Braunschweig, made the proposal. Emphasis added. Quoted in Reichelt, *Bericht . . . 1886*, 40. The group further decided, based on a proposal from teacher-director Karl Barthold in Mönchengladbach—"In consideration of the fact that idiocy is incurable—in the general sense of that word—both from the organic and from the mental side, and in consideration that the expression 'idiot-*curative*-care' [*Idioten-Heilpflege*] provokes many misunderstandings in the public and awakens unfulfillable hopes"— that the name of the conference should additionally be adapted. Henceforth it would be neutrally succinct and businesslike: "Conference for the Idiot-Sector" (*Konferenz für das Idiotenwesen*). See the debate in Reichelt, *Bericht . . . 1886*, 45–46.

30. Hermann Josef Ochs, Franz Sales Haus, Essen, in Bradl, *Anfänge*, 426–427.

31. J. P. Gerhardt, "Das Idiotenbildungswesen," in Gerhardt, *Zur Geschichte und Literatur*, 46–52, here 48.

32. See the informative overview of the most widely promoted positions that had evolved over the prior decades in A. Gündel, "Zur Klassifizierung der Idioten," *Zeitschrift für die Behandlung Schwachsinniger und Epileptischer* 12.5-6 (September 1896), 73–93. Rather than focusing primarily on gradations of severity, this author added two original dimensional emphases—the (in)ability to "concentrate" and / or the (in)ability to "conceptualize"—as diagnostic elements to consider in identifying proper categorization. See also the discussion of Sengelmann's own preferred categories—he distinguished between "feeblemindedness" (*Schwachsinn*), "imbecility" (*Blödsinn*), and "cretinism" (*Cretinismus*), even as he too stressed that the lines were blurry and that all of them could be summarily seen as forms of "idiocy" (*Idiotismus*), and as he additionally distinguished individuals' presenting types as describable either as "erethic" (choleric or irritable), "apathic" (melancholic), or "torpid" (phlegmatic). See Sengelmann, "Ontologie," *Idiotophilus* vol. 1, 1–23; and discussion in Hans-Walter Schmuhl and Ulrike Winkler, *Heinrich Matthias Sengelmann (1821–1899) und die Anfänge der Evangelischen Stiftung Alsterdorf* (Hamburg: Evangelische Stiftung Alsterdorf, 2021), 218. Addressing the institution directors' conference in 1889, Sengelmann noted that, of the "6000 idiots" then being served in residential institutions across Germany, the ones who were being "only occupied" had initially been taken in with the hope that they could be educated, and only when that proved not possible were they redirected to occupational divisions (*Beschäftigungsabteilungen*). Sengelmann, "Zur Orientierung," 6. In Sengelmann's compilation of statistics for the 1895 directors' conference, of the total by then of 8,803 residents—this time including also German-speaking Switzerland—3,399 were categorized as being "educated," 2,407 "only occupied," and 2,997 "solely cared for." Heinrich Matthias Sengelmann, *Die Idioten-Anstalten Deutschlands und der Deutschen Schweiz im Jahre 1895* (Norden: Soltau, 1895), 31.

33. Sengelmann, "Zur Orientierung," 5. See also the comments in the ensuing debates over distinctions and overlaps in Reichelt, *Bericht . . . 1889*: Inspector Piper, Dalldorf (31), Teacher Reichelt (32), Director Richter, Leipzig (34), Dr. Schaarschmidt, Braunschweig (35). The debates were never resolved. By 1900, remedial teacher Paul Tätzner in Dresden was continuing to insist that the "feebly-abled" should stay in public schools and only the "feeble-minded" be placed in remedial schools, even as he conceded that the boundaries were not clear. Paul Tätzner, "Die Entstehung des Gedankens, besondere Schulen für schwachsinnige Schüler zu errichten, und die Art, wie dieser Gedanke in der Nachhilfeschule zu Dresden-Altstadt Verwirklichung gefunden hat," *Zeitschrift für die Behandlung Schwachsinniger und Epileptischer* 16.4-5 (May 1900), 64–77, and 16.6-7 (July 1900), 81–120, here 102–104.

34. Ochs quoted in Bradl, *Anfänge*, 423.

35. See Sengelmann, "Zur Orientierung," 7; teacher-director Ochs in 1894 in Essen—arguing that individuals with significant cognitive disabilities could be placed in wards together with the "quiet insane"—quoted in Bradl, *Anfänge*, 428; the report that "Dalldorf has recently separated the ineducable idiots completely from its idiot-institution and transferred them to a

special ward of the insane asylum" in Wilhelm Weygandt, *Die Behandlung idiotischer und imbeciller Kinder in ärztlicher und pädagogischer Beziehung* (Würzburg: Stüber, 1900), 81–82; and—on the dilemmas of mixing "educable" or "trainable" residents with "idiots"—Ewald Meltzer, "Die staatliche Schwachsinnigenfürsorge im Königreich Sachsen," *Allgemeine Zeitschrift für Psychiatrie* 61.3 (1904), 370–385, and 61.4 (1904), 570–601, here 370–372.

36. Karl Barthold, "Die Notwendigkeit vermehrter Fürsorge für die Blöden in der Rheinprovinz (Referat bei der Eröffnung des Diakonissenmutterhauses in Sobernheim 1889," reprinted in Kaminsky, *Zwangssterilisation und "Euthanasie"*, 626–628, here 628.

37. Barthold in Reichelt, *Bericht . . . 1889*, 34.

38. A. Gündel, Rastenburg, at the directors' conference in 1904, quoted in Bradl, *Anfänge*, 545.

39. E.g., see "Zur reichsgesetzlichen Regelung des Irrenwesens," *Kölnische Zeitung*, 15 May 1902, 1.

40. As early as 1881, psychiatrist-director Dr. Karl Friedrich Kind, Langenhagen-Hannover, was summarized as arguing, in a speech "About the Idiot-Question," that "even those idiots best prepared and educated for life only so rarely come into such favorable circumstances that they can successfully pursue the battle with life. At every idiot-institution, even if it has been established solely for the so-called educable, an occupational institution [*Beschäftigungsanstalt*], or colony [*Colonie*] for permanent custody, should be attached. At the founding of every new idiot-institution the purchase of a larger complex of land must be considered." Summary of Dr. Kind, "Ueber die Idiotenfrage" (at the "Jahresversammlung des Vereins deutscher Irrenärzte zu Frankfurt a. Main am 8. u. 9. August 1881"), *Allgemeine Zeitschrift für Psychiatrie und psychiatrisch-gerichtliche Medicin* 38.5 (1882), 691–697, here 696. A Catholic version of related points is articulated by a Dr. Merscheim, who told the board of the Franz Sales Haus in Essen in 1909 that "soon also a workshop for the systematic work-training of adolescent idiots must be built" and that "under supervision of wardens those older male idiots who are work-capable and valuable for economic profitability, especially the sexually excitable ones, should be accommodated." Merschheim quoted in van der Locht, *Von der karitativen Fürsorge*, 191. In 1912, teacher-director Jacob Schwenk, Kalmenhof-Idstein, declared at that year's directors' conference that although "a great many German and non-German institutions for the feeble-minded have already annexed the . . . demanded work-colonies," it was "urgently necessary" to build yet more "work-colonies for the feeble-minded," both for institutional residents and for those graduates of the remedial schools who could not find other employment. Schwenk quoted in Thümmel, *Sozial- und Geistesgeschichte der Schule*, 52–53.

41. In 1904, Director Piper, Dalldorf, at a meeting in Berlin of the "Social Commission of the Training- and Welfare-Care Association for Mentally-Retarded (Feeble-Minded) Children," explained that masters should not be sought in Berlin but, rather: "It would be better to take the children out to the provinces," because there, as he said, "people are more upright and simple and occupy themselves more with the children without taking advantage of them." The subtext anxiety about potential exploitation was clear. "Berlin. (Erziehungs- und Fürsorgeverein.)," *Zeitschrift für die Behandlung Schwachsinniger und Epileptischer* 20.12 (December 1904), 188–189. By 1913, the remedial teacher Alwin Schenk in Breslau was arguing openly that the "work-teaching colonies" were training pupils for artisanal jobs (baking, gardening, basket-weaving) that were becoming outdated; he recommended that training for "simple and light industrial labor" would be far preferable and would prepare pupils for factory work. Alwin Schenk, "Was soll mit solchen unglücklichen Kindern geschehen, die zu schwach sind um an dem Unterrichte der Hilfsschule mit Erfolg teilzunehmen?," *Die Hilfsschule* 6.2 (February 1913), 34–37, here 34–35.

42. E.g., see Ochs in 1894 in Bradl, *Die Anfänge*, 427: "It is best for the female pupils, in the event that there is not a most careful mother available to advise and guide, to stay in

the institution for life." In 1904 Meltzer was already talking about heritability of feeble-mindedness and arguing that "feeble-minded girls are often sexually abused or fall into prostitution" and, more generally, that men and women alike benefited from continuing to provide small jobs in and around the institution. Meltzer, "Die staatliche Schwachsinnigenfürsorge," 597–598.

43. The phenomenon is especially well described for Bethel near Bielefeld, the largest of all the counter-worlds: Hans-Walter Schmuhl, *Friedrich von Bodelschwingh* (Reinbek: Rowohlt, 2005).

44. Sengelmann in Reichelt, *Bericht . . . 1889*, 6.

45. Kirmsse, "Die deutschen Anstalten," 81–82. Estimates in 1903 were that the actual need for residential institutional care Germany-wide was at least four times the number of people already then being served. Dr. med. Habermas, Inspektor Pfarrer Strebel, Oekonomieverwalter Bräuninger, *Fünfundfünfzigster Jahresbericht der Heil- und Pflegeanstalt für Schwachsinnige und Epileptische in Stetten i.R.* (Schorndorf: C.W. Mayer, 1903), 7. Also Stetten's *Jahresberichte* for the prior years report consistently that they received far more applications than they had room to accept. Notably, moreover, at the same historical juncture charitable institutions for physically disabled "cripples" also were both steadily expanding in size and described as not sufficiently meeting the extant need. Here too, contemporaries declared that optimistic claims that the majority could be made "employable" (*erwerbsfähig*) were delusional and that two-thirds would likely remain permanently institutionalized. See "Wieviel Krüppeln kann man helfen?," *Der alte Glaube* 27.9 (1907), 45.

46. The phrase "the better material" (*das bessere Material*) is in a retrospective summary of institution directors' previously expressed concerns by the Hubertusburg institution teacher E. Reichelt, "Welche Kinder gehören in die Hilfsklassen und welche in die Idioten-Anstalten," in Reichelt, *Bericht . . . 1889*, 32–36, here 32. The phrase "the invigorating elements" (*die belebenden Elemente*) is in Dr. Kind's summary of Karl Barthold's comments in the 1880 directors' conference discussion over whether remedial classes would be competition for residential institutions. Dr. Kind, "Idiotie und Cretinismus," *Bericht über die psychiatrische Literatur im 2. Halbjahre 1880. Zeitschrift für Psychiatrie 37. Supplement-Heft* (1881), 105–122, here 114.

47. Reichelt, "Welche Kinder."

48. E.g., see the engaged debates surrounding the presentation of Dr. Friedrich Bartels, director of municipal schools in Gera, in Reichelt, *Bericht . . . 1886*, 7, 35–37.

49. Barthold in Reichelt, *Bericht . . . 1880*, 26. For more on the continuing rivalrous discussions, see, e.g., Piper, "Ein Wort, die 'Hilfsklassen' bzw. 'Hilfsschule' betreffend," *Zeitschrift für die Behandlung Schwachsinniger und Epileptischer* 6.2 (April 1890), 26–29; Heinrich Kielhorn, "Ein Wort, die Hilfsklassen oder Hilfsschulen betreffend," *Zeitschrift für die Behandlung Schwachsinniger und Epileptischer* 6.3 (June 1890), 33–37; Piper, "Ein Wort, die Hilfsklassen oder Hilfsschulen betreffend," *Zeitschrift für die Behandlung Schwachsinniger und Epileptischer* 6.4 (October 1890), 49–52; E. Reichelt, "Mein Antrag auf der Braunschweiger Konferenz," *Zeitschrift für die Behandlung Schwachsinniger und Epileptischer* 7.3-4 (August 1891), 55–57; Karl Richter, "Erwiderung," *Zeitschrift für die Behandlung Schwachsinniger und Epileptischer* 14.1 (February 1898), 9–12; Karl Richter, "Bemerkungen," *Zeitschrift für die Behandlung Schwachsinniger und Epileptischer* 14.3 (April 1898), 43–47. The remedial teacher and activist on behalf of remedial schools Heinrich Kielhorn insisted that "the pupils of the remedial schools 'are no idiots,'" only to be rebuffed in response that "then they are half-idiots, feeble-minded—just as the institutions also have among their charges" (quoted in Richter, "Bemerkungen," 46). Then again, remedial teacher Arno Fuchs, in his guidebook on remedial education, declared unabashedly that "What a different, much more significant, more promising purpose the pedagogy of imbeciles has in comparison with the pedagogy of idiots!" Arno Fuchs, *Schwachsinnige Kinder, ihre sittliche und intellektuelle Rettung* (Gütersloh: Bertelsmann, 1899), v.

50. The phenomenon is summarized in Karl Ziegler, "Über das Ausstellen von Handarbeiten Schwachbegabter," *Die Hilfsschule* 6.1 (January 1913), 3–16.

51. Karl Ziegler, "Die Kinder können zu viel," *Zeitschrift für die Behandlung Schwachsinniger und Epileptischer* 14.3 (April 1898), 39–42, here 40–41. Related sentiments in Rudolf Fliedner, "Wie setzen wir uns mit den Anschauungen über die Nutzlosigkeit des Schwachsinnigen-Unterrichtes auseinander?," *Die innere Mission im evangelischen Deutschland* 9 (1910), 335–346, here 338.

52. All quotes and analysis in Garz et al., "Die 'Kielhorn-Rede,'" 34–39. See also Patrick Bühler, review of Musenberg, ed., *Kultur—Geschichte—Behinderung*, in *Erziehungswissenschaftliche Revue* 14.1 (January–February 2015), https://www.pedocs.de/volltexte/2018/15355/pdf/EWR_2015_1_Buehler_Rezension_Musenberg_Kultur_-_Geschichte_-_Behinderung.pdf.

53. "More than 200" teachers: Kielhorn remarks in the debate at the 1898 directors' conference in Breslau, following a presentation by Gottfried Heller, "Über Ermüdungsmessungen bei schwachsinnigen Kindern," in *Zeitschrift für die Behandlung Schwachsinniger und Epileptischer* 14.8 (December 1898), 136–150, here 147. On differential class sizes, see Leopold Laquer, *Die Hilfsschule für schwachbefähigte Kinder* (Wiesbaden: J. F. Bergmann, 1901), 15. On the history of the remedial teachers' self-organization, see F., "Cassel. (Zweiter Verbandstag der Hilfsschulen Deutschlands)," *Zeitschrift für die Behandlung Schwachsinniger und Epileptischer* 15.4-5 (May 1899), 102–104; and August Henze, "Vereinswesen," in Adolf Dannemann, ed., *Enzyklopädisches Handbuch der Heilpädagogik*, vol. 2 (Halle: Carl Marhold, 1911), 1835–1853.

54. See Fliedner, "Wie setzen wir uns," 340–341.

55. Adolf Arthur Grohmann, "Einiges über Schwachsinnige," *Zeitschrift für die Behandlung Schwachsinniger und Epileptischer* 15.4-5 (May 1899), 81–89, here 81–83, 88.

56. Tätzner, "Die Entstehung," 99, 115–117. It bears remembering that this was a time when sterilization, certainly on a mass scale, was not yet imaginable; lifelong institutionalization was *the* way to prevent reproduction. Tätzner did invoke heredity, calling for "the impeding and combating of conception of children among idiots and mentally and physically hereditary cripples of all kinds," and footnoting the Swiss psychiatrist and social reformer Auguste Forel, "Über Ethik," in *Die Zukunft* 7.53 (1899). Grohmann's essay had also attracted two earlier concerned responses: Editors' comment attached to Grohmann, "Einiges," 89; and E. Hasenfratz, "Herrn A. Grohmann—Zürich," *Zeitschrift für die Behandlung Schwachsinniger und Epileptischer* 15.10-11 (November 1899), 201–202. Grohmann's essay appeared as a short book as well and was reviewed favorably: Andernach, review of Grohmann, *Der Schwachsinnige und seine Stellung in der Gesellschaft* (Zürich: Ed. Rascher, 1900), in the *Zeitschrift für Psychologie und Physiologie der Sinnesorgane* 23 (1900), 238–239.

57. Fliedner, "Wie setzen wir uns."

58. Kirmsse, "Die deutschen Anstalten," 84; Schenk, "Was soll."

59. Kirmsse, "Die deutschen Anstalten," 84. The author was the teacher Max Kirmsse, from the Kalmenhof in Idstein / Taunus. Kirmsse can rightly be considered the first historian of cognitive disability in Germany, building an archive of 3,000 books and articles, working tirelessly to recover and publish information about pioneering experiments in remedial education, and— while so many other commentators engaged in intensified stigmatization—striving adamantly to defend the dignity of his pupils. On Kirmsse, see Richard von Premerstein, "Max Kirmsse, ein Historiker des Sonderschulwesens: Leben und Werk," *Zeitschrift für Heilpädagogik* 14.12 (1963), 688–695. The statistics Kirmsse cited in 1911 were for multiple reasons, as he himself explained, based on incomplete data (62–63, 82), but they constituted an under- rather than an over-estimate. A decade earlier, in 1900, psychiatrist Wilhelm Weygandt, while emphasizing for different reasons the shakiness and variability of the available statistics, had referenced already then circulating estimates of 60,000 Germans "suffering from inborn feeble-mindedness" and

suggested that this number was "far more likely to be too low than too high." Weygandt, *Die Behandlung*, 79–80.

60. One was an update, in 1891 (going into effect in 1893), to an earlier (1871) law; the update carried the cumbersome technical name "Law on the Implementation of the Federal Law on the Domicile of Assistance" (*Gesetz zur Ausführung des Bundesgesetzes über den Unterstützungswohnsitz*). It did not only mandate the placement of indigent individuals with disabilities (sensory, intellectual, and / or epileptic) or mental illness in "suitable institutions," insofar as they could not be cared for by their families. It additionally reorganized the financial subvention process to shift away from the municipality of birth (from which it had often been difficult to recover funds) to make the municipality of present residence responsible—while also providing for the regional provincial governments to subsidize a portion of the care fees. Many of the confessional charities negotiated care contracts with the provincial governments. The second, promulgated in 1900 and going into effect in 1901, was a law imagining and targeting a different category of individual for compulsory institutionalization, this time in residential correctional training institutes: "Law for the Welfare-Care-Training of Minors" (*Gesetz für die Fürsorgeerziehung Minderjähriger*). These were adolescents who were "difficult-to-manage" (*schwer erziehbar*) or "neglected" (*verwahrlost*), whether due to parental poverty or familial dysfunction, and hence in perceived danger of delinquency. The idea was considered progressive; the aim was to catch children early—some perhaps had already engaged in petty thievery—and to attempt rehabilitation rather than sending them directly to prison. In the first ten years, more than 70,000 minors were filtered through the "welfare-care-training" system. See "Zehn Jahre Fürsorge-Arbeit, ihr heutiger Stand," *Pädagogische Woche* 8.22 (1912), 342–343.

61. In the 1890s, facing overflowing asylums, uncertainty in treatment protocols, and an increasingly militant patients' rights movement, psychiatrists in Germany had not yet consolidated the cultural dominance to which they aspired. Concerned that Protestant and Catholic church–affiliated residential institution directors were not staying in their proper sphere and restricting themselves to care for those with mental disability and epilepsy but also making incursions into what psychiatrists thought was "their" domain of mental *illness*—and, not irrelevantly, successfully acquiring government subsidies as they did so—a national gathering of psychiatrists, meeting in Frankfurt / Main in 1893, was prompted to publish a manifesto demanding that not solely the asylums but *also* the residential institutions needed to be run by psychiatrists—or that at least all the intake, discharge, and treatment decisions needed to be made by them. An unrelated scandal of involuntary institutionalization at a Catholic asylum in 1894—sensationalized in the national press—impelled the Prussian government to act, promulgating a new policy regulation in September 1895 that formally mandated psychiatrists' oversight of *all* intake decisions and treatment plans, not just at institutions for the mentally ill but also—as psychiatrists had demanded—at institutions dedicated to care of epileptics and the mentally disabled. A full-blown turf war over control of the institutions ensued. Of the 48 most prominent residential institutions operating at the moment of the announced policy change, only 2 were run by psychiatrists (the latter had, after all, been fleeing the field of "idiocy" care for almost 50 years); the attack on pastors and pedagogues was direct and personal. See Ewald Reichelt, "Eine Gegenerklärung," *Zeitschrift für die Behandlung Schwachsinniger und Epileptischer* 10.1 (January 1894), 9–12, here 10. While initially the conflict was pitched to the public as one between contrasting worldviews (medical-scientific and "modern" versus practically "medieval" religious notions of "demon possession" as the causes of madness), the actual stakes were both more mundane and more serious. This was not actually about contrasting interpretations of mental disability or mental illness, but rather about power and money. Yet although both religiously oriented and remedial education–focused directors, forcefully reminding government bureaucrats about the long-elaborated distinctions between "insanity" and "idiocy,"

were able in June 1896 to achieve a modification retaining their authority at least for institutions for *children* with intellectual disabilities and / or with epilepsy, this proved to be a Pyrrhic victory; the debate kept escalating well into the first decade of the 1900s. See Benjamin Kocherscheidt, "Deutsche Irrenärzte und Irrenseelsorger: Ein Beitrag zur Geschichte von Psychiatrie und Anstaltsseelsorge im 19. Jahrhundert" (Dissertation, Medical Faculty, University of Hamburg, 2010).

62. See Pastor Krekeler, "Die Stellung und Aufgabe des Arztes in einer Idioten-Anstalt" at the Heidelberg directors' conference of September 17–20, 1895, in *Zeitschrift für die Behandlung Schwachsinniger und Epileptischer* 12.1-2 (February 1896), 1–7; Jacob Schwenk, "Wo stehen wir?," *Zeitschrift für die Behandlung Schwachsinniger und Epileptischer* 12.5-6 (September 1896), 93–101; Jacob Schwenk, "Die Bestimmungen vom 20. September 1895 und ihre Folgen für unsere Anstalten," *Zeitschrift für die Behandlung Schwachsinniger und Epileptischer* 15.1 (January 1899), 6–20; "Zum Ministerial-Erlass vom 20. September 1895," *Zeitschrift für die Behandlung Schwachsinniger und Epileptischer* 17.1-2 (February 1901), 22–25; "Zu der neuen preussischen 'Anweisung . . . ,'" *Zeitschrift für die Behandlung Schwachsinniger und Epileptischer* 17.9-10 (September 1901), 154–164; Jacob Schwenk, "Die Bestimmungen vom 26. März 1901," in P. Müller, ed., *Bericht über die X. Konferenz für Idiotenpflege und Schulen für schwachbefähigte Kinder* (1901), 157–163 (Kirmsse-Sammlung, Universität Marburg); Karl Ziegler, "Nochmals," *Zeitschrift für die Behandlung Schwachsinniger und Epileptischer* 18.9-10 (September 1902), 146–156.

63. A lightning rod in the ensuing conflicts was psychiatrist Emil Kraepelin, who had even made a point of showing up at the directors' conference in Heidelberg in 1895. Conceding there that "doctors have until now had little occasion to concern themselves with idiocy," he also insisted (in contradiction to decades of countervailing opinion) that "idiots" were, after all, "a subset of the mentally ill," and that only doctors could ever "finally discover the means to cure idiocy" (*endlich die Heilmittel der Idiotie zu finden*). Above all: "The doctor must be given an authoritative position in the institution." Kraepelin's remarks as recorded by P. Müller, in the discussion following Krekeler's presentation "Die Stellung," in *Zeitschrift für die Behandlung Schwachsinniger und Epileptischer* 12.1-2 (February 1896), 6–7. Teacher A. Gündel from Rastenburg, who was also present at the Heidelberg gathering, remembered Kraepelin's comments slightly differently: "We physicians must take over the leadership in the idiot-institutions so as to conduct experiments about the nature of idiocy." Gündel quoting Kraepelin in Bradl, *Anfänge*, 545. It is perhaps not irrelevant that Kraepelin's first reaction to people with psychiatric diagnoses was one of personal repulsion. As he wrote in his memoirs about his earliest assignment in 1878: "The first impressions I had of my new job were discouraging. The bewildering throng of innumerable stupefied, sometimes inaccessible, sometimes meddlesome sick persons, with their ridiculous or disgusting, pitiful or dangerous peculiarities, the impotence of medical intervention, which usually had to be limited to greetings and the most rudimentary physical care, the utter bafflement in the face of all these manifestations of insanity for which no scientific comprehension can be found, let me feel the entire weight of the profession I had chosen." What ultimately helped was "the numbing effect of habit" and "pleasant contact with like-minded colleagues." Emil Kraepelin, *Lebenserinnerungen* (Berlin: Springer, 1983), 12–13.

64. Proto-delinquent youth and mentally disabled youth turned out to be at least partially overlapping constituencies, and an individual could easily be considered both. Already by 1904—just three years after the "welfare-care-training" law went into effect—Pastor Paul Stritter was seriously asking his peers: "Is it necessary to establish specialized institutions for the feebly-abled among the welfare-care trainees?" Another pastor in 1908 who worked with youth in the correctional training institutes stated unequivocally that "feeble-mindedness" was "prevalent among the vast majority." Paul Stritter, "Ist die Gründung von besonderen Anstalten für schwachbegabte Fürsorgezöglinge notwendig?," *Bericht über die Konferenz des Vereins für Erziehung, Unterricht und Pflege Geistesschwacher* (Halle: Carl Marhold, 1904), 130–145; Pastor

Backhausen, Stephansstift, quoted in "II. Psychiatrie und Fürsorgeerziehung," *Mitteilungen des evangelisch-kirchlichen Erziehungs-Vereins der Provinz Westfalen* 9.1-2 (January–February 1909), 2–13, here 10.

65. "Psychopathic inferiority" had first been formulated in 1888 by the psychiatrist Julius Ludwig August Koch to describe a subset of his adult patients. Then—via the detour of philosopher and pedagogue Ludwig von Strümpell—it would be promoted most avidly by the remedial pedagogue Johannes Trüper, director of a charity institution in the Thuringian city of Jena and from 1896 on also main editor of *Die Kinderfehler* (The Defects of Children), one of several newly flourishing and much-consulted journals dedicated to the topics of disability and its remediation. "Psychopathic inferiority," as Trüper understood it, was meant to give a name to any perceived "irregularities" (*Regelwidrigkeiten*)—a vague term if ever there was one—whether inborn or acquired (and notably, he did *not* presume a heritable aspect), in behavior and / or personality, that did not quite meet the definition of mental illness, but did not fully indicate the presence of mental disability, either, but which above all appeared to harbor the danger of a slide into crime, or at least a disorderly lifestyle, unemployment and idleness, and hence, again—as with various middling levels of mental disability—to warrant institutionalization, close observation, and dedicated training into good comportment and solid work habits. See Johannes Trüper, *Psychopathische Minderwertigkeiten im Kindesalter* (Gütersloh: Bertelsmann, 1893), 3; Schotte, "Jena," 113–116. Kraepelin would become one of the most emphatic promoters of the term "psychopathic inferiority" or, simply, "psychopath," but he used the concept more loosely and generically than even Trüper had. See in this context Greg Eghigian, "A Drifting Concept for an Unruly Menace: A History of Psychopathy in Germany," *Isis* 106.2 (2015), 283–309. Kraepelin was also the primary promoter of the terms "moral insanity" and "moral feeble-mindedness"—sometimes as a diagnosis unto itself, and sometimes (since Kraepelin kept shifting the pieces of his own classificatory systems) as a subset of "psychopathic inferiority." (The coinage "moral insanity" had been borrowed from the English physician J. C. Prichard, for whom—in 1835—the concept had been meant to designate an abnormality in the emotional-affective as opposed to the cognitive realm; for Kraepelin, however, the adapted concept signaled something amoral or immoral in the more generic sense, such as compulsive lying and disobedient, unruly, unreliable behavior, more akin to what is now more likely to be called sociopathy.) On "moral feeble-mindedness" as one subtype of "inborn feeble-mindedness," but also as characterized by ruthlessness, egotism, and mendaciousness, see Emil Kraepelin, *Psychiatrie: Ein kurzes Lehrbuch für Studirende und Aerzte*, 3rd rev. ed. (Leipzig: Ambr. Abel, 1889), 562–563, 568. On "moral imbecility, moral feeble-mindedness.... born criminal types" (*moralische Imbecillität, sittlichen Schwachsinn.... geborene Verbrechernaturen*), see Emil Kraepelin, *Einführung in die psychiatrische Klinik* (Leipzig: Johann Ambrosius Barth, 1901), 308. And on "moral insanity," "moral imbecility," the "born criminal," and "moral stupidity," see A. Ross Diefendorf, *Clinical Psychiatry: A Text-Book for Students and Physicians, Abstracted and Adapted from the Seventh German Edition of Kraepelin's* Lehrbuch der Psychiatrie (New York: Macmilllan, 1923), 516–517. On the blurry as well as continually more elastic boundaries of what would come to count as "slightly abnormal," see Wilhelm Weygandt, *Leicht abnorme Kinder* (Halle: Carl Marhold, 1905). By 1914, the extraordinary elasticity of "psychopathy" was unapologetically conceded in the same breath as its "congenital" (*angeborene*) nature was asserted. See Otto Klieneberger, *Über Pubertät und Psychopathie* (Wiesbaden: J. F. Bergmann, 1914), 9: "Psychopathy covers the broad area of psychic borderline states (*Grenzzustände*). Borderline in the sense that psychopaths can be counted as normal individuals, yet they show a number of points of contact with the mentally ill. I summarize here under psychopathy all the manifestations which have been described in the literature as psychopathic inferiorities, as psychopathic constitutions, as psychasthenia, instability and degeneration, to which hysteria and neurasthenia are also closely related. These are congenital impairments. Often these are individuals, burdened

by the alcoholism, syphilis, mental illness and other physical or psychic abnormalities of their parents, who, due to an inferior disposition or at least a lowered capacity for resistance, carry within themselves the disposition to nervous disorders." See also the excellent analysis in Wolfgang Rose, Petra Fuchs, and Thomas Beddies, *Diagnose "Psychopathie": Die urbane Moderne und das schwierige Kind. Berlin 1918–1933* (Vienna: Böhlau, 2016).

66. The absurdity is commented on repeatedly in "II. Psychiatrie und Fürsorgeerziehung," 10–12. By 1912, psychiatric language had been fully absorbed. A large and impressive overview volume produced on behalf of the directors' conferences, providing narrative profiles and photos of more than 50 institutions, would be unselfconsciously titled: *Deutsche Anstalten für Schwachsinnige, Epileptische und Psychopathische Jugendliche* (German Institutions for Feeble-Minded, Epileptics and Psychopathic Youth). "Psychopathy" had, in short, cohered into a generally recognized condition, with ever more elastically defined components. In 1913, for instance, a new institution for "psychopathic" boys founded in Templin was celebrated as providing "a home for those who have gone astray in their feeling- and drive-life, whose drive for acquisitiveness has degenerated into thievery, drive for power into crudeness and brutality, drive for play into work-shyness, drive for wandering into vagrancy, [and] sexual drive into vice and perversity." Gnerlich, "Templin. Einweihung des Psychopathenheims," *Die Hilfsschule* 6.10 (October 1913), 286–288, here 287.

67. For example: Already in 1904, A. Gündel, a teacher-director from East Prussia, expressed the hope that doctors, who "naturally would need to be given free hand," would indeed manage "finally to arrive . . . at illumination of the darkness that is idiocy, namely via the anatomical foundations of the entire condition." In 1911, writing in a pamphlet published by the Catholic Caritas, the Franciscan Brother Josaphat, director of an "idiot-institution" in Linz am Rhein, was openly calling for more psychiatric research. Favorably invoking Kraepelin, he opined: "Children should not be sitting before me as psychological mysteries. The simple diagnosis: 'feeble-minded' is far too humble for a remedial pedagogue to be satisfied with, if he wants to salvage whatever can be salvaged. Only then, when we have discovered the true essence, the true nature, the actual source of the mental defects . . . Then we will also avoid false hopes, save ourselves from disappointment, avoid harmful experimentation and trial and error." Both quoted in Bradl, *Anfänge*, 545, 557.

68. Schotte, "Jena," 114.

69. Disselhoff, *Die gegenwärtige Lage*, 164 (Disselhoff even spoke of "nine-tenths" as poor); Brandes, *Der Idiotismus*, 75; Tätzner, "Die Entstehung," 69. Physician-director Oswalt Berkhan observed at the 1886 directors' conference, as though it were just incontestable baseline data, that of all the children produced by the rich, approximately 2 percent would turn out to be intellectually disabled. But among the—obviously far more numerous—poor, the rate would be 8 percent of all births. Berkhan in Reichelt, *Bericht . . . 1886*, 33–34. As Berkhan put it: "Yes, if we could alleviate poverty, then untold misery [i.e. disability] could be prevented." Yet he conceded that the enactment of a poverty-mitigating political vision "is, evidently, a task only for the future" (34).

70. A classic early summary statement of this insight is found in an 1868 book by Friedrich Barthold (brother of Sengelmann's frequent collaborator Karl Barthold and teacher-director at the Kuckenmühle institution in Stettin): *Der Idiotismus und seine Bekämpfung: Ein Beitrag zur praktischen Lösung der Idiotenfrage* (Stettin: Von der Nahmer, 1868), 27–28. Note also the remarks of teacher-director Hermann Josef Ochs at the Catholic Franz Sales Haus in Essen in 1881, who reported about the majority of his pupils that "the imbecility in most cases is not inborn [*nicht angeboren*], but rather must be seen as a result of untreated childhood diseases like encephalitis and meningitis [*Gehirnentzündung und Genickkrampf*]." Ochs quoted in Bradl, *Anfänge*, 366.

71. County school inspector Weichert in "Debatte," *Zeitschrift für die Behandlung Schwachsinniger und Epileptischer* 15.1 (January 1899), 16–20, here 18.

72. Discussed in Max Kirmsse, "Der Schwachsinnige und seine Stellung im Kulturleben der Vergangenheit und der Gegenwart," *Zeitschrift für die Behandlung Schwachsinniger* 42.6 (June 1922), 81–88, 103–110, here 86–88.

73. Indicatively, this reaction of Luther's was quoted and discussed by Sengelmann in 1885 in the context of grappling with the proposals of people in his own era who considered themselves "very enlightened" calling for individuals with severe disabilities to be killed. Sengelmann, "Gegen Luther," in *Idiotophilus*, vol. 3, 103–104.

74. John Locke, for instance, placed "idiots"—revealingly, he used the term interchangeably with "changelings"—as lesser than "savages," on a level with baboons, parrots, dogs. Stacy Clifford, "The Capacity Contract: Locke, Disability, and the Political Exclusion of 'Idiots,'" *Politics, Groups, and Identities* 2.1 (2014), 90–103.

75. Damerow, "Zur Cretinen- und Idiotenfrage," 505, 507–508. In the 1830s, Damerow had proposed that among cretins, "the spirit of the mind and the human soul do not exist" and that "they are more or less similar to and related to the aberrant types of the lowest human race"— and went on to compare cretins with the Papuans of New Guinea and with monkeys. Heinrich Damerow, "Ueber den Cretinismus in anthropologischer Hinsicht," *Medizinische Zeitung* 3.9 (1834), 39–40 and 3.10 (1834), 43–45. See also Horst Isermann, "Der Psychiater Heinrich Damerow (1798–1866) und sein Verhältnis zur Geistigen Behinderung," *Schriftenreihe der Deutschen Gesellschaft für Geschichte der Nervenheilkunde* 14 (2008), 135–142, here 137.

76. Key initiative came from the zoologist Ernst Haeckel. In 1868, in his popular textbook *Natürliche Schöpfungsgeschichte* (Natural History of Creation), Haeckel pointed to the ancient city-state of Sparta for inspiration, assuring readers that not only had its citizens left weak or deformed newborns out to die (in an uncanny echo with the folk mythologies justifying exposure of "changelings" on the grounds that then the fairies would take them back), but this habit had strengthened the Spartan race over the generations. The originality, in short, was that Haeckel claimed to find a causal connection between "euthanasia" and (what would soon be called) eugenics:

> Among the Spartans all newly born children were subject to a careful examination or selection. All those that were weak, sickly or affected with any bodily infirmity, were killed. Only the perfectly healthy and vigorous children were allowed to remain alive, and they alone later succeeded in procreation. Thus the Spartan race was not only preserved in exquisite strength and efficiency, but with each generation its physical perfection was increased. Certainly the people of Sparta owe their rare degree of manly strength and rugged heroism largely to this artificial selection or breeding. Häckel, quoted in Schmuhl, *Rassenhygiene*, 32.

Acute awareness that they had to form rebuttals to the death wishes is evident among directors and teachers at residential institutions: Sengelmann, "Gegen Luther"; Dr. med. Habermas, Inspektor Pfarrer Strebel, Oekonomieverwalter Bräuninger, *Neunundvierzigster Jahresbericht der Heil- und Pflegeanstalt für Schwachsinnige und Epileptische in Stetten i.R.* (Schorndorf: C.W. Mayer, 1897), 9–10 (these authors introduce the summary term "murder-thoughts" (*Mordgedanken*), and attempt an emphatic, heartfelt rebuke); and Karl Ziegler, "Über den Lebenszweck der Blödsinnigen," *Zeitschrift für die Behandlung Schwachsinniger und Epileptischer* 16.9-10 (October 1900): 156–163.

77. Otto Ernst [originally Otto Ernst Schmidt], "Ein Besuch," *Gedichte* (Leipzig: L. Staackmann, 1902), 132–138, here 135. That severe disability *did* raise significant doubts and confusion about God, Heaven, souls, bodies, and the purpose of care-provision—that the confrontation with disability was, around 1900, proving to be an especially vulnerable spot in the inherited edifice of Christian faith—is manifest with especially painful clarity in the muddled musings laid out in Ziegler, "Über den Lebenszweck der Blödsinnigen."

78. Heymann, responding to a talk by the Liberal politician Heinz Potthoff, quoted and discussed in "Fortschrittliche Damen," *Der alte Glaube* 9.7 (November 15, 1907), 163–165, here 164.

79. Friedrich Nietzsche, *Die fröhliche Wissenschaft*, in Nietzsche, *Werke in drei Bänden* (Munich, 1954), 84–85.

80. Adolf Jost, *Das Recht auf den Tod* (Göttingen: Dieterich, 1895), 6, 26.

81. Alfred Ploetz, *Die Tüchtigkeit unsrer Rasse und der Schutz der Schwachen* (Berlin: S. Fischer, 1895), esp. 5–8, 61–65, 143–147. At this point, Ploetz still expressed anti-antisemitic views, believing that Jews had intermarried especially effectively over the centuries, and that "the high mental capacity of the Jews and their prominent role in the developmental process of humanity must in view of the names Jesus, Spinoza, Marx be acknowledged with joy and no hesitation" (141); he would later change his mind. It has been said—though it is not verifiable—that Ploetz's book was among Hitler's prison readings; certainly Ploetz's proposals would prove notably inspirational for Nazis' efforts to reorganize sexual and reproductive mores and politics.

82. Martin Breitbarth, "Die Wechselbeziehungen zwischen geistiger Minderwertigkeit und sozialem Elend," *Die Hilfsschule* 8.11 (November 1915): 236–246, 259–264, here 236–237. The talk was initially addressed to an "Association for the maintenance and multiplication of the German Volk-strength" (*Bund zur Erhaltung und Mehrung der deutschen Volkskraft*).

83. Breitbarth, "Die Wechselbeziehungen," 237, 240, 242, 264.

84. This was hardly original with Breitbarth, but rather came straight from Kraepelin, who noted that causation was inevitably unclear and yet insisted that mental illness and mental disability were hereditarily linked—invoking the teachings on degeneration of French psychiatrist Bénédict Augustin Morel. See Kraepelin, *Psychiatrie*, 61–63. On Morel's influence on Kraepelin, see Roelcke, *Krankheit und Kulturkritik*. That Morel, for his part, actually had a quite differentiated understanding of the continually complex interplay of environmental and somatic factors and that in the nineteenth century in both France and Germany references to transgenerational "inheritance" and "predisposition" had consistently taken the possible impact of milieux and toxins into account, is well explained in Caroline Arni, *Of Human Born: Fetal Lives 1800–1950* (New York: Zone Books, 2024), esp. 130–133 and 224–227; and J. Andrew Mendelsohn, "Medicine and the Making of Bodily Inequality in Twentieth-Century Europe," in Jean-Paul Gaudillière and Ilana Löwy, eds., *Heredity and Infection: The History of Disease Transmission* (London: Routledge, 2001), 21–79, here 43–44.

85. Breitbarth, "Die Wechselbeziehungen," 239.

86. Breitbarth, "Die Wechselbeziehungen," 239–241. On the concept of "poverty porn" as critically described in present-day parlance, see Nathalie Dortonne, "The Dangers of Poverty Porn," *CNN Health* (December 8, 2016), https://www.cnn.com/2016/12/08/health/poverty -porn-danger-feat/index.html; Jennifer Lentfer, "Yes, Charities Want to Make an Impact. But Poverty Porn Is Not the Way to Do It," *The Guardian* (January 12, 2018), https://www .theguardian.com/voluntary-sector-network/2018/jan/12/charities-stop-poverty-porn -fundraising-ed-sheeran-comic-relief.

87. Breitbarth, "Die Wechselbeziehungen," 261.

88. Breitbarth, "Die Wechselbeziehungen," 239.

89. Breitbarth, "Die Wechselbeziehungen," 239.

90. Breitbarth, "Die Wechselbeziehungen," 244, 262–264.

91. Eleven years later, Breitbarth would say at the 1926 national gathering of the association of remedial school professionals: "The complete economic collapse, the immiseration of the entire population, the downfall [*Untergang*] of our Volk is bound to occur in the not too distant future, if we do not succeed in reducing the number of unproductive people to a tolerable level." Quoted and contextualized in Sieglind Ellger-Rüttgardt, "Hilfsschulpädagogik und Nationalsozialismus—Traditionen, Kontinuitäten, Einbrüche. Zur Berufsideologie der Hilfsschullehrerschaft im Kaiserreich und in der Weimarer Republik," *Pädagogik und*

Nationalsozialismus (Weinheim: Beltz, 1988), 147–165, here 157. The full text is Martin Breitbarth, "Die Berufs- und Erwerbsfähigkeit des Hilfsschülers," *Bericht über den XI. Verbandstag der Hilfsschulen Deutschlands zu München* (Halle, 1927), 47–67, here 50. Here also Breitbarth reminded listeners of the importance of keeping the "completely unemployable feeble-minded" in institutions, where the "more usable" (*brauchbareren*) among them could help to make institutional life more economic, and where they would not be tempted "to transfer their inferiority to the coming generation and through the multiplication of the feeble-minded contribute to the enlargement of the crisis of our Volk" (64).

92. For the city of Halle, Breitbarth had estimated that there were 2,000 individuals afflicted by "mental deficiency" out of a population of 200,000, i.e., 1 in a 100. Breitbarth, "Die Wechselbeziehungen," 237. In 1907, the remedial pedagogue Alwin Schenk had calculated that in his city of Breslau, 950 children had mental disabilities in an overall municipal population of 470,000. From this he went on to extrapolate that across the German lands, approximately 3 of every 10,000 in every birth year were mentally disabled, 18,000 per birth year (times 33 birth years for a total of 594,000) in an overall population of 60 million. Again, this came close to an estimate of 1 in 100 and was a group as large, Schenk noted, as "the standing army." He estimated that there were another 15,000 per birth year with mental disability in a population of 50 million in Austria-Hungary. See Alwin Schenk, "Die soziale Bedeutung der Hilfsschule," *Eos* 3.1 (1907), 17–22, here 19–20. However, Schenk's aim throughout these calculations was to underscore the value of remedial schooling and to call for yet more assistance for these individuals ("serious reflection and energetic love"), not to call for efforts to reduce their numbers. In less than a decade, the meanings of numbers had changed.

93. In 1914, physician Benno Laquer surveyed the state of debate around "The Degeneration-Question in Germany," and although he deliberately left open the question "Are we degenerated, does our race, our populace . . . require improvement," he also provided an overview of different estimates given by various authors with regard to the percentage of the German population that was deemed to be either "feeble-minded," "imbecilic," or "idiotic"—and found the range to be between 0.54% and 1.16%. (The number of "feebly-abled" children, meanwhile, was thought to be yet higher: between 13.1% and 14.7%.) In another calculation—here Laquer relied on the estimates of Alfred Grotjahn's *Soziale Pathologie* of 1912—if one considered the number of "mentally ill and idiots," "epileptics," "alcoholics," as well as individuals with sensory impairments of sight or hearing and those with tendencies toward asociality or criminality (for "2 / 3" of all of these, Laquer averred, their "inferiority was inherited"), then the evident conclusion, Laquer asserted, was that "One will therefore not go wrong, if one refers to an average rate of 1.5%–2% of the inhabitants of Germany as *permanently* substandard and *permanently* unsuitable for the production of offspring." Benno Laquer, *Eugenik und Dysgenik: Ein Versuch* (Wiesbaden: J. F. Bergmann, 1914), 22, 35–36. Emphases in the original. By 1933, when the Nazis were formulating their sterilization law, the estimates with regard to what percentage of the population should be sterilized would range from 10 to 20 percent and beyond. See, e.g., Fritz Lenz, *Menschliche Auslese und Rassenhygiene*, 3rd ed. (Munich: J. F. Lehmanns, 1931), 272–273; and the critical discussion in Paul Althaus, "'Unwertes' Leben im Lichte christlichen Glaubens," in Hans Meyer and Hans Duncker, eds., *"Von der Verhütung unwerten Lebens": Ein Zyklus von 5 Vorträgen* (*Bremer Beiträge zur Naturwissenschaft*, Sonderband 1933), 79–97, here 90–92.

Chapter Two: Love, Money, Murder

1. "Warum sind wir Brüder?" *Bote von Bethel* 31 (1902), 11–16, here 11–13. Emphasis added. In case either the corporeal or the emotional intensity of intellectual disability care and the imperative of recognizing the personhood of the individual being cared for was not clear enough to readers, von Bodelschwingh added his own experiences. "Do . . . the poor imbecile little ones

attach themselves to us?—Oh yes, they do, like burrs, and we must pull them to us, whether we like it or not, even if the mouth drips with saliva, and other infirmities make them very repugnant. . . . For by their guileless, heartfelt trust they force us to love." Moreover: "If one of these smallest ones turns away with the instinctive feeling: 'He doesn't love me back,' then we feel inwardly judged, quickly we lift the aggrieved little friend onto our lap: 'Hans I love you.'" The whole essay was, of course, a comment on the incident in the Gospel of John 9:1–3 in which Jesus rebukes his disciples for their assumption about the connections between disability and sin. The disciples had asked: "Rabbi, who sinned, this man or his parents, that he was born blind?" And Jesus replied: "Neither this man nor his parents sinned, but this happened so that the works of God might be displayed in him." An early version of some of the material in this chapter first appeared in Irene Kacandes, ed., *On Being Adjacent to Historical Violence* (Berlin: De Gruyter, 2022), 69–88; De Gruyter's permission to reuse this material is gratefully acknowledged here.

2. "Our Hans," quoted in Ludwig Schlaich, *Vernichtung und Neuanfang: Das Schicksal der Heil- und Pflegeanstalt in Stetten i. R., Anstalt der Inneren Mission, und ihrer Schwachsinnigen und Epileptischen während des Krieges und der Wiedereröffnung der Anstalt* (Stuttgart: Quell-Verlag, 1946), 5.

3. On the multiple intersections of "euthanasia" and the Holocaust, see: Annette Hinz-Wessels, "Antisemitismus und Krankenmord: Zum Umgang mit jüdischen Anstaltspatienten im Nationalsozialismus," *Vierteljahrshefte für Zeitgeschichte* 61.1 (2013), 65–92; Jörg Osterloh and Jan Erik Schulte, eds., *"Euthanasie" und Holocaust: Kontinuitäten, Kausalitäten, Parallelitäten* (Paderborn: Schöningh, 2021); Jörg Osterloh, Jan Erik Schulte, and Sybille Steinbacher, eds., *"Euthanasie"-Verbrechen im besetzten Europa: Zur Dimension des nationalsozialistischen Massenmords* (Göttingen: Wallstein, 2022). For basic orientation on the "euthanasia" killings, see the powerful classic studies in English: Michael Burleigh, *Death and Deliverance: "Euthanasia" in Germany c. 1900–45* (Cambridge, UK: Cambridge University Press, 1994); Henry Friedlander, *The Origins of Nazi Genocide: From Euthanasia to the Final Solution* (Chapel Hill: University of North Carolina Press, 1995). For the best overview of more recent research findings, see Uwe Kaminsky, "Die NS-Euthanasie: Ein Forschungsüberblick," in Klaus D. Henke, ed., *Tödliche Medizin im Nationalsozialismus: Von der Rassenhygiene zum Massenmord* (Köln: Böhlau, 2008), 269–290. See also the important fresh analyses in Götz Aly, *Die Belasteten: "Euthanasie" 1939–1945. Eine Gesellschaftsgeschichte* (Frankfurt / Main: Fischer, 2013); and Edith Sheffer, *Asperger's Children: The Origins of Autism in Nazi Vienna* (New York: W. W. Norton, 2018).

4. Impressive evidence of pride and confidence is collected in the handsome anthology ecumenically presenting dozens of Protestant and Catholic institutions (as well as one Jewish one): Paul Stritter and Ewald Meltzer, eds., *Deutsche Anstalten für Schwachsinnige, Epileptische und Psychopathische Jugendliche* (Halle: Carl Marhold, 1912).

5. On the pecking order between the physically and the mentally impaired, see Carol Poore, "Recovering Disability Rights in Weimar Germany," *Radical History Review* 94 (Winter 2006), 38–58; and Sieglind Ellger-Rüttgardt, *Geschichte der Sonderpädagogik*, 2nd ed. (Munich: Ernst Reinhardt, 2019), 278–290. For significant analyses of disabled veterans' self-advocacy during the Weimar years, see Greg Eghigian, *Making Security Social: Disability, Insurance, and the Birth of the Social Entitlement State in Germany* (Ann Arbor: University of Michigan Press, 2000); Deborah A. Cohen, *The War Come Home: Disabled Veterans in Britain and Germany* (Berkeley: University of California Press, 2001); Carol Poore, "Disability in the Culture of the Weimar Republic," in *Disability in Twentieth-Century German Culture* (Ann Arbor: University of Michigan Press, 2007), 1–66.

6. Friedrich Lensch, "Dennoch!," *Briefe und Bilder aus Alsterdorf* 55–56 (1931–32): 2–5, here 3.

7. For example, for Hadamar, see Monika Daum, "Arbeit und Zwang, das Leben der Hadamarer Patienten im Schatten des Todes," in Dorothee Roer and Dieter Henkel, eds., *Psychiatrie im Faschismus: Die Anstalt Hadamar 1933–1945* (Bonn: Psychiatrie-Verlag, 1986), 173–213. In

February 1943, in the midst of the second, decentralized murder phase at Hadamar, the head doctor, Adolf Wahlmann, wrote with special satisfaction to his superior Fritz Bernotat that all of the shoe repair and the sewing at the institution was already being done by patients, with no staff supervision needed at all, that a number of the grounds crews had patients as foremen (and there had been "no complaint"), that indeed an impressive 142 of the 171 male patients then in the clinic were steadily providing labor and, moreover, that "the fact that we have recently had patients take care of duties at the gate proves that we are endeavoring, wherever possible, to save personnel and thereby free up forces for the given tasks [i.e. "euthanasia"]. . . . Heil Hitler." Letter from Dr. Wahlmann to Landesrat Bernotat, February 22, 1943, reprinted in Gerhard Kneuker and Wulf Steglich, *Begegnungen mit der Euthanasie in Hadamar* (Rehburg-Loccum: Psychiatrie-Verlag, 1985), 99–100.

8. Also in the UK and the United States, the prospect of using a "lethal chamber" or of killing individuals with significant intellectual impairments, whether newborn or long-term institutionalized, by other means, was openly aired (and acquired support from such prominent figures as George Bernard Shaw and Helen Keller). But in neither nation did the idea gain the traction it would in post–World War I Germany. See Ian Dowbiggan, *A Concise History of Euthanasia: Life, Death, God, and Medicine* (Lanham, MD: Rowman & Littlefield, 2005); Volker Roelcke, "International and German Eugenics from ca. 1880 up to the Post-World War II Period: Medical Expertise—Political Ambition—Relations to Euthanasia in the Nazi Context," in Sheldon Rubenfeld and Daniel P. Sulmasy, eds., *Physician-Assisted Suicide and Euthanasia: Before, During, and After the Holocaust* (London: Lexington Books, 2020), 45–58. For the United States, note also the case of Chicago physician Harry Haiselden, who made the news recurrently in the 1910s for advocating deliberate non-treatment of newborns with disabilities. E.g., see "Surgeon Lets Baby, Born to Idiocy, Die," *New York Times*, July 25, 1917, 11.

9. Karl Binding and Alfred Hoche, *Die Freigabe der Vernichtung lebensunwerten Lebens: Ihr Maß und ihre Form* (Leipzig: Felix Meinen, 1920), 31–32, 53–55, 57. The text further expounded on a concept of "affection-value" (*Affektionswert*). The most severely disabled, the text argued, had no such value. Binding and Hoche distinguished here between long-beloved persons who in old age had lost their mental faculties to dementia and those who were from the start "on an intellectual level that we only find again very low down in the ranks of animals." The former group deserved to live until a natural death took them; the latter group should be helped into an early grave. The difference, Hoche said, was akin to that to be found between "the stone wreckage of a collapsed building" and "a random pile of stones lying around, on which no forming hand has ever lain"; the "total idiots," he further warned, might require care for the duration of "two generations or more." In Binding's words, the lives of such beings were "absolutely purposeless," although they themselves "do not experience them as unbearable." Binding suggested that the right to make a formal application to have these individuals killed should be granted to parents (or guardians)—but he also proposed in passing that *if* a mother wanted to keep such a child and was willing to take the responsibility for its care entirely on herself, she should be given the right of veto. Nonetheless, the main proposal endorsed by both men was for a commission (composed ideally of two physicians and one lawyer) which would be tasked by the state to evaluate which individuals were to be slain.

10. Binding and Hoche, *Die Freigabe der Vernichtung lebensunwerten Lebens*, 6.

11. Hermann Büchsel, "Euthanasie," *Aufwärts* 280 (30 November 1926), reissued 1927 as an offprint (and warmly recommended for education of deaconesses), Hauptarchiv der v. Bodelschwinghsche Stiftungen Bethel Kl. Erwerb. 189, 1–4, here 1. Also at the Alsterdorfer Anstalten in Hamburg (in 1927 under the director of Pastor Paul Stritter), this essay had been reprinted and recommended to the staff.

12. Sengelmann, 1871, quoted in Uwe Gleßmer und Alfred Lampe, *Mit-Leiden an Alsterdorf und seinen Geschichtsbildern von den Anstalten* (Norderstedt: Books on Demand, 2019); Heinrich

Matthias Sengelmann, *Idiotophilus. Systematisches Lehrbuch der Idioten-Heilpflege* (Soltau: Norden, 1885). At his death in 1899, there were 600 individuals with disabilities of various types living in the Alsterdorfer Anstalten, along with 140 staff.

13. Sengelmann's conference-concluding remarks in "III. Hauptversammlung," in E. Reichelt, ed., *Bericht über die V. Konferenz für das Idiotenwesen. Frankfurt a. M., vom 14.-16. September 1886* (Dresden: Kgl. Hofbuchhandlung von Hermann Burdach, 1886), 35–46, here 46.

14. "Die Du mir beschieden, / Man hat sie hienieden / Betrachtet wohl oft als den Kehricht der Welt; / Mir hat Dein Erbarmen / Die Aermsten der Armen / Als Deine Kleinode vor Augen gestellt." From Heinrich Matthias Sengelmann, *Abendklänge* (1894), reprinted on the inside cover of Hans-Walter Schmuhl and Ulrike Winkler, *Heinrich Matthias Sengelmann (1821–1899) und die Anfänge der Evangelischen Stiftung Alsterdorf* (Hamburg: Evangelische Stiftung Alsterdorf, 2021).

15. Friedrich von Bodelschwingh, "Christlicher Ratgeber für Epileptische," in *Friedrich von Bodelschwingh: Ausgewählte Schriften, Band II: Veröffentlichungen aus den Jahren 1872 bis 1910,* Alfred Adam, ed. (Bethel bei Bielefeld: Verlagshandlung der Anstalt Bethel, 1964), 67–82. Another feature of his piety was distinctive to his own searing experience of loss: In the course of two weeks, in January 1869, just a few years before he became the director of Bethel, he and his wife Ida had lost all four of their young children to diphtheria. Although in due time four more children (three sons and a daughter) would be born, this experience of catastrophic bereavement and sense of death's perpetual proximity intensified von Bodelschwingh's concern with obedience and deference to God's will. Hans-Walter Schmuhl, *Friedrich von Bodelschwingh* (Reinbek: Rowohlt Taschenbuch Verlag, 2005).

16. Three typical examples: Paul Althaus, "'Unwertes' Leben im Lichte christlichen Glaubens," in Hans Meyer and Hans Duncker, eds., *"Von der Verhütung unwerten Lebens": Ein Zyklus von 5 Vorträgen* (*Bremer Beiträge zur Naturwissenschaft*, Sonderband 1933), 79–97; Lensch, "Dennoch!," 5; Karl Stoevesandt, "Wann ist Leben 'lebenswert'?," *Aufwärts* 15.26 (January 31, 1933), 1–2, here 2.

17. See especially the insightful analyses in Matthias Benad, "Heilsanstalt Bethel: Sterbefrömmigkeit im 'Boten von Bethel' 1894–1900," *Theion* 7 (1996), 39–48; and Matthias Benad, "Religiöse Grundlagen," in Matthias Benad and Hans-Walter Schmuhl, eds., *Bethel-Eckardtsheim: Von der Gründung der ersten deutschen Arbeiterkolonie bis zur Auflösung als Teilanstalt (1882–2001)* (Stuttgart: Kohlhammer, 2006), 36–70. A typical message to his staff and to his wider reading public emphasized self-effacing humility and service: "Keep company with those at the bottom; the lowliest path is the safest, the most blessed path." (*Haltet Euch herunter zu den Niedrigen; der unterste Weg ist der sicherste, der seligste Weg.*) "Warum sind wir Brüder?," 11. (Whether this was an original concept coined by von Bodelschwingh or whether he "borrowed" it from the first head deaconess at the Bethel-linked deaconess training institution Sarepta, Emilie Heuser, can no longer be clarified. Church historian Ute Gause reports that Heuser's motto in life was: "I have always found that the lowliest path is the safest" and that this then "became a common saying within the deaconesses' institution." Ute Gause, *Töchter Sareptas: Diakonissenleben zwischen Selbstverleugnung und Selbstbehauptung* (Leipzig: Evangelische Verlagsanstalt, 2019), 20.)

18. Those working at Bethel were certainly not unaware that its defense of the value of disabled life was under attack. An example of the tenuous hold of the Hippocratic Oath among some doctors was evident as early as 1910 in frank remarks made by physician Walter Steinbiss, who joined the staff at Bethel to work in the on-site laboratory. Due to the extremity of his views, he did not last long and was encouraged to leave. But the remarks he made already upon receiving a tour—to the effect that hospitals for the disabled, in this case epileptics, were really not needed—was a sign of things to come. His reasoning? Because: "One or two spoonfuls of hydrocyanic acid [poison] would suffice" and, further (as Hermann Feldmann, the staff physician giving him a tour of the premises, recalled), "he was a[n] anatomic pathologist and could

not suppress the thought whenever he saw a sick person: 'Hopefully I will be soon getting your brain.'" Steinbiss quoted and paraphrased by Hermann Feldmann, "Denkschrift zu meinem Antrag vom 23. Januar 1910," Hauptarchiv Bethel, Akte 1-C 18h. On the Feldmann-Steinbiss conflict, see also Hans-Walter Schmuhl, *Ärzte in der Anstalt Bethel 1870–1945* (Bielefeld: Bethel-Verlag, 1998), 23–25.

19. The first example of what would become a regular genre is the photo with accompanying story about Käthe, clearly a favorite of von Bodelschwingh the elder, her caregiver deaconesses, and her peers: "Carmels Sonnenschein," *Bote von Bethel*, no. 15 (1898), 1–8 and photo on the back cover.

20. "Ein kleiner Prediger der Zufriedenheit," *Bote von Bethel*, no. 54 (1908), 10–16. Consigned to his bed with a tiny crippled body and paralyzed limbs and "the little hands with the long fingers" that "are so slender, weak, and chilled!," Christian M. had come to Bethel at age three, and by time of the story was twenty-one. "So he lies [for twelve years already in Nebo, one of Bethel's hospitals] in his child's bed, from year to year, and many a one who walks past him might think: Why does God permit this?" And yet: "His life is rich in joys . . . : he can rejoice and he can be thankful. Thankful people are always satisfied people. . . . He knows no fear and knows nothing of cares. . . . Only one thing the little heart demands: it yearns for love. He knows the Brother Deacon who cares for him exactly. . . . [His] dark eyes light up when the Brother can stay a bit by his bed and has some time to play with Christian. These games are of a very simple sort: a key-chain that one can drop through his sleeve, and then pull out again at his neck" (pp. 12–14). Without question a controlling paternalism toward an individual with severe disabilities is manifest here—as is didacticism toward the reader. But it is nonetheless of decisive significance that the von Bodelschwinghs, the son like the father, articulated deep love and appreciation for Christian in his unique individuality. Another especially significant example of a photo-story in the same year as that of Christian M. concerns the forty-four-year-old Margarete, whose decades of heavy epileptic seizures had damaged her cognition and made her deeply shy and withdrawn and who clutched a handful of wooden spools tightly at all times. "'Er liebt auch mich,'" *Bote von Bethel*, no. 57 (1908), 1–8.

21. In later years, stories especially popular with readers (who sent gifts and awaited regular updates on their doings) concerned the good friends Fritzchen and Mariechen, like Margarete residents of Patmos, the house in Bethel for the children (or very occasionally, as in Margarete's case, also adults) with the most severe disabilities. In his reports on Fritzchen and Mariechen, Fritz von Bodelschwingh articulated most directly the core idea for which Bethel stood. Describing Christmas in Patmos, he wrote: "There they sat again around the tree, all the ill children who with their seizures so often sink into the darkness and of whom so many are additionally lame or mute, blind or crippled. Most of them cannot learn anything and for this life they are wholly useless. There is only one thing that they can all do: to let themselves be loved and to be joyful." "Wie Fritzchen und Mariechen Weihnachten feierten," *Bote von Bethel*, no. 89 (1917), 7–14, here 9.

22. "Reise durch Bethels Geschichte," https://www.bethel.de/ueber-bethel/geschichte /zeitstrahl; Uwe Kaminsky, *Zwangssterilisation und "Euthanasie" im Rheinland: Evangelische Erziehungsanstalten sowie Heil- und Pflegeanstalten, 1933–1945* (Köln: Rheinland-Verlag, 1995), 53–59, 634–35; Lutz Kaelber, "Jewish Children with Disabilities and Nazi 'Euthanasia' Crimes," *Bulletin of the Carolyn and Leonard Miller Center for Holocaust Studies* 17 (Spring 2013), 1, 17–23; Hans-Ludwig Siemen, *Menschen blieben auf der Strecke: Psychiatrie und Nationalsozialismus* (Gütersloh: Jakob van Hoddis, 1987), 29–33.

23. Karl Bonhoeffer quoted (and interpreted and contextualized divergently) in Michael Seidel and Klaus-Jürgen Neumärker, "Karl Bonhoeffer und seine Stellung zur Sterilisierungsgesetzgebung," in Arbeitsgruppe zur Erforschung der Geschichte der Karl-Bonhoeffer-Nervenklinik, ed., *Totgeschwiegen 1933–1945: Zur Geschichte der Wittenauer Heilstätten seit 1957*

Karl-Bonhoeffer Nervenklinik (Berlin: Edition Hentrich, 1989), 269–282, here 270; and Uwe Gerrens, *Medizinisches Ethos und Theologische Ethik: Karl und Dietrich Bonhoeffer in der Auseinandersetzung um Zwangssterilisation und "Euthanasie" im Nationalsozialismus* (Munich: Oldenbourg, 1996), 63.

24. In addition to the provocation provided by their own text, an even more intemperate follow-up diatribe published in 1924 by the self-appointed Nietzsche-apostle and flagrant antisemite Gerhard Hoffmann (under the pseudonym Ernst Mann), articulated the urgency of killing the disabled even more forcefully. While Hoffmann in no way had the high professional prestige enjoyed by Binding and Hoche in their respective disciplines, the esteem in which *they* were held made his fulminations appear less chaotically wacky than they otherwise might have. Reflections on animal rights, artistic genius, and the dangers of communism jostled with phantasmatic conjurings of the "unnatural" sexual activities engaged in within "idiot-institutions." It was unacceptable, Hoffmann averred, that in the wake of "the collapse of 1918 . . . thousands of healthy, gifted children were abandoned to misery and impoverishment, in order to keep the mentally dead and felons alive." The "moral principles" that the "annihilation of life unworthy of life" supposedly violated were really not so inviolable, Hoffmann assured his readers, and he endorsed the idea that commissions of doctors should comb through all institutions to choose those who would be "consigned to painless annihilation." Ernst Mann [Gerhard Hoffmann], *Die Wohltätigkeit als aristokratische und rassenhygienische Forderung* (Weimar: Fritz Fink, 1924), 69–70, 72, 164. Far from simply ignoring Hoffmann, reviewers responding critically to Binding and Hoche engaged with Hoffmann's message as well, interpreting it (rightly) as an amplifier. Another enthusiastic follow-up author, taking the opportunity of the newly disinhibited atmosphere, was a municipal politician in the city of Liegnitz. Writing in a criminal justice periodical, he not only outlined his own preferred wording for a prospective law that would enable efficient disposition of applications for killing specifically those "mentally weak" persons who were "incurable," but also proposed that Binding and Hoche's numerical calculations were underestimations of the scope of the problem. According to his own quick math, in the German population of 60 million citizens, there were 83,400 imbeciles (13.9 percent). "If one calculates only 50% of these as unworthy of life, then 41,700 imbeciles are still left, who will be cared for their whole life long due to a false feeling of humanitarianism, without ever achieving anything productive for the whole." The author was disappointed about this remaining burden, but delighted to daydream about what could be done with the saved funds: old-age homes, adult education centers, orphanages. Martin Borchardt, Liegnitz, "Die Freigabe der Vernichtung lebensunwerten Lebens," *Deutsche Strafrechts-Zeitung* 9.7-8 (July–August 1922), 206–210, here 207–208.

25. In fact, he went on to say that "the suggestion always again heard, to get rid of these 'valueless existences' with a sufficient dose of morphine, can under current economic conditions hardly be justified"—pointing out, however awkwardly, that the disabled were at least, in a time of agricultural overproduction and reduced sales volumes, helping the economy in their function as "consumers" (*Konsumenten*). Lensch, "Dennoch!," 3.

26. Lensch, "Dennoch!," 2–5.

27. On conceptions of "biopolitics" and arguments developed by Foucault in 1975–1976 about "racism against the abnormal," see Michel Foucault, *Il faut défendre la société: cours au Collège de France, 1975–1976* (Paris: Gallimard / Seuil, 1997); Michel Foucault, *Les anormaux: cours au Collège de France, 1974–1975* (Paris: Gallimard / Seuil, 1999); Kim Su Rasmussen, "Foucault's Genealogy of Racism," *Theory, Culture and Society* 28.5 (September 2011), 34–51; and Bernard E. Harcourt, "Racism against the Abnormal" (5 / 13) and "'Society Must be Defended'" (6 / 13), both in *13 / 13: Michel Foucault's Collège de France Lectures (1970–1984)*, https://blogs.law .columbia.edu/foucault1313/513-2/ and https://blogs.law.columbia.edu/foucault1313/613-2/. For compelling reflections on the need to stop treating "racism" and "economic considerations"

as competing and instead integrate them in our understanding of Nazism—with evidence drawn from the Austrian case—see Herwig Czech, "Nazi Medical Crimes, Eugenics, and the Limits of the Racial State Paradigm," in Devin Pendas et al., eds., *Beyond the Racial State: Rethinking Nazi Germany* (New York: Cambridge University Press, 2017), 213–238; cf., on France, Paul-André Rosental, *A Human Garden: French Policy and the Transatlantic Legacies of Eugenic Experimentation* (New York: Berghahn, 2019).

28. Hans Harmsen quoted in Dirk Lampe, "Die Beiträge des Arztes Ewald Meltzer (Großhennersdorf) zur Debatte um Sterilisierung und Euthanasie (ca. 1914 bis 1939)" (Dissertation, Medizinische Hochschule Hannover, 1998), 30.

29. Karl Ernst Thrändorf, Ludwig Lemme, and Arthur Titius quoted in Ewald Meltzer, *Das Problem der Abkürzung "lebensunwerten" Lebens* (Halle: Carl Marhold, 1925), 78, 81, 82. Lemme's "biblical Pietism" in Paul Honigsheim, *The Unknown Max Weber*, ed. Alan Sica (London; New York: Routledge, 2017), 224–225. Titius said that, unlike nature, which sometimes produced mistakes, God was directed toward perfection. Thus, he wrote that if caregiving staff had tried, but "had the experience of being unable to awaken and nurture the personal life of an idiot, then one cannot in this case speak of a crime against a person." Titius, incidentally, soon thereafter was one of Dietrich Bonhoeffer's teachers. See the entry in the Dietrich Bonhoeffer website portal: https://www.dietrich-bonhoeffer.net/bonhoeffer -umfeld/arthur-titius/.

30. Büchsel, "Euthanasie," 2.

31. Martin Ulbrich, *Dürfen wir minderwertiges Leben vernichten? Ein Wort an die Anhänger und Verteidiger der Euthanasie* (Berlin-Dahlem: Wichern-Verlag, 1925), 3, 9–10, 12–14. This was the fourth text Ulbrich had written in response to Binding and Hoche; the first two are mentioned in the third: Martin Ulbrich, *Die Not der Anormalen und ihre Abwehr* (Hamburg: Überreich, 1923), 33. Ulbrich opened this third one with the observation that before World War I, life had been cheaper and "welfare-care for the abnormals" (*Anormalenfürsorge*) had not cost so much; but, adding the crippled veterans and those destabilized emotionally by war and revolution to the total of those who already suffered from sensory, physical, psychological, or intellectual disabilities, he calculated that one million Germans were in some way abnormal and that this indeed portended an enormous financial burden for the nation (3–4). The best prophylaxis would be to suppress alcohol sales and brothels and "all opportunities for fornication" (46).

32. Meltzer too (and even as he understood himself as an adamant opponent of Binding and Hoche's proposition, acknowledging that he would be deemed "backwards and sentimental" for being so), in the midst of an otherwise compelling anticapitalist excursus pointing out that the real "useless parasites of society" were not the disabled poor but the greedy rich, argued that if one really wanted to talk about the "waste of physical and psychic energy expended in the care of idiots," one should realize that "it is still nearly nothing against the energy that is spent these days on dirty literature and filthy art which so poison the life of the Volk that it only follows its carnal drives." Meltzer, *Das Problem*, 125, 51. Already in earlier writing, Meltzer had acknowledged that there were plenty of illnesses and unhappy circumstances that could cause progeny to be disabled, whether severely or moderately; "often enough," however, he continued, there were "relationships between idiocy and immoral fornication." Ewald Meltzer, *Zum Kampf gegen Unzucht und Unsittlichkeit!* (Dresden: C. Ludwig Ungelenk, 1917), 5.

33. Helmuth Schreiner, *Vom Recht zur Vernichtung unterwertigen Menschenlebens* (Schwerin: F. Bahn, 1928), 6. Schreiner was at this point director of the Protestant welfare institution Johannesstift in Berlin; later he became a theology professor in Rostock. Schreiner here told the story of a woman, born "in sorrow and misery, without arms and legs, the image of horror"—and as a child treated cruelly and abusively at home—but after being taken in to an institution of the Inner Mission having become for everyone around her, her fellow residents and the institution's

director, the greatest source of comfort and orientation. "This 'child'—she was such despite her 40 years," exuded "radiant peacefulness and inner strengthening for many of the ill people in her surroundings." She had learned to read, but learned "above all, that in the bond with Jesus there is a bliss and a strength in suffering that is not available to the imagination of healthy and strong people. Who could here dare to say that this life is less worthy?"

34. Schreiner, *Vom Recht zur Vernichtung unwertigen Menschenlebens*, 3, cf. 6.

35. Büchsel, "Euthanasie," 2–3.

36. "Die Treysaer Resolution des Central-Ausschusses für Innere Mission (1931)," in Jochen-Christoph Kaiser et al., eds., *Eugenik, Sterilisation, Euthanasie: Politische Biologie in Deutschland 1895–1945—Eine Dokumentation* (Berlin: Buchverlag Union, 1992), 106–10, here 106.

37. A typical summary view is provided by Pastor Friedrich Lensch, director of the Alsterdorfer Anstalten in Hamburg (participating in the conversations among pastors and doctors, 18–20 May 1931, that culminated in the Treysa Resolution): "After short holidays 50 percent of the girls return to us morally degenerated and abused. Is that the residents' libidinal urges, or the irresponsibility of their kin? . . . One vacation day is enough for them to go off the rails." Quoted in Harald Jenner, "Friedrich Lensch als Leiter der Alsterdorfer Anstalten 1930 bis 1945," in Michael Wunder et al., *Auf dieser schiefen Ebene gibt es kein Halten mehr: Die Alsterdorfer Anstalten im Nationalsozialismus*, 3rd ed. (Stuttgart: Kohlhammer, 2016), 185–245, here 210–211. On the pervasiveness of the cultural assumption that sexual exploitation of sterilized females was normative / expectable male behavior, see Gisela Bock, *Zwangssterilisation im Nationalsozialismus: Studien zur Rassenpolitik und Geschlechterpolitik* (1986, reprint Münster: MV Wissenschaft, 2010), 437–439.

38. Riveting minutes of the discussions as they unfolded in Treysa – including clear evidence of Harmsen's skillfully subtle steering of the conversation to achieve the group's support for sterilization despite initially rather widespread doubts and continual raising of a host of other issues by the participants – can be found in Jochen-Christoph Kaiser and Uwe Kaminsky, eds., *Biologiepolitik und Evangelische Kirche: Protokolle des "Ausschusses für eugenetische Fragen" des Centralausschusses für Innere Mission (seit 1933 "Ständiger Ausschuss für Rassenhygiene und Rassenpflege") 1931-1938* (Bielefeld: Verlag für Regionalgeschichte, 2024). Interestingly, some of the participants' formulations ultimately found their way into the text of the resolution, but in retrospect the most surprising and fascinating role in the discussions was played by psychiatrist Carl Schneider, then the head physician at Bethel (later one of the "selecting" doctors for the T4 murder program). In this rather private setting, Schneider kept casually indicating that eugenic viewpoints were based on a quite uncertain empirical foundation: "We know this and that about hereditary connections, but otherwise little about the extent of their significance." "A völkisch goal-setting program would only make sense if with it we could actually improve the hereditary health of our people. That is doubtful to me [*Eine völkische Zielsetzung würde doch nur Sinn haben, wenn wir die Erbgesundheit unseres Volkes bessern können. Das ist mir zweifelhaft*]." "We have no criterion for deciding whether mild feeble-mindedness is hereditary or not, even when it is familial." "We underestimate the range of variation in healthy people. Which characteristics do we want to eradicate?" "And what about the [claim that there has been an] increase in inferior people? It has not yet been proven." "The consequences would only become apparent after generations."

39. "Die Treysaer Resolution," 107–109. Within the Inner Mission, the most persistent critic of sterilization was not present at Treysa, but expressed his objections vehemently at a later meeting of Inner Mission representatives held in March 1933. There Paul Gerhard Braune urged: "Sterilization means renouncing an educational and ethical influence on people. . . . I reject sterilization in all cases, just as I reject the demands to eliminate hopelessly ill people from life." Quoted in Kaiser and Kaminsky, *Biologiepolitik und evangelische Kirche*. In July 1940 Braune would become the author of a memorandum challenging the Nazi regime about the T4 murder program; four weeks later he landed in Gestapo custody. Uwe Kaminsky, "'Wer ist gemeinschaftsunfähig?' Paul

Gerhard Braune, die Rassenhygiene und die NS-Euthanasie," in Jan Cantow and Jochen-Christoph Kaiser, eds., *Paul Gerhard Braune (1887–1954): Ein Mann der Kirche und Diakonie in schwieriger Zeit* (Stuttgart: Kohlhammer, 2005), 114–139.

40. Ewald Meltzer, "Gesetz zur Verhütung Erbkranken Nachwuchses," *Zeitschrift für die Behandlung Anomaler* 53 (1933): 113–119, here 115: "It is very gratifying that those who crafted the law have in section 12 declared the use of direct coercion permissible. It would be quite witless if people whom the hereditary health court has on the basis of sufficient documents declared to be hereditarily ill could now, for their part, make the law ineffective out of stubborn truculence."

41. Uwe Kaminsky, "Paternalistische Verschwiegenheit—Bethel, die Zwangssterilisation und NS-'Euthanasie,'" *Lippische Mitteilungen aus Geschichte und Landeskunde* (2020): 69–87, here 72–77; Ernst Klee, *"Die SA Jesu Christi": Die Kirche im Banne Hitlers* (Frankfurt / Main: Fischer, 1989), 92.

42. Michael Wunder, "Die Karriere des Dr. Gerhard Kreyenberg—Heilen und Vernichten in Alsterdorf," in Wunder et al., *Auf dieser schiefen Ebene*, 137–83, esp. 155–166; cf. "Die Treysaer Resolution," 108.

43. Paul Althaus, *Kirche und Volkstum* (Gütersloh: Bertelsmann, 1928), 33.

44. Disability, Althaus moreover noted, provided an incomparable opportunity also to encounter *God's* love. Althaus, "'Unwertes' Leben," 79, 82, 84, 86, 88, 91–92. Although the 1933 lecture had slipped into print in a scientific journal sandwiched between the lectures of his (uniformly pro-sterilization) co-panelists, Althaus was denied the right to republish it as he had planned, on grounds that it might discredit Nazi public health programming and state policy in the eyes of the public. Gotthard Jasper, *Paul Althaus (1888–1966): Professor, Prediger und Patriot in seiner Zeit* (Göttingen: Vandenhoeck & Ruprecht, 2015), 217–222. In no way, however, was his professorship endangered.

45. Karl Stoevesandt, "Medizin und menschliche Existenz," *Zwischen den Zeiten* 11.4 (1933), 326–344, here 334.

46. Karl Stoevesandt, "Rasse als Schöpfung und Weltanschauung," *Wort und Tat* 10.3 (1934), 65–76.

47. This is indicated in a letter to Barth, and discussed in Almuth Meyer-Zollitsch, *Nationalsozialismus und Evangelische Kirche in Bremen* (Bremen: Selbstverlag des Staatsarchivs der Hansestadt Bremen, 1985), 207. Thanks are due here to Uwe Gerrens for this information and his insights into Stoevesandt.

48. Fritz von Bodelschwingh quoted in Matthias Benad, "Bethels Verhältnis zum Nationalsozialismus," in Matthias Benad and Regina Mentner, eds., *Zwangsverpflichtet: Kriegsgefangene und zivile Zwangsarbeiter(-innen) in Bethel und Lobetal, 1939–1945* (Bielefeld: Verlag für Regionalgeschichte, 2002), 27–66, here 28.

49. Meltzer, "Gesetz," 115–116.

50. Photo from the Alsterdorfer Anstalten in Hamburg on the cover of Wunder et al., *Auf dieser schiefen Ebene*; photo with basket woven at Bruckberg, Neuendettelsau, in Alexander Mayer, ed., *50 Jahre Lebenshilfe Fürth—Jubiläumsdokumentation* (Nürnberg: NOVA-Druck, 2011), 17.

51. Gerhard Kunze, pastor in Hannover, and similar examples quoted in Kurt Nowak, *"Euthanasie" und Sterilisierung im "Dritten Reich": Die Konfrontation der evangelischen und katholischen Kirche mit dem Gesetz zur Verhütung erbkranken Nachwuchses und die "Euthanasie"-Aktion* (Göttingen: Vandenhoeck & Ruprecht, 1978), 98; see also Claudia Koonz, "Ethical Dilemmas and Nazi Eugenics: Single-Issue Dissent in Religious Contexts," *Journal of Modern History* 64 (Supplement: Resistance against the Third Reich) (December 1992), S8–S31.

52. Friedrich Lensch, "Die Alsterdorfer Anstalten im Dritten Reich," *Briefe und Bilder aus Alsterdorf* 58 (1934), 1–4, here 2.

53. Ernst Klessmann, "Auswirkungen des Gesetzes zur Verhütung erbkranken Nachwuchses für den seelsorgerlichen Dienst," in *Pastoralblätter* 77.6 (1935), 328–338, here 330, 334. Klessmann further explained that while "a great portion of hereditarily ill progeny" was indeed born of apparently healthy parents, this was misleading, for actually "they are carriers of hereditarily damaged assets" (331).

54. Wilhelm Wittneben, "Was muß der evangelische Erzieher von der Rassenpflege wissen und wie kann er sich in ihren Dienst stellen?," *Evangelische Jugendhilfe* 10.7-8 (July–August 1934), 171–185, here 171–172, 175, 177. Wittneben assured his listeners that while before World War I, in 1914, there had been approximately 300,000 "ill, inferior and achievement-incapable fellow members of the Volk," by 1934 the number had risen to approximately 500,000 (174–175). On Wittneben, see also Michael Nahm and Bruce Greyson, "The Death of Anna Katharina Ehmer: A Case Study in Terminal Lucidity," *Omega* 68.1 (2013–2014), 77–87.

55. As a leading member of the Catholic Caritas put it in 1924, regarding "the question recently raised, about whether it might not be permitted to rid the world painlessly of those with mental inferiority": "About the dreadfulness of such a question we do not need to waste a single word." Michael Fischer, "Die Entwicklung der Schwachsinnigenfürsorge," *Krankendienst* 5 (1924), 73–78.

56. Hermann Muckermann, "Eugenik und Katholizismus," in Günther Just, ed., *Eugenik und Weltanschauung* (Berlin: Alfred Metzner, 1932).

57. Uwe Kaminsky, "Joseph Mayer—Eugenik, Notstand, Euthanasie," *Römische Quartalschrift für christliche Altertumskunde und Kirchengeschichte* 109.1-2 (2014), 70–91.

58. Once the coercive Nazi sterilization law went into effect, Catholic physicians and nurses scrambled to get guidance from their bishops on what level of at least indirect participation might be permitted (handing over a sterile scalpel? comforting a person undergoing the procedure?) without damage to one's conscience. And, fully understanding the pressures their flocks were subjected to, Catholic religious authorities then did come up with individually adapted decisions to alleviate conflictedness—and in some cases actually urged that it was better for a Catholic doctor to perform the operation than to have it done by a nonbeliever. Excellent analysis of the complexities in Winfried Süß, "Antagonistische Kooperationen: Katholische Kirche und nationalsozialistisches Gesundheitswesen in den Kriegsjahren, 1939–1945," in Christoph Kösters, Erik Gieseking, and Karl-Joseph Hummel, eds., *Kirchen im Krieg: Europa 1939–1945* (Paderborn: Schoeningh, 2007), 317–341, here 319–320.

59. Franz Walter, "Die Vernichtung lebensunwerten Lebens (Euthanasie)," *Archiv für Rechts- und Wirtschaftsphilosophie* 16.1 (1923), 88–120, here 90. In the essay, Walter notes that the debate set in motion by the "euthanists" or "euthanasianists" (*Euthanatisten*), as he persistently calls them, does not only concern the acceptability of terminating this or that individual life, but that what is also at stake is the valuable asset of having a "moral order" in the first place (*in erster Linie steht das Gut der sittlichen Ordnung*). So the real question, he notes, is not whether the one or other life has lost its value, but rather whether it has so profoundly lost its value that this would justify the more general surrendering of that foundational moral asset (93; cf. 101). He further pinpoints the more or less acknowledged "egoism" (*Egoismus*) of wanting to avoid the sight of disability hiding inside the overhyped claims that one is motivated by mercy (102). And above all, he takes on the euthanasianists' tactic of accusing the Christian faithful of "sacrilegiously" opposing a "dignified notion of God" (*würdige Gottesidee*) as they misrepresent Christians as embracing passive endurance of suffering (rather than, as the euthanasianists recommend, alleviating that suffering by extinguishing it) (103). Turning to the practical matters of implementation, he calls attention to Binding and Hoche's own concession that the boundaries between the supposedly "total idiots" and the "middling states of mental enfeeblement" are fluid, discusses at length the inconsistencies in their economic calculations as well as in their

pseudo-mathematical discussions of "zero" versus "negative" life-value, and notes how transparently "brutal" it is to adjudicate the value of a life by its "usefulness" alone (109–111, 117).

60. Franz Walter, "Euthanasie und Volkswirtschaft," in *Die Euthanasie und die Heiligkeit des Lebens* (Munich: Max Hueber, 1935), 478–497, here 480, 485, 488–489. The remark in double quotes is an appreciative restatement of a point made by the physician Ferdinand Straßmann in his critical analysis of Binding and Hoche published in 1921. See Ferdinand Straßmann, "Die Freigabe der Vernichtung lebensunwerten Lebens," *Ärztliche Sachverständigen-Zeitung* 27 (1921), 7–10, here 9. Hoche himself, Walter also observed, had only called for killing those he deemed "mentally fully dead," whose numbers he had estimated at 3,000–4,000. As Walter acerbically notes: "But 3,000–4,000 idiots fewer in Germany would not have much of a measurable effect on the national budget" (483). Walter additionally cited Berlin-Buch psychiatrist Eugen Wauschkuhn. Aside from the extraordinarily eloquent self-advocate Rudolf Kraemer's countertext to Binding and Hoche published in 1933, Wauschkuhn's 1922 review was arguably the most brilliantly snarky contemporaneous takedown of Binding and Hoche, mocking not just their math (with its "cheap games"), but also their grandiose self-ascriptions as bravely "heroic" in daring to break with the traditional respect for life. Eugen Wauschkuhn, "Die Freigabe der Vernichtung lebensunwerten Lebens," *Psychiatrisch-Neurologische Wochenschrift* 24 (1922), 215–217, here 215–216.

61. Stadtarzt Dr. Schröder (Essen), "Hat die Arbeit der Hilfsschule rassenhygienische Bedeutung?," *Die Hilfsschule* 17.4 (April 1924), 49–53, here 49–50.

62. Albert Griesinger, "Muß die Hilfsschule um ihre Berechtigung kämpfen?," *Die Hilfsschule* 1926, 188–192, here 188, 191.

63. H. Schnitzer, "Die Auslese der Hilfsschulkinder," in Erwin Lesch, ed., *Bericht über den Dritten Kongress für Heilpädagogik in München, 2.-4. August 1926* (Berlin: Springer, 1927), 40–51, here 40, 42.

64. Ignaz Kaup, "Volksentartung und Staatswirtschaft," in Erwin Lesch, ed., *Bericht über den Zweiten Kongress für Heilpädagogik in München 29. Juli bis 1. August 1924* (Berlin: Springer, 1925), 45–58, here 52, 57. The very fact that several US states had already passed sterilization laws (Indiana was the first in 1907), would prove to be a major talking point also for promoters of the Nazi sterilization law, even though the net cast by the German law would be far wider. On sterilization in the United States, see Johanna Schoen, *Choice and Coercion: Birth Control, Sterilization, and Abortion in Public Health and Welfare* (Chapel Hill: University of North Carolina Press, 2005); Alexandra Minna Stern, *Eugenic Nation: Faults and Frontiers of Better Breeding in Modern America* (Berkeley: University of California Press, 2005); and Molly Ladd-Taylor, *Fixing the Poor: Eugenic Sterilization and Child Welfare in the Twentieth Century* (Baltimore, MD: Johns Hopkins University Press, 2017). By the 1930s, Nazi presentation of Germany as simply being one among multiple nations implementing or considering sterilization legislation was especially well expressed in an illustration headlined "We are not alone" (or "We're in good company"): "Wir stehen nicht allein," *Neues Volk* 4.3 (1936), 37.

65. Binding and Hoche were clearly part of the frame of reference for journalists as well. Thus, for instance, when the traditional institution directors' conference was held in Kassel in 1927, and a local newspaper reported with enthusiasm on a film shown there about a unique, praxis-oriented pedagogical technique developed by the teacher-director of the institution at Chemnitz-Altendorf, Reinhold Gürtler—Gürtler was famous for using ordinary daily-use objects, like a footstool or a handkerchief, and creatively building an entire hour's lesson around these—the paper emphasized how joyful life at Chemnitz-Altendorf apparently was, how brilliantly Gürtler's approach stimulated both the cognition and the "vital imagination" also of the "feeble-minded." The reporter concluded—an obvious reference to Binding and Hoche—that such education and care provided within institutions was "proof, that effort and concern for

that only apparently 'life unworthy of life' can bear rich fruit." On the other hand, in his preceding summary of another film shown at the conference—this one about Alsterdorf—the reporter reflexively described the residents in terms blending theology and biology as "those who pay with their bodies for the sins of mankind." See "Die Erziehung der Geistesschwachen. (Öffentlicher Lichtbildervortrag.)" (reprint of report from "Kasseler Tageszeitungen"), in *Bericht über die 19. Konferenz des Vereins für Erziehung, Unterricht und Pflege Geistesschwacher von 26. bis 28. September 1927 in Kassel und Hephata bei Treysa* (Halle: Marhold, 1929), 6–7. See also Reinhold Gürtler, *Triebgemäßer Erlebnisunterricht - Ein Beitrag zur Praxis der Heilpädagogik und der Arbeitsschule* (Halle: Marhold, 1924).

66. In 1928, Karl Ziegler—in prior decades more noteworthy for meditative reflections on remedial pedagogy—called on his fellow teachers to catch up with the latest eugenic research and emphatically endorsed sterilization. Karl Ziegler, "Halbe Arbeit? Ein rassenhygienisches Mahnwort an die Hilfsschullehrer," *Die Hilfsschule* 21 (1928), 245–264.

67. Gustav Lesemann, "Heilpädagogik und Eugenik," *Die Hilfsschule* 26 (1933), 141–154, here 153. Emphases in the original.

68. Lesemann quoted and discussed in Ellger-Rüttgardt, *Geschichte der Sonderpädagogik,* 270, 272–273.

69. Erich Gossow, "Erbgesund oder Erbkrank?," *Die deutsche Sonderschule* 1.12 (1934), 651–659, here 659.

70. A famous exception that proves the rule is Frieda Stoppenbrink-Buchholz, a more generally remarkable counter-example to the predominant trends of acquiescence to, if not more fervent complicity with, the Nazi regime among remedial education professionals. She fought valiantly to protect one of her students from sterilization—and was additionally a significant reformer emphasizing a holistic approach to each child and the value of a community among peers. Frieda Buchholz, *Das brauchbare Hilfsschulkind—ein Normalkind* (Weimar, 1939); Sieglind Ellger-Rüttgardt, *Frieda Stoppenbrink-Buchholz (1897–1993): Hilfsschulpädagogin* (Weinheim: Deutscher Studienverlag, 1997).

71. Wolfgang Jantzen, *Sozialgeschichte des Behindertenbetreuungswesens* (Munich: DJI Verlag, 1982), 154. Another indicative vernacular term for the remedial school was "sterilization school" (*Sterilisationsschule*). Werner Brill, "Sonderpädagogik und Behinderung im Nationalsozialismus: Spezifika der Situation in Berlin," in Rüdiger vom Bruch and Rebecca Schaarschmidt, eds., *Die Berliner Universität in der NS-Zeit*, vol. 2 (Stuttgart: Franz Steiner, 2005), 229–241, here 238.

72. Max Bittrich, "Das Hilfsschulwesen in Großdeutschland," *Weltanschauung und Schule* 6 (1942), 76–85, here 77.

73. The incredulity and dismay expressed—both in the moment and retrospectively—that individuals who were quite able and willing to provide labor were also nonetheless included among the targets for murder reveals just how well understood by the public this element of the decision-making process either for or against killing was. See, e.g., the letter of Archbishop Conrad Gröber of Freiburg to Chief of the Reich Chancellery Hans Lammers, August 1, 1940, in which he volunteered, remarkably, that Catholic charities would be willing to cover all costs of care that might arise for those who had been destined for death, while also noting that "euthanasia" had claimed "a very large number of mentally ill and mentally weak individuals already," despite the fact that "many of those who died had been absolutely work-capable." Letter reprinted in Johann Neuhäusler, *Kreuz und Hakenkreuz: Der Kampf des Nationalsozialismus gegen die katholische Kirche und der kirchliche Widerstand, Erster Teil* (München: Katholische Kirche Bayerns, 1946), 356. No less wrenching is a memory-essay collected in the late years of the GDR, when a woman in anguish recalled the story of her uncle, mentally impaired due to a serious disease in childhood, who had been much loved and appreciated not just by his family and fellow villagers but also his employers in the bakery in which he—when so many men had been pulled into military service—was "ever more indispensable" as he performed a great deal of heavy labor

and was "eager and industrious . . . hardworking, strong." His manner, she recalled, was "completely normal" and he "did not stand out as 'mentally weak.'" Nonetheless—villagers assumed it was due to denunciation from "a few especially fanatic Nazis"—he was institutionalized against the family's wishes and the news of his death followed. Frau Dr. Maltry, "Unentbehrlich in der Bäckerei," in Wolf-Dieter Talkenberger, ed., *"Euthanasie"—Familienerinnerungen aus Ostdeutschland an die Verbrechen der Nazi-Zeit* (Evangelischer Pressedienst, Dokumentation Nr. 52 (December 7, 1992), 34, Evangelisches Landesarchiv Berlin 55.5 / 468.

74. Philipp Rauh, "Medizinische Selektionskriterien versus ökonomisch-utilitaristische Verwaltungsinteressen: Ergebnisse der Meldebogenauswertung," and Gerrit Hohendorf, "Die Selektion der Opfer zwischen rassenhygienischer 'Ausmerze', ökonomischer Brauchbarkeit und medizinischem Erlösungsideal," both in Maike Rotzoll et al., eds., *Die nationalsozialistische "Euthanasie"-Aktion "T4" und ihre Opfer: Geschichte und ethische Konsequenzen für die Gegenwart* (Paderborn: Schöningh, 2010), 297–309 and 310–324, esp. 317. Cf. Ludwig Schlaich, *Lebensunwert? Kirche u. innere Mission Württembergs im Kampf gegen die "Vernichtung lebensunwerten Lebens"* (Stuttgart: Quell-Verl., 1947), 75–76.

75. Jakob Rupp quoted in Ernst Klee, *"Euthanasie" im NS-Staat: Die "Vernichtung lebensunwerten Lebens"* (Frankfurt / Main: Fischer, 1983), 237.

76. Karl-Adolf Bauer, "Aus der Geschichte der Diakonie-Anstalten Bad Kreuznach," in Evangelische Akademie Mülheim / Ruhr, ed., "Diakonie im Dritten Reich: Tagung in Zusammenarbeit mit dem Diakonischen Werk der Evangelischen Kirche im Rheinland und den Diakonie-Anstalten Bad Kreuznach, 16.-17. Mai 1987, Außentagung in Maria Laach," *Begegnungen* 5 (Mülheim / Ruhr, 1987), 61–70, here 68.

77. The survivor—Robert Kuttler—had been a resident at Stetten and returned there in 1950, living until 1983, to the ripe age of eighty-five. The perpetrator physician—Horst Schumann, among whose additional crimes can be counted "sterilization and castration experiments on young Greek women and gypsy children in the concentration camps of Ravensbrück and Auschwitz," and who was never convicted—died in the same year at the age of seventy-six. Werner Müller, ". . . als die 'grauen Busse' kamen: Wie sich der 'Kampf gegen alles Kranke und Wertlose' im unteren Remstal zugetragen hat," *Rems-Murr Rundschau* 279 (December 3, 1983).

78. Frank Janzowski, *Die NS-Vergangenheit in der Heil- und Pflegeanstalt Wiesloch: . . . so intensiv wenden wir unsere Arbeitskraft der Ausschaltung der Erbkranken zu* (Ubstadt-Weiher: Verlag Regionalkultur, 2015), 292–93.

79. Klee, *"Euthanasie,"* 445, 410.

80. Daum, "Arbeit und Zwang," 204–205; Christoph Schneider, ed., *Hadamar von Innen: Überlebendenzeugnisse und Angehörigenberichte* (Berlin: Metropol, 2020), 36–40; Andrea Berger and Thomas Oelschläger, "'Ich habe sie eines natürlichen Todes sterben lassen': Das Krankenhaus im Kalmenhof und die Praxis der nationalsozialistischen Vernichtungsprogramme," in Christian Schrapper and Dieter Sengling, eds., *Die Idee der Bildbarkeit: 100 Jahre sozialpädagogische Praxis in der Heilerziehungsanstalt Kalmenhof* (Weinheim: Juventa, 1988), 269–336, here 335.

81. Kneuker and Steglich, *Begegnungen,* 100–103; Leo Waltermann, "Diakonie im Dritten Reich: Aus der Geschichte Konsequenzen für heute," in Evangelische Akademie Mülheim / Ruhr, "Diakonie im Dritten Reich," 85–117, here 87.

82. Werner Müller, "Existenzängste noch heute wach," *Rems-Murr Rundschau* 279 (December 3, 1983). For an account of the devastating losses at the very oldest Catholic institution for individuals with mental impairments—Ecksberg in Bavaria, founded in 1852—see Hans Wollasch, *Ein Jahrhundert der Sorge um geistig behinderte Menschen,* vol. 2 (Freiburg: Verband katholischer Einrichtungen für Lern- und Geistigbehinderte e.V., 1980), 108–111. In the first phase of "euthanasia," 245 of Ecksberg's 288 residents were deported to their deaths in the gas at the T4 center of Hartheim in Austria, and Wollasch reproduced wrenching images from a postwar chronicle (between pages 128 and 129, and between 144 and 145) in which photographs

of lovingly remembered residents were coupled with typed or handwritten notations indicating, over and over, "gassed" or "all gassed." In the second phase of the killings, not only were residents from Ecksberg taken to Eglfing-Haar, a psychiatric clinic near Munich, where they were subjected to deliberate starvation in Eglfing-Haar's "hunger houses." Ecksberg itself—its administration taken over by the Nazis—became a kind of relay station at which deportees from other institutions were temporarily held before being moved on to another site to be killed. For the names of those killed at Hartheim, see the website, "Die Behindertenanstalt Ecksberg," http:// www.geschichtswerkstatt.de/ecksberg.html.

83. An early postwar document that evocatively describes this experience of confronting impossible non-choices facing institutional administrators is by a physician at the Catholic institution of Rottenmünster in Württemberg: Dr. Josef Wrede, "Euthanasie und Rottenmünster" (April 15, 1947), reproduced in Carl Becker, "Die Durchführung der Euthanasie in den katholischen caritativen Heimen für geistig Behinderte," *Jahrbuch der Caritaswissenschaft* (1968), 104–119, here 111–115.

84. Martin Kalusche, *"Das Schloß an der Grenze": Kooperation und Konfrontation mit dem Nationalsozialismus in der Heil- und Pflegeanstalt für Schwachsinnige Stetten i. R.*, 2nd ed. (Hamburg: Martin Kalusche, 2011), 184.

85. See his seven principles criticizing the idea of "usability" in 1937 in Kalusche, *"Das Schloß an der Grenze,"* 129.

86. Schlaich, *Lebensunwert?*, 72, 77.

87. Hans, quoted in Schlaich, *Vernichtung und Neuanfang*, 5.

88. Schlaich, *Lebensunwert?*, 79. And—notably—quoted as epigraph in Ernst Klee, ed., *Dokumente zur "Euthanasie"* (Frankfurt / Main: Fischer, 1985).

Chapter Three: How Does One Recognize a Crime?

1. Gisela Bock, "Gutachten speziell zur Frage der Zwangssterilisation im Nationalsozialismus," printed in *Wiedergutmachung und Entschädigung für nationalsozialistisches Unrecht: Öffentliche Anhörung des Innenausschusses des Deutschen Bundestages am 24. Juni 1987*, Zur Sache 3 / 87 (Bonn: Deutscher Bundestag, Referat Öffentlichkeitsarbeit, 1987), 258–265, here 260.

2. Martin Niemöller, "Ansprache an die Vertreter der Bekennenden Kirche in Frankfurt a. M., am 6. Januar 1946," in *Die deutsche Schuld, Not und Hoffnung* (Zollikon-Zürich: Evangelischer Verlag, 1946), 1–19, here 5–6.

3. Michael S. Bryant, *Confronting the "Good Death": Nazi Euthanasia on Trial, 1945–1953* (Denver: University Press of Colorado, 2017), 101, 127, 147–169. For a detailed contemporaneous discussion of how courts resolved the dissonance between physicians' participation in murders and their claims that they both had been opposed to the killings and had succeeded in saving considerable numbers of patients, see Anton Roesen, "Gewissen und Gesetz: Zum Euthanasie-Prozeß in Düsseldorf," *Rheinischer Merkur* 7 (February 11, 1950), 3.

4. Christoph Schneider, "Die Bilanz kann nicht zufriedenstellen: Ein Gespräch mit OStA a.D. Johannes Warlo," *Kritische Justiz* 48, no. 3 (2015): 340–350.

5. Discussed and quoted in Ernst Klee, *"Euthanasie" im NS-Staat: Die "Vernichtung lebensunwerten Lebens"* (Frankfurt/ Main: Fischer, 1983), 384–385.

6. Brenske, "Tötungen aus eugenischen und aus Euthanasiegründen," *Juristische Rundschau* 7 (July 1952): 275–278, here 275. See also Brenske's follow-up essay, assuring readers that other legal theorists shared his views and also reminding readers of three Christian theologians of the 1920s who had provided religious arguments to justify "euthanasia" of individuals with profound disabilities—he expressly named Thrändorf, Lemme, and Titius (all of whom had been cited by Ewald Meltzer)—thereby carrying their perspectives into the post-Nazi era. Brenske, "Nochmals zum Thema: Euthanasie," *Juristische Rundschau* 6 (June 1953), 215–216.

7. See, for instance: Hans Otto Wesemann, "Der Hörer hat das Wort" (radio broadcast, March 26, 1950, Nordwestdeutscher Rundfunk), with listeners' letters. Archive of the Nordwestdeutscher Rundfunk, Köln. The host noted that there was no simple division between Christians and "rationalists," but rather differences of opinion within each side, and that Christians too were torn between the commandment not to kill and the demands of "mercy" (*Barmherzigkeit*). As for Binding and Hoche before, so too in many of the letters sent in, the topic of assisted suicide was blurred with the topic of murder. One letter-writer, living near Bethel ("where one is proud that one has saved several hundred people from death"), raised the question of whether it would not be "more humane" for the children with disabilities to be killed and instead to allow the "most valuable" children to live in the institution, as they might later become "useful people, who have work and can earn their bread." Anon. listener letter, March 15, 1950.

8. Schneider, "Die Bilanz kann nicht zufriedenstellen," 344.

9. For a detailed account of Walther Schmidt's energetic organization of the killing processes at the Eichberg, see Peter Sandner, *Verwaltung des Krankenmordes: Der Bezirksverband Nassau im Nationalsozialismus* (Gießen: Psychosozial, 2003), 535–539. For the prosecution's case against Schmidt and its initial success in the courts, see the summary in: Revisions-Urteil des Oberlandesgerichts Frankfurt gegen Dr. Walter Eugen Schmidt und Oberschwester Helene Schürg (Dezember 1946) - Bd. 72, Blatt 1–34, Landesarchiv Baden-Württemberg, Wü 29 / 3 T 1 Nr. 1759/03 / 01, https://www.deutsche-digitale-bibliothek.de/item/TQ2LXPYNQ2QH DA623DESQKBWWVM4A75D. A succinct overview of the pattern of dropped charges is also provided in Ernst Klee's testimony to the Hessischer Landtag in 2000: Hessischer Landtag, Bericht des Präsidenten des Landtags über das Symposium zur Antwort der Landesregierung auf die Große Anfrage der Fraktion BÜNDNIS 90 / DIE GRÜNEN betreffend Verfolgung und Vernichtung durch das NS-Regime in Hessen, Drucksache 13 / 7176 zu Drucksache 13 / 1595 (February 7, 2000), https://starweb.hessen.de/cache/DRS/15/1/01001.pdf.

10. The best documentation and analysis is in Christoph Schneider, "Strafverfolgung," *Der Kalmenhof in Idstein—NS-"Euthanasie" und ihre Nachgeschichte* (Paderborn: Schöningh, 2023), 185–210. See also petition signature list and photo of Mathilde Weber Muthig (after the war, she married the former concentration camp doctor Julius Muthig) in Christian Schrapper and Dieter Sengling, "Sozialpädagogik im Nationalsozialismus—Die Heilerziehungsanstalt Kalmenhof / Idstein 1888–1988: Ein Beispiel," in Christina Vanja and Martin Vogt, eds., *Euthanasie in Hadamar: Die nationalsozialistische Vernichtungspolitik in hessischen Anstalten* (Kassel: LWV Hessen, 1991), 113–122, here 119; and Rudolf Müller, "Das Heim des Todes," *Stern* 45 (1987), IIIa / 2. See also Lutz Kaelber, "Gedenken an die NS-'Kindereuthanasie'—zwei Fallbeispiele (Eichberg, Kalmenhof) und allgemeine Folgerungen zur Gedenkkultur," in Arbeitskreis zur Erforschung der nationalsozialistischen "Euthanasie" und Zwangssterilisation, ed., *Den Opfern ihre Namen geben—NS-"Euthanasie"-Verbrechen, historisch-politische Verantwortung und Erinnerungskultur—Fachtagung vom 13. bis 15. Mai 2011 in Kloster Irsee* (Ulm and Münster: Klemm & Oelschläger, 2011), 201–232.

11. See Gerhart Hermann Mostar, "'Ich klage an!'" *Schwäbische Illustrierte* 6.33 (August 18, 1951), 1004–1005, 1016; and "Darum sterben Tausende!" *Die 7 Tage* (August 1, 1952), 1, 3. The *Schwäbische Illustrierte* in Stuttgart, with film stars Ingrid Bergman and Cary Grant on the cover (which gives a good sense of the intended audience), provided a multipage spread under the urgent plea: "We demand freedom for Dr. Walther Schmidt." Schmidt, readers were told, had "a strong belief in Hitler" but also was "church-attached" and had a deep "religious faith." These tendencies had not come into contradiction until 1941, when he was told at a high-level meeting of fifty doctors involved in the "euthanasia" program what was expected. This created "The Conflict" within him (as the caption to his portrait announced): to kill or not to kill. First, the "temptation was great" to think that "euthanasia" might in fact be the right course when he

saw what monstrosities the children were. The magazine included a drawing of hydrocephaly and also lingered upon lurid, deliberately disgust-invoking descriptions (of children who were only 90 cm long but with a head circumference of 120—and under dissection it turned out they had no brain at all, but rather 8–10 liters of water in their heads, or, in another case, a 1-year-old, 60 cm long with a head circumference of 150 and on the forehead one huge gangrenous abscess; this child's head didn't move at all, but the child's kicking made the neck continually get twisted and the breathing blocked, so one nurse had to spend all her time changing its position every 3 minutes; also there were 11-year-olds, skeletal, emaciated, deaf, dumb, and blind, lying in their own feces, forced due to the abscesses to lie for months in water, fed since birth by tube . . . (the description continues). But Schmidt did not succumb, "even when the parents wished for [the child's] death." Thirteen times Schmidt begged to be transferred to the front to escape this great conflict of conscience, but instead he was promoted to head doctor of the clinic. He solved his crisis by choosing a third path: healing the children. His faith had "driven" him to "circumvent" the "euthanasia-actions ordered by the Reich chancellery." He had saved "at least 1200" children. He introduced "80 new treatment methods"—with machines bought at his own expense. He succeeded in "spontaneous" cure of multiple sclerosis. Meanwhile, the poor man in prison had been "extraordinarily worn down" by the years spent there (at this point five); "his mouth trembled"; he was "'finished.'" And it was so unfair, the magazine contended, comparing his case to those of all the other doctors who had been accused of participation in "euthanasia" a few years later and had been either acquitted or at most had gotten two years behind bars. As a concluding afterthought, the magazine did mention that there had been circa sixty cases when Schmidt had been able to reconcile his faith with a decision to kill, as the children in question had been so very close to death already. Thirty times he had a nurse give the injection, thirty times he did it himself. A year later, 1952, a women's magazine, *Die 7 Tage*, took up the case: "This is why thousands are dying!," the front page screamed. "Incurably ill sick people are waiting for Dr. Schmidt to be released." (The theory was that Schmidt was a curative genius—having developed a panoply of amazing treatments with which he could cure "tens of thousands" who suffered from multiple sclerosis, he could also "beat back polio in its early stages," and repair glandular disorders.) And here were photos of his father and his little daughter, pining for him "with identical yearning." Yet he remained in prison—with "murderers, pimps, thieves . . . con artists, manslaughterers, and sex criminals." Once again, horrific images of monstrous children were described, while Schmidt was styled as a widely revered humanitarian. All of this might seem so ludicrously preposterous that it could not possibly work. Yet the campaign was successful; prominent politicians demanded Schmidt's release, more than 550 citizens signed a petition pleading for him, and the Hessian Minister of Justice in 1953 succumbed against his own better judgment and set Schmidt free. When challenged, the minister invoked the massive public pressure. See Günter Dahl, "Sollen ehemalige KZ-Ärzte wieder praktizieren dürfen?," *Die Zeit* (February 27, 1958).

12. James Q. Whitman, *Hitler's American Model: The United States and the Making of Nazi Race Law* (Princeton, NJ: Princeton University Press, 2018).

13. Dagmar Herzog, "Post-Holocaust Antisemitism and the Ascent of PTSD," *Cold War Freud: Psychoanalysis in an Age of Catastrophes* (New York: Cambridge University Press, 2017), 89–122.

14. "Drittes Gesetz zur Änderung des Bundesergänzungsgesetzes zur Entschädigung für Opfer der nationalsozialistischen Verfolgung," *Bundesgesetzblatt* 31 (June 29, 1956), 559–596, here 563.

15. Hans Lewenstein in "Frage der Entschädigung für Zwangssterilisierte; Anhörung von Sachverständigen," Deutscher Bundestag, Protokoll No. 34, April 13, 1961 (https://www.euthanasiegeschaedigte-zwangssterilisierte.de/dokumente/bt-protokoll-13-04-1961.pdf), 16–24, here 17–18.

16. Helmut Ehrhardt in "Frage der Entschädigung für Zwangssterilisierte," 25, 29.

17. Hans Nachtsheim in "Frage der Entschädigung für Zwangssterilisierte," 3, 7, 9.

18. Werner Villinger in "Frage der Entschädigung für Zwangssterilisierte," 13, 15. As Villinger summarized it, Kemp had shown, in a study evaluating the previously born children of mothers who had subsequently been sterilized (the Danes had a sterilization law since 1929), that of their existing children, 50–60 percent had severe cognitive or emotional problems, many had moderate ones, and only 5 percent were healthy "without flaw" (*ganz einwandfrei*) (15). Villinger's role as one of the T4 "assessors" would be publicized only a month after the Bundestag testimony, in the pages of *Der Spiegel*. Shortly thereafter, Villinger tumbled to his death on a vacation in the mountains (whether by accident or by suicide was never resolved). "Die Kreuzelschreiber," *Der Spiegel* 19 (May 2, 1961).

19. Hans Nachtsheim, "Warum Eugenik?," *Fortschritte der Medizin* 81 (1963), 711–714, here 711–713. Nachtsheim's crimes would not be exposed until after his death, in the 1980s.

20. Henning Tümmers, "Schon wieder 'vergessene Opfer'?," *Ärzteblatt Baden-Württemberg* 7 (2010): 286–89, here 287.

21. "Stellungnahme Pastor Friedrich v. Bodelschwinghs (III.) am 21. Januar 1965 vor dem Wiedergutmachungsausschuss," reprinted in Bernward Wolf, ed., *Lebenslang als Minderwertig abgestempelt: Das Mahnmal zum Gedenken an die Opfer von Zwangssterilisationen während der NS-Zeit in Bethel: Dokumentation, Hintergründe, Fragen an gegenwärtiges Handeln*, Bethel-Beiträge 56 (Bielefeld: Bethel-Verlag, 2001), 47.

22. Uwe Kaminsky, "Zwischen Rassenhygiene und Biotechnologie: Die Fortsetzung der eugenischen Debatte in Diakonie und Kirche, 1945 bis 1969," *Zeitschrift für Kirchengeschichte* 116.2 (2005), 204–41, here 215–218; Uwe Kaminsky, "Vom eugenischen Dunkel am Fuße des anti-euthanatischen Leuchtturms: Zur Nachgeschichte von Eugenik und 'Euthanasie' am Beispiel der Evangelischen Kirche nach 1945," in Justizministerium des Landes NRW, ed., *Justiz und Erbgesundheit: Zwangssterilisation, Stigmatisierung, Entrechtung* (Düsseldorf: Justizministerium des Landes NRW, [2009]), 195–210.

23. Interview with Werner Catel by Hermann Renner: "Aus Menschlichkeit töten? Spiegel-Gespräch mit Professor Dr. Werner Catel über Kinder-Euthanasie," *Der Spiegel*, February 18, 1964, 41–47, here 41, 43.

24. Werner Catel, *Grenzsituationen des Lebens: Beitrag zum Problem der begrenzten Euthanasie* (Nuremberg: Glock und Lutz, 1962), 9–10. See also Hans-Christian Petersen and Sönke Zankel, "'Ein exzellenter Kinderarzt, wenn man von den Euthanasie-Dingen einmal absieht'—Werner Catel und die Vergangenheitspolitik der Universität Kiel," in Hans-Werner Prahl, ed., *Uni-Formierung des Geistes: Universität Kiel im Nationalsozialismus* (Kiel: Malik, 2007), 133–178.

25. Ursula Weber, "Lüttich und die Euthanasie," *Deutsches Zentralblatt für Krankenpflege* 7 (1963), 198; Jochen Fischer, "Von der Utopie bis zur 'Vernichtung lebensunwerten Lebens' (September 1963)," in Hans Christoph von Hase, ed., *Evangelische Dokumente zur Ermordung der 'unheilbar Kranken' unter der nationalsozialistischen Herrschaft in den Jahren 1939–1945* (Stuttgart: Evangelisches Verlagswerk, 1964), 35–65, here 62; Hans Schomerus, "Euthanasie und manipuliertes Leben," *Christ und Welt* 17.11 (1964), 13.

26. E.g., see Fischer, "Von der Utopie," 59–62; Albert Hartmann, "Das ethische Urteil über das Töten mißgebildeter Kinder," in *Aktuelle Probleme des Lebensschutzes durch die Rechtsordnung* (Würzburg: Echter, 1964), 101–132, here 121–122; Georg Siegmund, "Begrenzte Euthanasie? Dürfen mißgebildete Kinder getötet werden?," *Theologie und Glaube* 56.6 (1966), 469–486; E. Wolf, "Das Problem der 'Euthanasie' im Spiegel evangelischer Ethik," *Zeitschrift für Evangelische Ethik* 10.1 (1966), 345–361. Catholics also felt compelled to tackle Catel's provocation systematically. The annual conference of the "Association of Catholic Institutions for the Mentally Disabled" in 1964 was launched with a keynote entitled "Euthanasia as a Timely Problem." Albert Hartmann SJ, "Euthanasie als aktuelles Problem," *Jahrestagung der "Vereinigung katholischer*

Einrichtungen für geistig Behinderte" vom 21. bis 24. September in Königstein im Taunus. Sonderdruck aus dem Caritasbrief für das Bistum Limburg 4 (1964), 6–16.

27. Ludwig Schlaich, "Zur Frage der 'Euthanasie,'" *Zeitschrift für evangelische Ethik* 1962, 48–51, here 48–49. See also the scathing review of the book, calling out Catel's "bluffing with alleged scientificity," full of "muddledness" and "deviousness." The book "does not satisfy … the most primitive scholarly requirements" and "deserves no tolerance, but at best pitying puzzlement." Ludwig Schlaich, review of Werner Catel, *Grenzsituationen des Lebens,* in *Blätter der Wohlfahrtspflege* 1 (1963), 32.

28. "Aus Menschlichkeit töten?," 42–44.

29. Ewald Meltzer, *Das Problem der Abkürzung "lebensunwerten" Lebens* (Halle: Carl Marhold, 1925).

30. Udo Dittmann, "Fritz Bauer und die Aufarbeitung der NS-'Euthanasie,'" *Forschungsjournal Soziale Bewegungen* 28.4 (2015), 208–229, here 210.

31. Thomas Vormbaum, ed., *"Euthanasie" vor Gericht: Die Anklageschrift des Generalstaatsanwalts beim OLG Frankfurt / M. gegen Dr. Werner Heyde u.a. vom 22. Mai 1962* (Berlin: Berliner Wissenschafts-Verlag, 2005), 431–435, esp. 433–434. The primary authors of the indictment were the state prosecutors Wilhelm Wentzke and Karl-Heinz Zinnall; Johannes Warlo joined Bauer's "euthanasia" prosecution team when the bulk of the text was done.

32. Helmuth Ehrhardt, *Euthanasie und Vernichtung "lebensunwerten" Lebens* (Ferdinand Enke Verlag: Stuttgart, 1965), 1. Emphasis mine.

33. Schneider, "Die Bilanz kann nicht zufriedenstellen," 349.

34. Gerhard Schmidt, *Selektion in der Heilanstalt 1939–1945* (Stuttgart: Evangelisches Verlagswerk, 1965), book flap.

35. Presentation by Gerhard Schmidt on the occasion of receiving the Griesinger Medaille in 1986, printed as "Das unerwünschte Buch," in Gerhard Schmidt, *Selektion in der Heilanstalt* (Berlin: Springer, 2011), 119–126, here 119–120. See also the reflections on the postwar role of Schmidt's former mentor Kurt Schneider, along with the possible motives for his complicity in urging that the text be suppressed, in Dirk Blasius, "Psychiatrischer Mord in der Zeit des Nationalsozialismus: Perspektiven und Befunde," in Vanja and Vogt, *Euthanasie in Hadamar,* 51–57.

36. Schmidt, *Selektion in der Heilanstalt* (1965), cover.

37. Schmidt, *Selektion in der Heilanstalt* (1965), 18, 17, 18, 24.

38. Schmidt, *Selektion in der Heilanstalt* (1965), 24, 33, 30, 19–20. "The man of the master race [*Herrenmensch*], agitated propagandistically by this [hallucinated] heredity-demon, as soon as he saw the grimace of the monstrosity in the flesh, had to perceive it as a dishonor for his racial pride [*Rassenstolz*]." "What a surprise that despite having coddled the heredity-demon, in these weakened times there is still such an impressive reservoir of master race-men available." "Many an SS or Lebensborn man may, seeing malformed or idiotic people, discover—in addition to a slight pressure of discomfort—an opportunity for self-deification [*Selbstvergötterung*]" (26, 30, 28).

39. Schmidt, *Selektion in der Heilanstalt* (1965), 19, 24, 26, 25. "Psychologically," Schmidt noted, "the hereditary-health-complex, once instilled and always again induced, develops a compulsion to overcompensation—a leap from exclusion from reproduction to exclusion from life" (26).

40. Schmidt, *Selektion in der Heilanstalt* (1965), 30, 35. See also Schmidt's sharp critique of Helmut Ehrhardt's "euthanasia"-apologetic remarks in his book of 1965 (34).

41. Letter quoted in Klee, *"Euthanasie" im NS-Staat,* 13.

42. See "Tötung von Geisteskranken—Mord im Sinne des Strafgesetzes," *Münchener Jüdische Nachrichten,* Nr. 1736 (1967), 5–6.

43. The case made international news, repeatedly. See "Three doctors acquitted of complicity in Nazi mercy killings, ordered retried," *Jewish Telegraphic Agency Daily News Bulletin* 37.154

(August 11, 1970), 3; "The World," *Los Angeles Times* (November 15, 1985). The doctors—Heinrich Bunke, Aquilin Ullrich, and Klaus Endruweit—were in fact re-tried, but soon declared "unfit," even as they continued to practice medicine.

44. Deutscher Bildungsrat, *Zur pädagogischen Förderung behinderter und von Behinderung bedrohter Kinder und Jugendlicher* [Empfehlungen der Bildungskommission] (Stuttgart: Ernst Klett Verlag, 1974).

45. See the excellent analysis in Raphael Rössel, "'Das muss ertragen werden': Die Serie 'Unser Walter' (ZDF 1974) und die Familiarisierung von Behinderungen," *Zeithistorische Forschungen* 19 (2022), 388–397, here 389.

46. Bericht über die Lage der Psychiatrie in der Bundesrepublik Deutschland—Zur psychiatrischen und psychotherapeutisch/psychosomatischen Versorgung der Bevölkerung, Deutscher Bundestag, 7. Wahlperiode, Drucksache 7 / 4200, 14.

47. Already in his early publications as a freelance journalist, Klee had been drawn to writing about individuals ostracized by society. In all cases, he made a point of directly living in the conditions he described—including spending nights in jail and in the squalid barracks that housed immigrant laborers—and while a student of theology and social work in the late 1960s, he had deliberately experimented with the loss of self-ownership of one's body and (what he reported experiencing as) a distressing dependence on helpers for getting dressed and undressed, in order to understand at least a small bit of the corporeal and subjective experiences of (some kinds of) physical disability. He also sought to experience firsthand the barriers throughout a typical city confronting any user of a wheelchair (and in one of his activist stints, put a municipal politician in a wheelchair as well to make the point unambiguous to him). By 1971, Klee had turned his journalistic attention to the issue of intellectual disability, producing a critical radio program for the Hessischer Rundfunk on the contradictions structuring daily life at Bethel with its several thousand citizens carrying diagnoses of epilepsy and / or mental impairment. The program captured, powerfully (with numerous clips of on-site talk), Bethel's then-typical treacly-pious self-presentation, as well as the patronizing tone used by staff members toward those in their care. Klee excoriated as "zoo"-like the tours Bethel provided (50,000 visitors annually) that gave the public the "frisson" of briefly immersing themselves among the "abnormals," but which did nothing to work to educate these visitors to the humanity of Bethel's residents. Starting in 1973, Klee joined Gusti Steiner, a social worker and wheelchair user living with muscular dystrophy, in teaching a praxis-oriented course for individuals with disabilities at the community college in Frankfurt / Main on "Mastering the Environment," and in 1975, Klee helped coordinate a protest in the city center using wheelchairs to force a massive traffic jam, just at rush hour, to call attention to the need for curb-cutting. But by 1981, Klee was increasingly determined to cede leadership in activism to disability self-advocates, and casting about for a different kind of project while maintaining his commitment to the topic of disability, he turned to investigating the national past. See Ernst Klee, "Gottes Stadt in Deutschland: Ein Bericht über Bethel," Hessischer Rundfunk, October 30, 1971 (typed transcript), 35–36, in Gedenkstätte Hadamar, Slg., N Klee, 186; Georg Gabler, "Erinnerungen an Ernst Klee," *kobinet-nachrichten*, March 14, 2022, https://kobinet-nachrichten.org/2022/03/14/erinnerungen-an-ernst-klee/; and Dagmar Herzog, "Die Subjektivität der Täter:innen," in Knud Andresen et al., eds., *Vom Ich zum Wir und wieder zurück? Subjektverständnisse zwischen Politisierung und Entradikalisierung seit den 1960er Jahren* (Göttingen: Wallstein, 2023), 20-39.

48. Klee, "Euthanasie", 385.

49. Klee, "Euthanasie", 150, 162, 336, 401, 427–428, 449–450.

50. Klee, "Euthanasie", 12.

51. Klee, "Euthanasie", 154, 425, 450, 447–448, 254.

52. Klee's concept of perpetrator motivation, intuitively arrived at in the 1980s, has become very much of a piece with contemporary perspectives. E.g., Wendy Lower, *Hitler's Furies:*

Women in the Nazi Killing Fields (New York: Houghton Mifflin, 2013); Omer Bartov, *Anatomy of a Genocide: The Life and Death of a Town Called Buczacz* (New York: Simon & Schuster, 2018); Edward B. Westermann, *Drunk on Genocide: Alcohol and Mass Murder in Nazi Germany* (Ithaca, NY: Cornell University Press, 2020).

53. Klee, *"Euthanasie"*, 28, 51.

54. Klee, *"Euthanasie"*, 71, 223, 244–247, 268–273, 338–339.

55. Klee, *"Euthanasie"*, 454.

56. Klee, *"Euthanasie"*, 320, 391.

57. Klee, *"Euthanasie"*, 196, 286, 292.

58. Klee, *"Euthanasie"*, 278.

59. See Hans-Josef Wollasch, "'Euthanasie' im NS-Staat: Was taten Kirche und Caritas?," *Themen des Deutschen Caritasverbandes*, May 15, 1984, 1–12; "'. . . von der Schuldfrage über die Ursachenfrage zur Strukturfrage'" (interview by Manfred Hellmann of Kurt Nowak), *Der Ring: Informationsblatt der v. Bodelschwingschen Anstalten* 4 (April 1985), 10–15.

60. E.g., "Gespräch mit dem Soziologen Ernst Klee über seine Forschungen zur Euthanasie," *Westdeutscher Rundfunk*, July 12, 1984 (audio recording).

61. The 1988 TV documentary "Alles Kranke ist Last" ("All that is sick is a burden"—a quote from a psychiatrist employed at the prominent Protestant charity institution Neuendettelsau in Bavaria, which had ended up giving 1,911 of its 2,137 residents over to the Nazi killing machinery) brought Klee's research to an even wider audience. Ernst Klee and Gunnar Petrich, "'Alles Kranke ist Last': Die Kirchen und die 'Vernichtung lebensunwerten Lebens'" (film, 1988), https://www.youtube.com/watch?v=w0ZMw4dequI; cf. the text in *Krüppel-Stolz: Selbstbestimmtes Leben*, October 25, 2010, http://cripplepride.blogspot.com/2010/10/alles-kranke-ist-last.html.

62. Vatican remarks quoted in Gerhard Fetka, "Der Zorn des an der Kirche Mitleidenden," *Neue Zeit* (Graz), March 24, 1992.

63. Animus: Waltraut Sax-Demuth, "'Unrichtiges und Halbwahrheiten: Material aus Bethel manipuliert,'" *Westfalen-Blatt*, July 28, 1988, 2; Norbert Trippen, "Falsches Bild von der Wirklichkeit," *Rheinischer Merkur* 18 (May 3, 1991), 21. Plaudits, while summing attacks on Klee: Ellen Presser, "Mitleid mit den Mördern: Ein wichtiges Buch von Ernst Klee über kirchliche Hilfe für Nazis," *Frankfurter Jüdische Nachrichten* (Rosh Hashanah, 1991), 32.

64. "Erklärung zu den Geschehnissen in den Diakonie-Anstalten Bad Kreuznach, die im Zusammenhang mit dem nationalsozialistischen Programm der 'Vernichtung lebensunwerten Lebens' stehen" (September 25, 1984), *Offene tür*, March 1985; and Landessynode der Evangelischen Kirche im Rheinland, "Erklärung zu Zwangssterilisierung, Vernichtung sogenannten lebensunwerten Lebens und medizinischen Versuchen an Menschen unter dem Nationalsozialismus" (January 12, 1985), *Evangelische Theologie* 45/5 (1985), 459–462. In addition to the important contributions of Pastor Jürgen Seim in the context of the working group *Kirche und "Euthanasie"*, pioneering leadership in encouraging further Protestant church critical self-interrogation was played by: Jörn-Erik Gutheil, "Die evangelische Kirche stellt sich ihrer Vergangenheit: Bericht aus der Rheinischen Landeskirche," in Evangelische Akademie Bad Boll, "Vergessene Opfer: Wiedergutmachung für die Betroffenen der Zwangssterilisation und des nationalsozialistischen Euthanasie-Programms, Tagung vom 27. bis 29. März 1987 in Bad Boll," *Protokolldienst* 14/87 (Bad Boll, 1987), 70–82;. See also: Jürgen Seim, ed., *Mehr ist eben nicht: Kranksein, Behindertsein, Menschsein* (Gütersloh: Verlag Jakob van Hoddis, 1988); Ingrid Genkel, "Du bist nichts, Dein Volk ist alles—Gibt es eine kirchliche Mitschuld an der Vernichtung lebensunwerten Lebens?," *Deutsches Allgemeines Sonntagsblatt* 31 (July 31, 1988), 13–14. Controversy continued: "'Persilscheine und falsche Pässe': Half die evangelische Kirche alten Nazis? Kirchenhistoriker Hans Prolingheuer zu den falschen Wahrheiten der Reinwasch-Ökumene," *Norddeutscher Rundfunk*, October 9, 1992, https://kirchengeschichten-im-ns.de/wp-content/uploads/2022/07/reinwasch_oekumene.pdf.

65. See the discussion in Klee,*"Euthanasie"*, 48–51, including the sidebar with the story of the deaf woman.

66. Klaus Dörner, "Brief an den Petitionsausschuß des Deutschen Bundestages, 26.01.1984," in Klaus Dörner, ed., *Gestern minderwertig, heute gleichwertig?: Folgen der Gütersloher Resolution* (Gütersloh: Hoddis, 1985), 1–3, here 1, 3. Other concerned professionals also understood sterilization survivors as belonging to the category of the racially persecuted. Two young doctors in Bremen documented and analyzed both the decisions of Nazi sterilization courts and postwar experts' continuing insistence on the necessity of sterilizations, even as, these doctors noted, a semantic restructuring at the point of Germany's military defeat in 1945 meant that ideals of "racial hygiene" were no longer explicitly referenced and the purported need for sterilization was presented as a strictly "unpolitical" matter—while at the same time expansively derogatory and stigmatizing rhetoric continued unchecked. The two doctors were convinced that the 1933 law needed to be understood "as a Nazi-law," that the "extent of the arbitrariness" in the practice of the sterilization courts would need to be shown yet more clearly, and that the "intimate connection between the sterilization law and the mass murders referred to as euthanasia" remained to be more fully demonstrated. But, although the politician formally endorsing their book when it was published in 1984 insisted as a foundational point that "the sterilizations in the time of National Socialism were a direct expression of the then-prevailing racism with its contempt for human beings" (*unmittelbarer Ausdruck des damaligen menschenverachtenden Rassismus*)— Herbert Brückner, Senator für Gesundheit und Sport, "Vorwort"—the most persuasive conceptual framing for making this case had evidently not yet been identified. See Hans-Georg Güse and Norbert Schmacke, *Zwangssterilisiert—Verleugnet—Vergessen: Zur Geschichte der nationalsozialistischen Rassenhygiene am Beispiel Bremen* (Bremen: Brockkamp, 1984), 136, 167, 172.

67. Gisela Bock, "Racism and Sexism in Nazi Germany: Motherhood, Compulsory Sterilization, and the State," *Signs* 8, no. 3 (Spring 1983): 400–421.

68. Gisela Bock, *Zwangssterilisation im Nationalsozialismus: Studien zur Rassenpolitik und Geschlechterpolitik* (1986, reprint Münster: MV Wissenschaft, 2010), 49.

69. Schmidt, *Selektion in der Heilanstalt* (1965), 30.

70. Bock, *Zwangssterilisation im Nationalsozialismus*, 12, 35, 51, 53.

71. Bock, "Gutachten," 260. See also her testimony in *Wiedergutmachung und Entschädigung*, 52–56, 102–104. A comparable phrasing is in her book: *Zwangssterilisation*, 12. The idea is prefigured in Hannah Arendt: "The Nazis did not think that the Germans were a master race, to whom the world belonged, but that they should be led by a master race, as should all other nations, and that this race was only on the point of being born." Hannah Arendt, "Totalitarianism in Power," in *The Origins of Totalitarianism*, 2nd ed. (Cleveland and New York: Meridian, 1958), 389–459, here 412.

72. Helmut E. Ehrhardt in *Wiedergutmachung und Entschädigung*, 137–138, 265–288, here 269. Emphasis added.

73. Helmut E. Ehrhardt, "Weitere Entschädigung für NS-Unrecht. - Öffentliche Anhörung am 24.6.1987 (Protokoll Nr. 7). - Ergänzende Stellungnahme" (1987), 2, 4–5, 9. Archiv Gisela Bock.

74. Nowak, who had been in training to become a nurse, landed in a psychiatric ward after having a concussion from a fall down a flight of stairs; there she was subjected to brutal and unnecessary treatments, including insulin shocks, which damaged her health further. She again came to the attention of medical authorities when she—supposedly—behaved publicly in an unruly manner during an attempted visit to her brother, who had been hospitalized at the Charité (the fever dreams he had after a serious bout of angina were taken as signs of mental illness); both she and her brother soon thereafter received the summons to the sterilization court, where they were confronted with the alternatives of either agreeing to be sterilized or being returned to institutions; two weeks later, both were operated on; her brother later served

in the Wehrmacht and died in the war. Nowak would suffer from searing abdominal pain for years and after the war underwent further operations. Repeated efforts to achieve legal recognition of the violation were rebuffed by the authorities with the remark that the harm caused by a sterilization was "immaterial." But Nowak did not give up, and the Federation she had co-organized spawned local branches in multiple cities and had 600 members already within the first two years; it became a highly successful organization, engaging in compelling lobbying and public awareness campaigns well into the twenty-first century. Matthias von Hellfeld, "Agonie ohne Ende," *Die Zeit* 8 (February 17, 1989); and Frank Schneider et al., *Registered, Persecuted, Annihilated: The Sick and the Disabled under National Socialism* (Heidelberg: Springer Medizin, 2014), 184–191. Niemand had labored as a warehouse stocker and driver for a large grocer and as a metal-fitter and locksmith at various ports, but had several nervous collapses marked by exhaustion and severe depressions that had made him unable to work for months at a time and which prompted hospitalizations in psychiatric wards. Horst Illiger, *"Sprich nicht drüber!" Der Lebensweg von Fritz Niemand* (Neumünster: Paranus, 2004).

75. The history is recounted in "Wir über uns," https://www.euthanasiegeschaedigte -zwangssterilisierte.de/wir-ueber-uns/.

76. Fritz Niemand and Klara Nowak in *Wiedergutmachung und Entschädigung*, 107–111, 137, 145–146, 157, 256–258.

77. Ehrhardt, "Weitere Entschädigung," 1. For an outstanding contextualization and emphasis on different details of the Bundestag committee debate, see Henning Tümmers, *Anerkennungskämpfe: Die Nachgeschichte der nationalsozialistischen Zwangssterilisationen in der Bundesrepublik* (Göttingen: Wallstein, 2011), 272–296.

78. Gisela Bock in *Wiedergutmachung und Entschädigung*, 265. Social Democratic Bundestag member Renate Schmidt, one of the most devoted advocates of the survivors, was sincerely worried that Ehrhardt's follow-up statement would undo the good that Bock's testimony had done and give Christian Democrats grist for continuing to block a more satisfactory resolution. Bock's retorts to Ehrhardt's assertions would ultimately be persuasive, but for the near future the government resisted acknowledgment of injustice and—not least on fiscal grounds—was only prepared to create a hardship fund to which survivors, under strict limits, could apply for support. Kathrin Braun and Svea Luise Herrmann, "Unrecht zweiter Ordnung: Die Weitergeltung des Gesetzes zur Verhütung erbkranken Nachwuchses in der Bundesrepublik," in Sonja Begalke, Claudia Fröhlich, and Stephan Alexander Glienke, eds., *Der halbierte Rechtsstaat: Demokratie und Recht in der frühen Bundesrepublik und die Integration von NS-Funktionseliten* (Baden-Baden: Nomos, 2015), 223–241.

79. Michael Burleigh and Wolfgang Wippermann, "Hilfloser Historismus: Warum die deutsche Geschichtswissenschaft bei der Erforschung der Euthanasie versagt hat," in Karl Ludwig Rost, Till Bastian, and Karl Bonhoeffer, eds., *Thema: Behinderte* (Stuttgart: Hirzel, 1991), 11–23. Toward the right side of the political spectrum, there were obviously countless motives for avoiding attention to National Socialist crimes. But also liberals and leftists had, with an intensity and force that is itself suspect, been exceedingly wary of paying attention to "ideology"—believing it to be somehow less "real" than economic relations or structures, or the machinations of high politics. Dörner himself had for several years been taking his cue from younger leftist independent scholars Karl Heinz Roth and Götz Aly and their coinage of the formula (in 1983) referring to the killings of the disabled as the "final solution to the social question." While this was meant as a welcome effort to get the crimes against the disabled taken more seriously by echoing the famous Nazi term for the mass murder of European Jewry, the phrase was problematic, as Bock would soon point out. In Dörner's use especially, as with many other efforts on the political left to treat Nazi antisemitism as somehow purely instrumental rhetoric covering over an "actual" preoccupation with repressing the working class, racisms of all kinds were viewed as somehow solely a matter of superstructural ideas floating around in the

air, without genuine efficacy. This is why Bock consistently emphasized *implementation*: the ways racism turned into politics, becoming all too real and consequential in the realms of laws, institutions, and practices. See Gisela Bock, "Krankenmord, Judenmord und national-sozialistische Rassenpolitik: Überlegungen zu einigen neueren Forschungshypothesen," in Frank Bajohr, Werner Johe, and Uwe Lohalm, eds., *Zivilisation und Barbarei: Die wider-sprüchlichen Potentiale der Moderne—Detlev Peukert zum Gedenken* (Hamburg: Christians, 1991), 285–306; and cf. Jürgen Matthäus, "'The Axis around which National Socialist Ideology Turns': State Bureaucracy, the Reich Ministry of the Interior, and Racial Policy in the First Years of the Third Reich," in Devin Pendas et al., eds., *Beyond the Racial State: Rethinking Nazi Germany* (New York: Cambridge University Press, 2017), 241–271.

80. Dirk Blasius, *"Einfache Seelenstörung": Geschichte der deutschen Psychiatrie, 1800–1945* (Frankfurt / Main: Fischer, 1994), 145.

81. With his dogged persistence, Dörner had succeeded impressively in convincing Chancellor Helmut Kohl, Federal President Richard von Weizsäcker, and (on behalf of the Catholic church) Cardinal Joseph Höffner to acknowledge Nazi crimes against the disabled formally—even if only in passing—at the occasion of their speeches marking the fortieth anniversary of the war's end in 1985. The texts are reprinted in Dörner, *Gestern minderwertig.*

82. Rolf Surmann, *Abgegoltene Schuld? Über den Widerspruch zwischen entschädigungspoliti-sichem Schlusstrich und interventionistischer Menschenrechtspolitik* (Hamburg: Unrast, 2005), 108. Already in February 1986, in response to the application of an individual sterilized in 1936, whose earlier effort to have the NS sterilization court's verdict reversed had been rejected in 1957, a court in Kiel—basing its decision on the facts of the case, but also on a transformed understanding that the sterilization campaign had been a manifestation of NS injustice, and among other things inspired by critical research conducted by a team of young physicians investigating the complicity of the University of Hamburg's medical clinic in the NS sterilization program—for the first time declared the NS sterilization law to be incompatible with West Germany's constitution and its guarantee of bodily integrity for all citizens. See Susanne Knoop, "Recht auf Fortpflanzung und medizinischer Fortschritt" (Dissertation, University of Konstanz, 2005), 182–183; Friedemann Pfäfflin, "Anfänge der Auseinandersetzung mit der NS-Psychiatrie in Hamburg" (lecture delivered at the conference, "Hamburger Universitätspsychiatrie im Nationalsozialismus. Zukunft der Erinnerung," January 27, 2023).

83. Arbeitsgemeinschaft Bund der "Euthanasie"-Geschädigten und Zwangssterilisierten, "Zeittafel zur Entschädigungspolitik für Zwangssterilisierte und "Euthanasie"-Geschädigte (Stand 20.2.2022)," https://www.euthanasiegeschaedigte-zwangssterilisierte.de/themen /entschaedigung/zeittafel-entschaedigungspolitik-fuer-zwangssterilisierte-und-euthanasie -geschaedigte/.

84. "Antrag der Abgeordneten Dr. Jürgen Gehb et al., Ächtung des Gesetzes zur Verhütung erbkranken Nachwuchses vom 14. Juli 1933" (Deutscher Bundestag, Drucksache 16 / 3811) (13.12.2006), 3, https://dserver.bundestag.de/btd/16/038/1603811.pdf.

85. "Beschlussempfehlung und Bericht des Rechtsausschusses" (Deutscher Bundestag, Drucksache 16 / 5450, 23.05.2007), 1, http://dip21.bundestag.de/dip21/btd/16/054/1605450 .pdf. This involved some sleight of hand as, in so designating the sterilization law, the politicians were—whether out of ignorance or out of eager support for the cause of disability rights—eliding the fact that the "Law for the Restoration of the Civil Service," passed in April 1933, i.e., a few months prior to the sterilization law in July 1933—the law that had driven "non-Aryans" (as well as leftist political opponents of Nazism) out of the civil service—was actually the Nazis' "first racial law."

86. On the preparatory activist prehistory to the establishment of the memorial, see Sigrid Falkenstein, "Gedenk- und Informationsort für die Opfer der 'Euthanasie'-Morde," https://www .euthanasie-gedenken.de/t4_erinnerungsort.htm; and the DFG-sponsored "Erinnern heißt

gedenken und informieren: Die nationalsozialistische Euthanasie und der historische Ort Berliner Tiergartenstraße 4. Ein Erkenntnistransfer-Projekt," directed by the medical historians and psychiatrists Gerrit Hohendorf and Maike Rotzoll, https://gepris.dfg.de/gepris/projekt /234017019?language=de. See also the pioneering book by Sigrid Falkenstein about her murdered aunt, Anna Lehnkering, which did a great deal to shift the public terms of conversation about the persecution of people with disabilities during the Third Reich and the postwar silences within families: *Annas Spuren: Ein Opfer der NS-"Euthanasie"* (Munich: Herbig, 2012).

87. "Antrag der Fraktionen CDU / CSU, SPD, FDP und Bündnis 90 / Die Grünen: Gedenkort für die Opfer der NS-'Euthanasie'-Morde" (Deutscher Bundestag, Drucksache 17 / 5493, 13.04.2011), 1, https://dserver.bundestag.de/btd/17/054/1705493.pdf.

Chapter Four: The Fascism in the Heads

1. "Die Lebenshilfe in ihrem Verhältnis zu Anstalten und Vollzeiteinrichtungen," in *Lebenshilfe für geistig Behinderte: Rückblick—Ausblick* (Marburg: Lebenshilfe für geistig Behinderte e.V., 1983), 60–61, here 60.

2. Wolfgang Jantzen, "Faschismus und Behinderung," in Studienkreis zur Erforschung und Vermittlung der Geschichte des deutschen Widerstandes, *Informationen* 1 (1981), 1–4, here 3.

3. Conditions were also bleak in large-scale residential institutions in the UK and the United States and Canada. See Maureen Oswin, *The Empty Hours: A Study of the Week-end Life of Handicapped Children in Institutions* (London: Allen Lane, 1971); Deborah Cohen, "Children Who Disappeared," in *Family Secrets: Shame and Privacy in Modern Britain* (New York: Oxford University Press, 2013), 87–123; Rubahanna Amannah Choudhury, "The Forgotten Children: The Association of Parents of Backward Children and the Legacy of Eugenics in Britain, 1946–1960" (Ph.D. thesis, Oxford Brookes University, 2015); Burton Blatt and Fred Kaplan, *Christmas in Purgatory: A Photographic Essay on Mental Retardation* (orig. 1966; reprint, New York: Human Policy Press, 1974); David J. Rothman and Sheila M. Rothman, "The Litigator as Reformer," in Steven Noll and James W. Trent Jr., eds., *Mental Retardation in America: A Historical Reader* (New York: New York University Press, 2004), 445–465; Kate Rossiter and Jen Rinaldi, "Introduction," *Institutional Violence and Disability: Punishing Conditions* (New York: Routledge, 2019), 1–22.

4. For the medical profession, see esp. Volker Roelcke, "Medical Ethics in Post-War Germany: Reconsidering Some Basic Assumptions," *Wiener klinische Wochenschrift* 130 (2018), Supplement 3, S180–S183; Heiner Fangerau, Sascha Topp, and Klaus Schepker, eds., *Kinder- und Jugendpsychiatrie im Nationalsozialismus und in der Nachkriegszeit: Zur Geschichte ihrer Konsolidierung* (Berlin: Springer, 2017).

5. Wilhelm Hofmann, "Zum Problem der heilpädagogischen Betreuung schwachsinniger Kinder," *Zeitschrift für Heilpädagogik* (1959), 248–250, here 248. Numerous similar quotes and critical analysis in Siegfried Gehrecke, "'Strukturwandel' der Hilfsschule?," in *Hilfsschule heute—Krise oder Kapitulation?* (Berlin: Marhold, 1971), 37–46.

6. See, e.g., Johann Neuhäusler, "Antichrists Wüten gegen das 'unwerte Leben,'" in *Kreuz und Hakenkreuz: Der Kampf des Nationalsozialismus gegen die katholische Kirche und der kirchliche Widerstand, Erster Teil* (München: Katholische Kirche Bayerns, 1946), 307–315; Paul Gerhard Braune, "Der Kampf der Inneren Mission gegen die Euthanasie," *Innere Mission* 37.5-6 (1947), 12–44.

7. On neglect and abuse at numerous institutions—including beatings, straitjacketing, and other forms of fixation, as well as pharmaceutical experimentation—see Heiner Fangerau et al., eds., *Leid und Unrecht: Kinder und Jugendliche in Behindertenhilfe und Psychiatrie der BRD und DDR 1949 bis 1990* (Köln: Psychiatrie-Verlag, 2021). On systemic abuses at one of the largest Catholic institutions for the "educable mentally feeble," see Bernhard Frings, *Heimerziehung im Essener Franz-Sales-Haus 1945–1970* (Münster: Aschendorff, 2012) and Uwe Kaminsky and

Katharina Klöcker, *Medikamente und Heimerziehung am Beispiel des Franz Sales Hauses: Historische Erklärungen—ethische Perspektiven* (Münster: Aschaffendorf, 2020). For contemporaneous statements on the overcrowding and understaffing in Catholic and Protestant institutions alike, see: Bernhard Rüther, "Werden die Ärmsten vergessen?," *Jahrbuch für Caritaswissenschaft und Caritasarbeit* (Freiburg: Lambertus, 1957), 28–34; Roger Anderson, "Ein hilfloser Schrei: Kristall besuchte die unglücklichen Menschen von Bethel," *Kristall* 14 (1964), 10–17; Bernhard Rudolph, "Hier können Sie helfen!" *Bild* 17 (March 24, 1972), 7. For a memory-essay by a former conscientious objector describing "the shocking situation" when he arrived in 1975 to begin his alternative service at a Protestant residential institution on "the ward for the severely-disabled" (*Schweb*—the institution's internal shorthand for *Schwerbehindertenstation*), his own strong sense of shame at what residents had to endure, his fury at acquaintances who suggested that the residents would be "better off dead," and his dawning realization that the conditions there represented "massive human rights violations in the West Germany of that time," see Werner Brill, "Veränderung durch Aufklärung: Zur Bedeutung von Ernst Klee für die Disziplin der Sonder- und Heilpädagogik," *Behindertenpädagogik* 52.4 (2013), 389–401, here 389–390. The encounter was life-changing for Brill—as it was for so many other conscientious objectors of that era who did their alternative service in residential institutions for people with disabilities; he became a radical disability pedagogy professor and researched and wrote extensively also on the history of special pedagogy in the Weimar and Nazi periods.

8. It is conspicuous with what regularity, for twenty years into the postwar era, institution directors and staff remark on the continuance of broad-based popular hostility, even of overtly expressed death wishes. See, e.g., the original version of the speech given by pastor-director Johannes Klevinghaus at the occasion of the postwar reopening of the Wittekindshof, printed as "Dokument," in Hans-Walter Schmuhl and Ulrike Winkler, *"Der das Schreien der jungen Raben nicht überhört": Der Wittekindshof—eine Einrichtung für Menschen mit geistiger Behinderung, 1887 bis 2012* (Bielefeld: Verlag für Regionalgeschichte, 2012), 553–562, here 556–558; Rea Kulenkampff, *Die kleine Patmos-Schule* (Bethel: Verlagshandlung der Anstalt Bethel, 1954), 5–6; Ludwig Schlaich, "Zur Frage der 'Euthanasie'," *Zeitschrift für evangelische Ethik* (January 1962), 48–51, here 48; Johannes Klevinghaus, "Der geistig behinderte Mensch in der heutigen Gesellschaft" (speech delivered in Alsterdorf, October 18, 1963), *Hundert Jahre Dienst an Geistesschwachen in Alsterdorf* (Hamburg: Alsterdorfer Anstalten, 1963), 12–17, here 13–14; Friedrich von Bodelschwingh, *Lebensunwert? Eine Stellungnahme* (special reprint of *Bote von Bethel* 66 (June 1964)), 5. Notably, even a standard postwar religious encyclopedia entry on "welfare-care for the feeble-minded" (*Schwachsinnigenfürsorge*) commented on the "fatalistic, if not downright hostile-rejecting stance" of the public toward the mentally disabled, and on the "still existing remnants of unmerciful intolerance." K. Janssen, "Schwachsinnigenfürsorge," *Die Religion in Geschichte und Gegenwart*, 3rd rev. ed., vol. 5 (Tübingen: Mohr, 1961), 1586–1587.

9. Frau Brüning quoted in Heiko Gebhardt and Dieter Heggemann, "Das grausame Dorf," *Stern* 45 (1969), 34–38, here 37. Cf. Karlheinz Eckert, "Burgfrieden in der ausgebrannten Aumühle," *Süddeutsche Zeitung* 254 (October 23, 1969), 17; Hannelore Schütz-Doinet, "Dorf ohne Deppen," *Die Zeit* 44 (October 30, 1970); Oskar Neisinger, "Heile Welt auf altbayrisch: Stirbt der Fall Aumühle in den Akten?," *Publik* 4.14 (April 2, 1971), 1; "Eh hinten dran," *Der Spiegel* 22 (May 27, 1973). See also the brilliant film by Alexeij Sagerer, *Aumühle* (1973), which uses deliberate vulgarity to make profound moral-political points. The film highlighted the stupefied and brutish provinciality of the villagers through an ingenious enactment in which senseless killing of chickens and geese—and later a pig—is juxtaposed with in-person interviews with both the suavely unapologetic Catholic priest and the still-shaken home manager with yet a third element: documentary footage of happy children and youth with intellectual impairments. The priest and villagers had, in egging on the violence, called the (non-Jewish) home manager a "Jew-pig" (*Judensau*). Eva-Elizabeth Fischer, "Sagerers Schlachtfest," *Süddeutsche Zeitung*

(April 28, 2017). The film provides implicit commentary both on the "euthanasia" murders and on the Holocaust—signaled not least by an intertextual moment that is recognizably referencing Sidney Lumet, *The Pawnbroker* (1965).

10. "Hinterwäldler": Regierungsrat Müller quoted in Gebhardt und Heggemann, "Das grausame Dorf," 38; "nicht ganz zu Unrecht": Kai Hermann, "'Was nützt uns ein soziales Gewissen?'" *Der Spiegel* 44 (October 26, 1969); "einen ungünstigen moralischen Einfluß": Landrat Fritz Gerstl's views summarized in "Pfarrer seines Amtes enthoben," *Bremer Nachrichten* 249 (October 22, 1969), 12.

11. Roswin Finkenzeller, "Die Fürstenecker hüllen sich in Schweigen," *Frankfurter Allgemeine Zeitung* (October 27, 1969), 8.

12. Hermann, "'Was nützt uns.'"

13. See the saddened summary remarks by Federal President Gustav Heinemann in his Christmas message to the nation in December 1970: "kurz berichtet," *Bundesarbeitsblatt* 2 (February 1971), 133.

14. Helmut von Bracken, *Vorurteile gegen behinderte Kinder, ihre Familien und Schulen* (Berlin: Carl Marhold, 1976), 361; see also—summarizing and commenting on von Bracken's initial findings—Helmut A. Paul, "Das behinderte Kind—ein Sonderproblem?" in Theodor Hellbrügge et al., *Probleme des behinderten Kindes* (Munich: Urban & Schwarzenberg, 1973), 15–33, here 22–25.

15. Von Bracken, *Vorurteile*, 61–62, 85, 114, 128, 362.

16. Von Bracken, *Vorurteile*, 82, 358.

17. "'Das Image von behinderten Kindern bei der Bevölkerung der Bundesrepublik,'" *Lebenshilfe* 10.1 (1971), 1–7, here 7. In this study, 78 out of 100 individuals questioned opined that mentally disabled children should be sent to live in an institution (1, 5). Several years later, then-Federal President Walter Scheel of the Free Democratic Party took the occasion of the International Day of the Disabled to cite a study that had found 90 percent of the populace claiming not to know how to behave in relation to the disabled and 70 percent endorsing the isolation of the disabled in closed institutions. See Walter Scheel, "16. Welttag der Behinderten," *Bulletin. Presse- und Informationsamt der Bundesregierung* 41 (March 26, 1975), 393–395, here 393. A wealth of press clippings at the archive of the Christian Democrats' Konrad-Adenauer-Stiftung make clear that both the breadth and the stubborn persistence of ordinary citizens' prejudices against and discomfort around people with any kinds of disability were a constant concern, regularly aired by politicians and by the media all through the 1970s—and into the 1980s. Pressearchiv, Konrad-Adenauer-Stiftung, Thema "Behinderte."

18. For a concise summary of these conditions, see "So fing es an," *Lebenshilfe für geistig Behinderte: Rückblick—Ausblick*, 6–8.

19. Werner Villinger had, it was revealed in 1961, been a "selector" for the T4 killings. His younger associate Hermann Stutte, like Villinger an NSDAP member since 1937, continued into the postwar years unselfconsciously to refer to the "dissociality [*Dissozialität*]" and "sociobiological inferiority [*sozialbiologische Unterwertigkeit*]" of the patients that juvenile psychiatrists most frequently dealt with and persisted in interpreting "criminal behavior," "immoral lifestyle," or "lack of giftedness" as transgenerationally genetically transmitted conditions. See, on both men, Volker Roelcke, "Erbbiologie und Kriegserfahrung in der Kinder- und Jugendpsychiatrie der frühen Nachkriegszeit: Kontinuitäten und Kontexte bei Hermann Stutte," in Fangerau et al., *Kinder- und Jugendpsychiatrie*, 447–464, here 449–452.

20. Gesetz über die Schulpflicht im Deutschen Reich, July 6, 1938, https://www.verfassungen .de/de33-45/schulpflicht38.htm.

21. For a balanced account that honors the courage of those teachers who found ways to keep children with more significant intellectual disabilities in a caring school setting despite the 1938 law, see Manfred Höck, *Die Hilfsschule im Dritten Reich* (Berlin: Carl Marhold, 1979), 170–188.

22. Heinz Bach, "Grundsätzliche Überlegungen zur Sonderschule für praktisch Bildbare," *Lebenshilfe* 4.4 (1965), 196–199, here 197. See also Wilfried Rudloff, "Überlegungen zur Geschichte der bundesdeutschen Behindertenpolitik," *Zeitschrift für Sozialreform* 49.6 (2003), 863–886, here 870–874; Jan Stoll, "'Behinderung' als Kategorie sozialer Ungleichheit: Entstehung und Entwicklung der 'Lebenshilfe für das behinderte Kind' in der Bundesrepublik Deutschland in den 1950er und 1960er Jahren," *Archiv für Sozialgeschichte* 54 (2014), 169–191.

23. Franz-Lorenz von Thadden's son Ernst-Dietrich, born 1952, had physical and mental disabilities brought on by encephalitis and high fever at age 6 weeks. Not only did von Thadden succeed in launching the needed school in Saarbrücken; he made the cause of disability rights and improved care and education central to both his journalistic and his subsequent political career, publishing recurrently on the subject, launching a working group on "Protection of the Weak" (*Schutz der Schwachen*) within the CDU-CSU party in December 1969 almost immediately upon his entry into the Bundestag; and working closely with politicians from other parties to advance government support for the needs of people with disabilities, psychiatric patients, and the elderly. See esp. Franz-Lorenz von Thadden, "Unser geliebtes, unglückliches Kind," *Saarbrücker Landeszeitung* [date unknown, 1958–1959], reprinted in Marielisa von Thadden et al., eds., *Die Welt ist weit, und ich bin jung: Das Leben des Franz-Lorenz v. Thadden* (Bonn: Verlag Franz Schön, 2015), 435–438; and Franz-Lorenz von Thadden, "Die im Schatten leben," *Deutsches Monatsblatt* 12 (1969), 9. In 1961, for instance, he wrote: "We Germans have a heavy duty of conscience towards those whom the National Socialist regime denied even the right to live by killing them by the tens of thousands. . . . Their murder can admittedly no more be undone than that of the Jews, but at least the shameful remembrance of the 'euthanasia' crimes should make us look for ways and means to help the sufferers of our time to the best of our ability." Franz-Lorenz von Thadden, "Auch diesen Kindern helfen!," *Saarbrücker Landeszeitung* [date unknown, 1961], Archiv Maresa von Fürstenberg. The von Thadden family's battle to found the Saarbrücken school made national news: "'Nicht laufen, nicht sprechen, nicht hören,'" *Der Spiegel* 13 (March 21, 1971). Over the decades, the original initiative evolved into a successful multidimensional service organization, encompassing communally integrated residential settings and a broad array of professional training opportunities. See "Historie," reha gmbh, https://rehagmbh.de/unternehmen/historie.

24. In 1970, in the midst of the Bundestag discussion which sparked the plan for the Psychiatrie-Enquête, von Thadden in his opening remarks addressed his colleagues "as the father of a child who is mentally disabled." See "Dritte Beratung," Deutscher Bundestag 44. Sitzung (April 17, 1970), 2263–2278, here 2276; and see also the remarks of representative Picard, "Dritte Beratung," 2263–2267; as well as "Schriftlicher Bericht des Ausschusses für Jugend, Familie und Gesundheit über den Antrag der Abgeordneten Picard [et al.] . . . betr. Situation der Psychiatrie in der Bundesrepublik (June 9, 1971), Deutscher Bundestag, 6. Wahlperiode, Drucksache VI / 2322; and Felicitas Söhner, *Psychiatrie-Enquete: mit Zeitzeugen verstehen. Eine Oral History der Psychiatrie-Reform in der BRD* (Köln: Psychiatrie-Verlag, 2020). The representatives' core message, as von Thadden reported, was that a psychiatric illness was "'neither a flaw, nor an arbitrary or irreversible fate, but rather suffering—suffering that requires our care and assistance just as much as a physical illness.'" Franz-Lorenz von Thadden, "Die im Dunkeln leben," *Deutschland Union-Dienst* 24.75 (April 21, 1970), 3–4, here 3.

25. Ulrich Bleidick, "Die Entwicklung und Differenzierung des Sonderschulwesens von 1898 bis 1973 im Spiegel des Verbandes Deutscher Sonderschulen," *Zeitschrift für Heilpädagogik* 24.10 (1973), 824–845, here 825.

26. "'Nicht laufen.'"

27. Karl-Peter Gerschlauer, "Aktiver Streik—Vorlesungsboykott der Studenten der Studiengangseinheit Heil- und Sonderpädagogik, Marburg," in *Behindertenpädagogik in Hessen* 12.1 (1973), 32–34, here 34.

28. Helmut von Bracken, *Entwicklungsgestörte Jugendliche* (Munich: Juventa, 1965), 73. See also the critical analysis in Manfred Gerspach, "Zum Jahr der Behinderten 1981: Die Enthistorisierung eines sozialen Phänomens," *Behindertenpädagogik* 20.4 (1981), 330–342, here 335.

29. Bericht über den Stand der Maßnahmen auf dem Gebiet der Bildungsplanung, Deutscher Bundestag, 5. Wahlperiode, Drucksache V / 2166, October 13, 1967, 17.

30. Ernst Begemann, "Zum Problem der Einschulung der 'Hilfsschüler,'" *Zeitschrift für Heilpädagogik* 21.4 (1970), 173–192, here 183; W. Ferdinand and R. Uhr, "Sind Arbeiterkinder dümmer oder letztlich nur 'die Dummen'?," *Die Grundschule* 5.4 (August 1973), 237–239.

31. Ulf Preuss-Lausitz, "Probleme der Integration von Sonderschülern in die Gesamtschule," *Zeitschrift für Heilpädagogik* 22.3 (1971), 183–193.

32. Jakob Muth, "Lernbehinderte Kinder in der Grundschule—Aussonderung oder Integration?," *Die Grundschule* 5.4 (August 1973), 231–236; Rudloff, "Überlegungen," 112.

33. Begemann, "Zum Problem," 183, 188–189.

34. Johanna Aab et al., *Sonderschule zwischen Ideologie und Wirklichkeit: Für eine Revision der Sonderpädagogik* (Munich: Juventa, 1974), 80–81; Gerspach, "Zum Jahr," 334; Gerschlauer, "Aktiver Streik," 34.

35. Karl-Heinz Grothe, "Die Bundesrepublik—Volk der Sonderschüler?," *Sonderpädagogik* 4.1 (1974), 41–43.

36. Ferdinand und Uhr, "Sind Arbeiterkinder dümmer," 237.

37. Compare the contrasting perspectives in: *Die Anstalt*, December 20, 2022, https://www .zdf.de/comedy/die-anstalt/die-anstalt-vom-20-dezember-2022-100.html; and the Niedersachsen FDP campaign to retain segregated Förderschulen, https://fdp-nds.de/offene -foerderschulen-offene-chancen.

38. Deutscher Bildungsrat, *Zur pädagogischen Förderung behinderter und von Behinderung bedrohter Kinder und Jugendlicher* [Empfehlungen der Bildungskommission] (Stuttgart: Ernst Klett Verlag, 1974), 15–16, 24.

39. Deutscher Bildungsrat, *Zur pädagogischen Förderung*, 16, 18, 27–28. One historian has aptly referred to Muth's *Recommendation* as "highly regarded, oft invoked, complied with only to a limited extent." Rudloff, "Überlegungen," 873. That has proven true up to the present, as resistance also against the guidelines mandating integration (now called inclusion) in the UN Convention on the Rights of Persons with Disabilities, ratified by Germany in 2009, persists. But in its moment, Muth both forced a new conversation and legitimated the radicals, who saw an opening and ran with it.

40. Bleidick, "Die Entwicklung," 837–838.

41. Ulrich Bleidick, *Einführung in die Behindertenpädagogik. Band I Allgemeine Theorie und Bibliographie* (Stuttgart: Kohlhammer, 1977), 31, 33–34.

42. Karl-Heinz Berg, "Separierung der Heilerziehung, eine Chance für die Behinderten," *betrifft: erziehung* 9.5 (May 1976), 21–23. See also the critique of Berg's views as "definitely in proximity to faschistoid thought," in Barbara Rohr et al., "Fünf Thesen und eine Frage," *betrifft: erziehung* 9.5 (May 1976), 23, 25, here 25.

43. Georg Feuser, "Integration statt Aussonderung Behinderter?," *Behindertenpädagogik* 20.1 (February 1981), 5–17.

44. Georg Feuser, "Integration = die gemeinsame Tätigkeit (Spielen/ Lernen/ Arbeit) am gemeinsamen Gegenstand/ Produkt in Kooperation von behinderten und nichtbehinderten Menschen," *Behindertenpädagogik* 21.2 (May 1982), 86–105, here 89.

45. A. S. Neill, *Summerhill: A Radical Approach to Child Rearing* (New York: Hart, 1960).

46. Wolfgang Jantzen, "Aufbewahrung oder Therapie?," *Zeitschrift für Heilpädagogik* 23.4 (1972), 267–271; Wolfgang Jantzen, "Nein zur Macht—ein Exkurs zu Freiheit und Befreiung," *Jahrbuch der Luria-Gesellschaft* 2020, 28–38.

47. Jantzen, "Aufbewahrung," 270; cf. 267.

48. Wolfgang Jantzen, "Kritische Psychologie in der Behindertenpädagogik," in Günter Rexilius, ed., *Psychologie als Gesellschaftswissenschaft* (Opladen: Westdeutscher Verlag, 1988), 352–372, here 353; Wolfgang Jantzen, "Die Freiheit ist eine Tat . . . Biographische Reflexionen" (Vortrag bei der Fachtagung der Luria-Gesellschaft e.V.: "Das andere nicht nur zu denken, sondern es zu machen." Kulturhistorische Theorie und ihre Weiterentwicklung zur Gegenhegemonie. Darmstadt, 1. Oktober 2016), in *Jahrbuch der Luria-Gesellschaft* 2017, 46–71. The Brecht text was the antiwar poem for children, *Die drei Soldaten* (1932), with illustrations by George Grosz.

49. Georg Feuser, "Es ging immer um das Mögliche, das im Wirklichen nicht sichtbar ist!," *Jahrbuch der Luria-Gesellschaft* 2017, 72–109; "Interview mit Georg Feuser," in Frank J. Müller, ed., *Blick zurück nach vorn—WegbereiterInnen der Inklusion. Band 2* (Gießen: Psychosozial, 2018), 57–146.

50. Feuser, "Es ging immer," 8, 10–11.

51. An oft-cited reference was the German translation of an essay by Vygotsky from 1924, not least because it makes clear that the "defect" lies in us, the teachers: "Possibly the time is no longer far away in which the field of pedagogy will find it embarrassing to speak of a defective child, because that could imply that there is some insurmountable deficiency within it. . . . It lies in our hands to act in such a way that the deaf, the blind, and the feeble-minded child are not defective. Then also the word itself will disappear, the true sign of our own defect." L. S. Wygotski, "Zur Psychologie und Pädagogik der kindlichen Defektivität," *Die Sonderschule* 2 (1975), 65–72, here 72. For the fullest summary of the cultural-historical school's relevance to Jantzen and Feuser, see Wolfgang Jantzen, *Allgemeine Behindertenpädagogik: Sozialwissenschaftliche und psychologische Grundlagen* (Weinheim: Beltz, 1987).

52. It was fitting that in subsequent years, and not least because of his revulsion at traditional Christianity, Jantzen in particular would be drawn to various forms of liberation theology, from the German feminist Dorothee Sölle to the Argentine philosopher-theologian Enrique Dussel. The tagline for a book series he would later edit with the Psychosozial Verlag was adapted from Dussel (even as it, unmistakably, also echoed Buber): "The only sacred thing that counts is the existence of the Other." (*Das einzig Heilige, das zählt, ist die Existenz des Anderen*).

53. Wolfgang Jantzen, "Theorien zur Heilpädagogik," *Das Argument* 15.80 (1973), 152–169; Wolfgang Jantzen, "Materialistische Erkenntnistheorie, Behindertenpädagogik und Didaktik," *Demokratische Erziehung* 2 (1976), 15–29, here 16.

54. Wolfgang Jantzen, "Behinderung und Faschismus," *Behindertenpädagogik in Hessen* 14.4 (November 1975), 150–169, here 162; Jantzen, "Faschismus und Behinderung," 2.

55. Wolfgang Jantzen, *Sozialgeschichte des Behindertenbetreuungswesens* (Munich: DJI, 1982), 10; Karl Marx, "Zur Kritik der Hegelschen Rechtsphilosophie. Einleitung" (1843), http://www.mlwerke.de/me/me01/me01_378.htm.

56. Bleidick, "Die Entwicklung," 832; Arbeitsgemeinschaft Sonderschulen des Kreises Gelnhausen und der Stadt Gießen, "Schreiben an den hessischen Kultusminister," *Zeitschrift für Heilpädagogik* 24.2 (1973), 131–132, here 131. Emphasis in the original.

57. Wolfgang Jantzen, *Sozialisation und Behinderung: Studien zu sozialwissenschaftlichen Grundfragen der Behindertenpädagogik* (Gießen: Focus-Verlag, 1974), 1–2, 4. Jantzen is without question responding directly to the petition letter, as he quotes select passages from it on p. 3. The book became an underground classic, read by special education students at universities across West Germany.

58. Wolfgang Jantzen, "Überlegungen zu Gegenstand und Methode der Behindertenpädagogik als Sozialwissenschaft," *Behindertenpädagogik in Hessen* 13.3. (August 1974), 134–140.

59. Wolfgang Jantzen, "Materialistische Behindertenpädagogik und Therapie," *Behindertenpädagogik* 17.2 (May 1978), 78–107, here 89.

60. Georg Feuser, "Erziehung und Unterricht geistigbehinderter Kinder," *Zeitschrift für Heilpädagogik* 21.1 (1970), 1–17, here 1. Emphasis in the original. Jantzen had picked up on this

element in Feuser from the start, insisting that the mentally disabled child be "recognized as a fully valuable, equally entitled human partner, who just like everyone else has the right to a fulfilled life." Jantzen, "Aufbewahrung," 267.

61. Feuser, "Integration = die gemeinsame Tätigkeit," 89.

62. "Denn der echte Erzieher hat nicht bloß einzelne Funktionen seines Zöglings im Auge, wie der, der ihm lediglich bestimmte Kenntnisse oder Fertigkeiten beizubringen beabsichtigt, sondern es ist ihm jedesmal um den ganzen Menschen zu tun, und zwar um den ganzen Menschen sowohl seiner gegenwärtigen Tatsächlichkeit nach, in der er vor dir lebt, als auch seiner Möglichkeit nach, als was aus ihm werden kann." Martin Buber, "Über Charaktererziehung," in *Reden über Erziehung* (Heidelberg: Lambert Schneider, 1964), 53–73, here 53.

63. "Er wird zu dem Ich, dessen Du wir ihm sind." https://www.georg-feuser.com/. See also Georg Feuser, "Ich bin, also denke ich! Allgemeine und fallbezogene Hinweise zur Arbeit im Konzept der SDKHT," *Behindertenpädagogik* 40.3 (2001), 268–350, here 285; Martin Buber, "Ich und Du," in *Das Dialogische Prinzip* (Heidelberg: Lambert Schneider, 1965), 7–121, here 32. Feuser had elaborated: "A human being is in his presentness already that which is momentarily possible, with regard to potential changes; competent, in short, no matter how disabled he may appear to us. [*Ein Mensch ist seiner Gegenwart nach das momentan Mögliche hinsichtlich der möglichen Veränderungen; also kompetent, wie behindert er uns auch erscheinen mag.*]" (285).

64. Georg Feuser, *Gemeinsame Erziehung behinderter und nichtbehinderter Kinder im Kindertagesheim: Ein Zwischenbericht* (Bremen: Diakonisches Werk Bremen, 1987).

65. Feuser, "Ich bin," 268, 271.

66. Georg Feuser, "Integration—eine Frage der Didaktik einer allgemeinen Pädagogik," in *Behinderte in Familie, Schule und Gesellschaft* 1 (1999).

67. Georg Feuser, "Zur Konzeption und Praxis der Substituierend Dialogisch-Kooperativen Handlungs-Therapie," *Psychiatrische Pflege Heute* 27 (2021): 70–75. To be clear: Feuser never sentimentalized disability itself, never romanticized what integration could achieve, and never pretended that even the best educational intervention could magically make disability go away. He also—almost unique in his field—never blamed parents ("They [families] do not break . . . over the fact of the so-called 'disabledness' of their child, but over the lovelessness and contempt of this society.") But he was certain that rejection of the disabled—and rejection of those who worked with the disabled—was a sign of the impoverishment and psychic crippling of the nondisabled. And much of what passed for special education, he argued, was an "ideology . . . that oppresses those whom it promises to liberate." Feuser, "Integration statt Aussonderung," 6, 14.

68. Jantzen, "Behinderung und Faschismus," 152; Karl Tornow and Herbert Weinert, *Erbe und Schicksal: Von geschädigten Menschen, Erbkrankheiten und deren Bekämpfung* (Berlin: Metzner, 1942), 156–157.

69. Jantzen, "Faschismus und Behinderung," 3.

70. Parent activism for integration began around 1975; by 1984 there was a formal network, Eltern für Integration. See Manfred Rosenberger, "Die Entwicklung zur Schule ohne Aussonderung aus Elternsicht," in Peter Heyer et al., eds., *Zehn Jahre wohnortnahe Integration: Behinderte und nichtbehinderte Kinder gemeinsam in der Grundschule*, 2nd, rev. ed. (Frankfurt / Main: Arbeitskreis Grundschule, 1994), 38–42.

71. E.g., see Klaus Pramann, "Die 'Übergangsstation' im Kloster Blankenburg: Von der Langzeitpsychiatrie zurück in die Stadt - Erfahrungen nach 18-monatiger Arbeit im Modellprojekt auf der Station I," *Jahrbuch für Psychopathologie und Psychotherapie* 4 (1984), 221–226.

72. For an earlier use of the term antipostfascist in a different context, see Dagmar Herzog, *Sex after Fascism: Memory and Morality in Twentieth-Century Germany* (Princeton, NJ: Princeton University Press, 2005).

73. By 1984, the critical pressure from activists would lead the Lebenshilfe's Wohnstätten- and Werkstatt-Ausschüsse to recommend that the Lebenshilfe's long-standing custom of

distinguishing between "mentally disabled" and "severely mentally disabled" be dropped, and that access to the dormitories be opened to everyone. Hans-Walter Schmuhl and Ulrike Winkler, *Wege aus dem Abseits: Der Wandel der Wohnformen für Menschen mit geistiger Behinderung in den letzten sechzig Jahren (1958–2018)* (Lebenshilfe-Verlag, 2018), 23.

74. E.g., see R. Z., "Laurien: Behinderte Kinder dürfen Gesunde nicht in ihrer Entwicklung hemmen," *Berliner Morgenpost*, November 15, 1981, Pressearchiv, Konrad-Adenauer-Stiftung, Thema "Behinderte." The case of Jenny Lau exemplified with particular clarity the absurdity of politicians' and bureaucrats' resistance to integration. See Gisela Lau and Wolf-Dieter Lau, *Jenny darf nicht in die Oberschule: Dokumentation* (Berlin: Selbstverlag, 1987); Gisela Lau and Wolf-Dieter Lau, "Was kommt nach der Schule, oder was ist eigentlich aus Jenny Lau geworden?" *Gemeinsam leben—Zeitschrift für integrative Erziehung* 8.1 (2000), 30–32, http://bidok.uibk.ac.at /library/gl1-00-lau.html.

75. Although West (and East) Germans had picked up on the "normalization" principle— formulated by the Danish reformer Niels Erik Bank-Mikkelsen and ensconced in Danish welfare policy in 1959, soon amplified also by the Swedish parent-activist Bengt Nirje—about ten years later than did welfare professionals in Denmark, Sweden, the Netherlands, the UK, or the United States (the aim was to structure the daily lives of individuals with mental disabilities as "normally" as possible, including by replacing institutions with family-scale, communally integrated supported living situations), the concept did at least begin to inspire efforts at restructuring and reform *within* those West German institutions that had the resources and the motivation to modernize, often under pressure from younger staffers, sometimes under pressure from politicians, already by the later 1960s and certainly by the mid-1970s. Educational excursions by directors and staff, to Denmark and the Netherlands in particular, to see how alternate models could work, made clear to the West Germans just how antiquated and repressive their own modus operandi had generally been, and prompted reorganizations in style and substance upon return. But there were also instances in which medical or care staff—painfully aware of how retrograde and undignified the conditions in a particular institution were—passionately pleaded with the administrators to upgrade their approach, only to be ignored. Compare, for instance, the situations in Bethel and Alsterdorf in the 1970s: Hans-Walter Schmuhl, "Transnationale Beziehungsnetze und Reformimpulse: Die Rezeption des Normalisierungsprinzips in den v.Bodelschwinghschen Anstalten Bethel in den 1970er Jahren," *Westfälische Forschungen* 70 (2020), 135–161; Gerda Engelbracht and Andrea Hauser, "Normalisierungsprinzip im behindertenpolitischen 'Entwicklungsland' Deutschland," in *Mitten in Hamburg: Die Alsterdorfer Anstalten, 1945–1979* (Stuttgart: Kohlhammer, 2013), 258–263. See also the classic statement: Bengt Nirje, "The Normalization Principle and its Human Management Implications," in Robert Kugel and Wolf Wolfensberger, eds., *Changing Patterns in Residential Services for the Mentally Retarded* (Washington, DC: President's Committee on Mental Retardation, 1969), 181–195.

76. Presentation at the "Humanes Wohnen" conference of the Lebenshilfe in Aachen, November 1981: R. Woch, V. Schmid, M. Wamsler, C. Bradl, and R. Nathow, "Ausgliederung geistig Behinderter aus Einrichtungen der Psychiatrie," in *Humanes Wohnen—seine Bedeutung für das Leben geistig behinderter Erwachsener: Bericht der 10. Studientagung der Bundesvereinigung Lebenshilfe für geistig Behinderte e.V.* (Marburg, 1982), 88–97, here 91, 94.

77. Sil Schmid, *Freiheit heilt: Bericht über die demokratische Psychiatrie in Italien* (Berlin: Wagenbach, 1977); John Foot, *The Man Who Closed the Asylums: Franco Basaglia and the Revolution in Mental Health Care* (London: Verso, 2015); Chantal Marazia et al., "'Visions of another world': Franco Basaglia and German Reform," in Tom Burns and John Foot, eds., *Basaglia's International Legacy: From Asylum to Community* (New York: Oxford University Press, 2020), 227–244.

78. Michael Göhlich, "Politische Zeiten, sachbegeisterter Mittler," in Jutta Schöler, ed., *Normalität für Kinder mit Behinderung: Integration. Texte und Wirkungen von Ludwig-Otto Roser* (Berlin: Luchterhand, 1998), 54; cf. "4 agosto: la legge 517 compie 40 anni," *disabili.com*,

August 4, 2017, https://www.disabili.com/scuola-a-istruzione/articoli-scuola-istruzione/oggi
-4-agosto-la-legge-517-compie-40-anni-lunga-vita-all-integrazione; Giuseppe Adernò, "Compie
40 anni la legge 517 sull'integrazione," *La tecnica della scuola*, August 1, 2017, https://www
.tecnicadellascuola.it/compie-40-anni-la-legge-517-sull-integrazione; Daniela Casaccia, "Un
po' di cronistoria tra tanti voti e poco giudizio," *Insegnare*, June 2020, https://www.insegnare
online.com/rivista/opinioni-confronto/cronistoria-voti-giudizio.

79. "Interview mit Jutta Schöler," in Frank J. Müller, ed., *Blick zurück nach vorn—WegbereiterInnen der Inklusion. Band 1* (Gießen: Psychosozial, 2018), 115–142.

80. Ludwig-Otto Roser, "Schule ohne Aussonderung in Italien," in Helga Deppe-Wolfinger, ed., *behindert und abgeschoben: Zum Verhältnis von Behinderung und Gesellschaft* (Weinheim and Basel: Beltz, 1983), 155–161. See also Jutta Schöler, "Die Arbeit von Milani-Comparetti und ihre Bedeutung für die Nicht-Aussonderung behinderter Kinder in Italien und in der Bundesrepublik Deutschland," *Behindertenpädagogik* 26.1 (1987), 2–16.

81. Ludwig-Otto Roser, "Integration Behinderter in Italien: Anspruch und Realität," *Behinderte in Familie, Schule und Gesellschaft* 3 (1981), 28–33.

82. For further imaginative examples of collaborative research projects, see Christa Eck et al., "Uckermark-Grundschule, Berlin: Schule ohne Aussonderung – eineinhalb Jahre Schulversuch," in Renate Valtin, Alfred Sander und Anton Reinartz, eds., *Gemeinsam leben – gemeinsam lernen: Behinderte Kinder in der Grundschule* (Frankfurt / Main: Arbeitskreis Grundschule e.V., 1984), 139-188.

83. E.g., Ulf Preuss-Lausitz, *Fördern ohne Sonderschule: Konzepte und Erfahrungen zur integrativen Förderung in der Regelschule* (Weinheim and Basel: Beltz, 1981); Martin Rudnick, *Laßt uns mit Euch leben! Behinderte und Nichtbehinderte lernen gemeinsam* (Weinheim and Basel: Beltz, 1983); Wolfgang Podlesch, "Kinder mit geistiger Behinderung und mit schwerer Mehrfachbehinderung in Integrationsklassen," in Heyer et al., *Zehn Jahre*, 58–63. For an early systematization of the baseline conditions needed for effective integration, as well as of the concrete obstacles all too often encountered on the local levels by the first experimenters, see Wolfgang Jantzen, *Allgemeine Behindertenpädagogik: Band 2 Neurowissenschaftliche Grundlagen, Diagnostik, Pädagogik und Therapie* (Weinheim: Beltz, 1990), 249–251.

84. On the inventive, communal solidarity-based approach of the PRIMUS-Schule Berg Fidel-Geist in Münster, building on the critical "pedagogy of the oppressed" developed in the 1960s by Brazilian educator and philosopher Paulo Freire, see: Reinhard Stähling and Barbara Wenders, *Worin unsere Stärke besteht. Eine inklusive Modellschule im sozialen Brennpunkt* (Gießen: Psychosozial, 2021), 313–315, 349–363. On the Antonius von Padua Schule in Fulda, see: "Jakob Muth-Preisträger 2017: Antonius von Padua Schule" (Bertelsmann Stiftung, 2017), https:// www.bertelsmann-stiftung.de/de/unsere-projekte/abgeschlossene-projekte/jakob-muth-preis/2017/antonius-von-padua-schule; and "Pionier in Sachen Inklusion: Padua-Schulleiter Hanno Henkel geht," *osthessen-zeitung.de*, July 20, 2023, https://www.osthessen-zeitung.de /einzelansicht/news/2023/juli/pionier-in-sachen-inklusion-padua-schulleiter-hanno-henkel-geht.html. And on the historic "oldest integrated school in Germany," the Fläming-Grundschule in Berlin, see: "Fläming-Grundschule – inklusive Schwerpunktschule," https://flaeming-grund-schule.de/; and Holger Twele, *Filmheft KLASSENLEBEN* (Bundeszentrale für politische Bildung, 2005), 19, https://www.bpb.de/shop/materialien/filmhefte/34067/klassenleben/.

85. Bericht über die Lage der Psychiatrie in der Bundesrepublik Deutschland—Zur psychiatrischen und psychotherapeutisch/psychosomatischen Versorgung der Bevölkerung, Deutscher Bundestag, 7. Wahlperiode, Drucksache 7 / 4200, 14–15. On any given day in West Germany, depending on the state one was in, somewhere between 15 and 25 percent of the more than 94,000 human beings filling the beds in psychiatric wards did not belong there—and yet had been there for years. Cf. on the Psychiatrie-Enquête and its aftermath: Christian Bradl, "Der Mythos vom harten Kern," *Sozialpsychiatrische Informationen* 13.1 (1983), 7–25; Christian Bradl,

"Keine neuen Grosseinrichtungen für Geistigbehinderte mehr—Erfahrungen aus der DGSP-Initiativen," *Jahrbuch für Psychopathologie und Psychotherapie* IV (1984), 218–221; Christian Bradl, "Leben und Hilfen für geistig Behinderte in der Gemeinde, ein Beitrag zur Diskussion um s.g. psychiatrische Langzeitpatienten," *DGSP-Rundbrief* 28 (April 1985), 9–12.

86. As one hospital director had opined in protest back in 1965 when a regional administrator recommended that the mentally disabled really should be sorted into their own spaces: "If all the feeble-minded patients were to be transferred from the existing regional hospitals, the most important operations would collapse; the regional hospitals have always depended on the active assistance of feeble-minded patients." Years later, just as the Enquête authors were deliberating, this administrator recalled in a letter to an acquaintance "the storm" of objections with which he had been met: "I was told unanimously that the mentally disabled could not be dispensed with because of their labor. They were needed in the kitchen, the residence hall, the garden and the fields." Udo Klausa, notes on a meeting with the hospital directors, June 23, 1965, in Bonn; Udo Klausa, letter to Wegener, March 12, 1974. Both sources quoted and analyzed in Uwe Kaminsky and Thomas Roth, *Verwaltungsdienst, Gesellschaftspolitik und Vergangenheitsbewältigung nach 1945. Das Beispiel des Landesdirektors Udo Klausa* (Berlin: Metropol, 2016), 225, 252. On Klausa, see also Mary Fulbrook, *A Small Town Near Auschwitz: Ordinary Nazis and the Holocaust* (New York: Oxford University Press, 2012). Both books provide assessments of Klausa's self-transformation from a behind-the-scenes facilitator of the Holocaust in occupied Poland to a welfare administrator engaged in "conservative modernization" and successfully suppressing his past in the postwar era.

87. Another stimulus prompting the formation of the Fachausschuß in Hamburg in August 1979 was a particularly dramatic scandal-exposé of conditions at the Alsterdorfer Anstalten published as a cover story in *ZEIT-Magazin* in April 1979; there had been a prior informal gathering at a DGSP meeting in Rickling to develop a "problem catalogue" of issues to address. Invitation letter from Gudrun Podzuk, August 6, 1979, Archiv Christian Bradl. On the DGSP, see Christian Reumschüssel-Wienert, *Psychiatriereform in der Bundesrepublik Deutschland: Eine Chronik der Sozialpsychiatrie und ihres Verbandes—der DGSP* (Bielefeld: transcript, 2021).

88. Deutsche Gesellschaft für Soziale Psychiatrie/Rheinische Gesellschaft für Soziale Psychiatrie, Einladung und Programm: "Mit geistig Behinderten leben—aus der Anstalt in die Gemeinde," Tagung in Köln, 3.-5. April 1981; Deutsche Gesellschaft für Soziale Psychiatrie, Einladung und Programm: "Der Mythos vom harten Kern—den Teufelskreis der Ausgrenzung durchbrechen," Internationaler Workshop Wuppertal, den 28./29. Oktober 1982; Deutsche Gesellschaft für Soziale Psychiatrie, Einladung und Programm: "(Irr-)Wege aus der Isolation. Lebensräume geistigbehinderter Menschen zwischen Anstaltsreform und Integration in die Gemeinde," Tagung . . . 11.4. bis 13.4.1986 in Osnabrück. Archiv Christian Bradl. Examples of media coverage: Gabriele Krüper, "Behinderte aus Getto in sozialen Alltag führen," *Kölner Stadt-Anzeiger* 84 (1981); Bea Füsser-Novy, "Der harte Kern—ein Mythos," *Tageszeitung*, November 3, 1982; Gusti Steiner, "raus aus den Ghettos," *Luftpumpe* 5.12 (1982), 14–15; Susanne Walia, "Der Mythos vom 'harten Kern,'" *Psychologie Heute* (March 1983), 58–59.

89. Christian Bradl, "Wider die Spaltung der Behinderten," *Behindertenpädagogik* 26.1 (1987), 66–78.

90. Rainer Nathow, "Die Entsorgung findet in den Anstalten statt" (1981), in Michael Wunder and Udo Sierck, eds., *Sie nennen es Fürsorge: Behinderte zwischen Vernichtung und Widerstand*, 2nd ed. (Frankfurt/Main: Mabuse, 1987), 129–132, here 129–130. Emphases in the original.

91. Klaus von Lüpke, "Familienentlastende und ambulante Dienste—Beispiele aus Essen und Fröndenberg," presentation at the "(Irr-) Wege" conference in Osnabrück. DGSP, Einladung und Programm: "(Irr-) Wege," 9. See also Klaus von Lüpke, *Nichts Besonderes: Zusammen-Leben und Arbeiten von Menschen mit und ohne Behinderung* (Essen: Klartext Verlag, 1994). Over time, the model projects developed in Essen would provide ever more imaginative integrative

opportunities and services, from shared church worship to youth leisure activities to cultural offerings open to everyone, integration assistants placed in kindergartens, abled-disabled pairings pursuing "tandem work projects," vacation accompaniment for people with disabilities, and a variety of experiments in assisted and shared living. See "Menschenstadt Essen," *Evangelische Kirche in Essen—Nachrichten*, December 2023, https://www.kirche-essen.de/index.php?file =gue-dienste-menschenstadt-essen.

92. Jenny Schmehl and Rainer Woch, "Gründung einer Regionalgruppe" (letter to "DGSP-Mitglieder und Interessierte"), April 6, 1981, Archiv Christian Bradl; cf. "Das Projekt ist völlig umstritten und hat ein überholtes Konzept," *Bonner Rundschau*, September 13, 1983.

93. Deutsche Gesellschaft für Soziale Psychiatrie / Arbeitsgruppe Heilpädagogisches Heim Bonn, Dokumentation: Gemeindeorientierte Wohnformen für Geistigbehinderte statt Grossheim in Bonn-Vilich (September 1985), 9. Archiv Christian Bradl.

94. Pastor Klaus von Lüpke, the inspirational director of disability services for the city of Essen, quoted appreciatively in Bradl, "Wider," 70–71.

95. Ulrich Bleidick, *Betrifft Integration: Behinderte Schüler in allgemeinen Schulen* (Berlin: Marhold, 1988).

96. Christian Gaedt, "Einrichtungen für Ausgeschlossene oder 'Ein Ort zum Leben': Überlegungen zur Betreuung Geistigbehinderter," *Argument-Sonderband* 73 (1981), 96–109; Christian Gaedt, "Die Anstalt ist kein Ort zum Leben: Erwiderung auf die Kritik Michael Wunders," *Jahrbuch für Kritische Medizin* 9 (1983), 154–167; Christian Gaedt, "What is a 'place to live'? Sociological and Psychological Prerequisites for Life in the Community." Paper presented at the International Conference, "A Place to Live Outside the Mainstream," September 1994, Blankenberge, Belgium, http://www.christian-gaedt.com/Seite5.html.

97. Peter Schlaich's remarks at the roundtable on "Anstaltsreform oder Gemeindeintegration?" at the "(Irr-) Wege" conference in Osnabrück 1986 quoted and summarized in Bradl, "Wider," 71.

98. A recent anthology on deinstitutionalization notes that as late as the mid-1990s, 142,000 people in by-then-reunified Germany lived in 3,000 institutions or homes of some kind. Of these, only 14 percent lived in a more independent or small-group situation; only a quarter of the total lived in institutions with fewer than 50 residents. Another quarter continued to live in institutions that housed more than 300 residents. (In Sweden, by contrast, as of 1997, 95 percent of people with mental disability lived in assisted living situations in neighborhoods, or with their families; only 5 percent lived in facilities with more than 5 residents; Norway's numbers were similar.) See Wilfried Rudloff et al., "Krise der Anstalten, Deinstitutionalisierung und gesellschaftlicher Wandel in Deutschland," in Wilfried Rudloff et al., eds., *Ende der Anstalten? Großeinrichtungen, Debatten und Deinstitutionalisierung seit den 1970er Jahren* (Paderborn: Brill Schöningh, 2022), 3–34, here 9–10. For a profound analysis of deleterious conditions still prevailing in a large Protestant institution into the 1990s, see the "Lilienthaler Memorandum" of 1993, available online at http://bidok.uibk.ac.at/library/jantzen-de-institut2.html#idm29.

99. Nati Radtke and Udo Sierck, "Lieber Lebendig als Normal!" and Udo Sierck, "Die Entwicklung der Krüppelgruppen," both in Wunder and Sierck, *Sie nennen es Fürsorge*, 149–156; Swantje Köbsell, "Towards Self-Determination and Equalization: A Short History of the German Disability Rights Movement," *Disability Studies Quarterly* 26.2 (Spring 2006); Jan Stoll, "Neue soziale Bewegungen von Menschen mit Behinderungen—Behinderten- und Krüppelbewegung in den 1970er und 1980er Jahren," in Gabriele Lingelbach and Anne Waldschmidt, eds., *Kontinuitäten, Zensuren, Brüche: Lebenslagen von Menschen mit Behinderungen* (Frankfurt/ Main: Campus, 2016), 214–238; Jonas Fischer, "Umstrittene Interessenvertretung von Menschen mit Behinderungen: Zur Geschichte von Kriegsopferverbänden, Elterninitiativen, Clubs, VHS-Kursen und Krüppelgruppen," in Theresia Degener and Marc von Miquel, eds., *Aufbrüche und Barrieren: Behindertenpolitik und Behindertenrecht in Deutschland und Europa seit den 1970er Jahren* (Bielefeld: transcript, 2019), 213–242.

100. Rudloff, "Überlegungen," 867–868; Elsbeth Bösl, *Politiken der Normalisierung: Zur Geschichte der Behindertenpolitik in der Bundesrepublik Deutschland* (Bielefeld: transcript, 2009); Jan Stoll, *Behinderte Anerkennung? Interessenorganisationen von Menschen mit Behinderungen in Westdeutschland seit 1945* (Frankfurt / Main: Campus, 2017).

101. Silke Boll et al., *Geschlecht: Behindert, besonders Merkmal: Frau* (Munich: AG Spak, 1985); Günther Cloerkes, *Einstellung und Verhalten gegenüber Behinderten: Eine kritische Bestandsaufnahme internationaler Forschung* (Berlin: Marhold, 1985).

102. Franz Christoph, *Krüppelschläge: Gegen die Gewalt der Menschlichkeit* (Reinbek: Rowohlt, 1983). For background on the postwar persistence of the concept of an emotionally deformed "cripple-soul" (*Krüppelseele*) purportedly common to people with physical impairments, along with its pernicious consequences for pedagogy, see "Die Lehrerinnen und Lehrer," in Hans-Walter Schmuhl and Ulrike Winkler, *Gewalt in der Körperbehindertenhilfe: Das Johanna-Helenen-Heim in Volmarstein von 1947 bis 1967* (Bielefeld: Verlag für Regionalgeschichte, 2013), 245–257.

103. Susanne von Daniels et al., eds., *Krüppel-Tribunal: Menschenrechtsverletzungen im Sozialstaat* (Köln: Pahl-Rugenstein, 1983).

104. Ernst Klee, *Behinderte im Urlaub? Das Frankfurter Urteil: Eine Dokumentation* (Frankfurt / Main: Fischer, 1980); Theresia Degener, "Juristische (Vor-)Urteile," in Gusti Steiner, ed., *Hand- und Fußbuch für Behinderte* (Frankfurt / Main: Fischer, 1988), 39–48.

105. Carol Poore, *Disability in Twentieth-Century German Culture* (Ann Arbor: University of Michigan Press, 2007), 278.

106. In an otherwise excellent book, Britta-Marie Schenk considers the cross-identification between the cripple-activists of the 1980s and people with mental disabilities as a presumptuous appropriation. I here disagree with that assessment. Britta-Marie Schenk, *Behinderung verhindern: Humangenetische Beratungspraxis in der Bundesrepublik Deutschland (1960er bis 1990er Jahre)* (Frankfurt / Main: Campus, 2016), 309–310, 318. See also Kirsten Achtelik, "Schrecken humangenetischer Beratung" (review of Schenk, *Behinderung verhindern*), *Gen-ethisches Netzwerk, e.V.* (August 2017), https://www.gen-ethisches-netzwerk.de/behinderung/rezension-schrecken-humangenetischer-beratung.

107. Horst Frehe, "Die Helferrolle als Herrschaftsinteresse nichtbehinderter 'Behinderten-(Be-)Arbeiter,'" in Wunder and Sierck, *Sie nennen es Fürsorge*, 157–163, here 157; cf. Horst Frehe, "Konfrontation oder Integration," *Forum für Medizin und Gesundheitspolitik* 18 (1982), 7–21; Udo Sierck, "Wer integriert wen?—Anmerkungen zur Integrations-Diskussion," in *Das Risiko nichtbehinderte Eltern zu bekommen* (München: AG-SPAK, 1989), 9–12.

108. Franz Christoph, "Unterdrückung Behinderte durch Nichtbehinderte—Begründung eines Antrages auf Asyl," in *Behindertenpädagogik* 18.4 (1979), 344–365.

109. "Heimliches Wirken," *Der Spiegel* 41 (October 7, 1984).

110. Udo Sierck and Nati Radtke, *Die WohlTÄTER-Mafia: Vom Erbgesundheitsgericht zur Humangenetischen Beratung* (Hamburg: Selbstverlag, 1984).

111. In the self-published edition of 1984, Sierck and Radtke already called attention to the Lebenshilfe's role. *Die WohlTÄTER-Mafia*, 67. By the time they published updates, Lebenshilfe's enmeshment was far clearer. Udo Sierck and Nati Radtke, "Nachtrag zur 2. Auflage" (January 1985), in *Die WohlTÄTER-Mafia: Vom Erbgesundheitsgericht zur Humangenetischen Beratung*, 5th ed. (Frankfurt / Main: Mabuse, 1989), 123–133.

112. "Sterilisation bei Jugendlichen mit Behinderung," *Panorama* (October 2, 1984), https://daserste.ndr.de/panorama/archiv/1984/-,panorama16124.html.

113. Gusti Steiner quoted in Martin Theben, "8. Mai 1980: Erinnerung an Demo gegen Frankfurter Reiseurteil," *kobinet-nachrichten* (May 8, 2020), https://kobinet-nachrichten.org/2020/05/08/8-mai-1980-erinnerung-an-demo-gegen-frankfurter-reiseurteil/.

114. See Udo [Sierck]'s comments on "contradicting identifications" (*Identifikations-Gegensätze*) and on cross-checking before making public statements in "Zwischen Widerstand

und Anpassung," in *Krüppel-Zeitung* (October 1983), 18–19. See also Lothar Sandfort, "Gruene und Behinderte," *Krüppel-Zeitung* (October 1983), 15–16. The Green Party became a major scene for disability rights activism, attracting many "cripple" self-advocates and members of the Fachausschuß.

115. Swantje Köbsell, *Eingriffe: Zwangssterilisation geistig behinderter Frauen* (Munich: AG Spak, 1987), 7, 87–110.

116. For background, see "Zur Frage der Sterilisation geistiger Behinderter," *Pro Familia Informationen* (May 1976), 18–19.

117. Michael Wunder, "Die Sterilisation Behinderter und der Schatten der Geschichte," *Kritische Justiz* 21.3 (1988), 309–314; Jürgen Seim/ Peter Caesar, "Dürfen Behinderte Kinder haben? Zur Sterilisierung Behinderter," *Evangelische Kommentare* 9 (1989), 39–42; Klaus Dörner, "Was unterscheidet die heutigen Überlegungen zur Sterilisation von Menschen mit geistiger Behinderung von den Zwangssterilisationen der NS-Zeit?," in Theodor Strohm and Jörg Thierfelder, *Diakonie im "Dritten Reich": Neuere Ergebnisse zeitgeschichtlicher Forschung* (Heidelberg: Heidelberger Verlagsanstalt, 1990), 323–337.

118. See, e.g., Udo Sierck and Nati Radtke, "Arbeit ohne Aussonderung: Das Röpers-Hof-Café in Hamburg," *Puls: Drucksache aus der Behindertenbewegung* 34 (1992), 38–42.

119. "Bedrohung der Kinder," *Der Spiegel* 16 (April 12, 1987).

120. Two other cripple-movement activists who had physical disabilities and who advocated vigorously on behalf of the rights of people labeled intellectually impaired were Swantje Köbsell and Lothar Sandfort. See the speeches given by these two and other activist professionals—a group including, notably, the Nazi coercive sterilization survivor Klara Nowak—at a hearing called by the Green Party in May 1988. Die Grünen, ed., *Sterilisation Behinderter—Hilfe statt Zwang* (Bonn: Selbstverlag, 1988).

121. Franz Christoph, "(K)ein Diskurs über 'lebensunwertes Leben'!," *Der Spiegel* 23 (June 4, 1989); Dagmar Herzog, *Unlearning Eugenics: Sexuality, Reproduction, and Disability in Post-Nazi Europe* (Madison: University of Wisconsin Press, 2018), 56–58.

Chapter Five: Socialist Humanism Confronts Disabled Life

1. "Bericht des Präsidiums des Bundesvorstandes des FDGB über die Lebensbedingungen, Betreuung und Pflege älterer Bürger in Feierabend- und Pflegeheimen zum Ministerratsbeschluß vom 08.08.1973," Bestand Politbüro ZK der SED—Internes Parteiarchiv, Bundesarchiv (Berlin), quoted in Monika Kohnert, "Pflege und Umgang mit Behinderten in der DDR," in Deutscher Bundestag, ed., *Materialien der Enquete-Kommission "Überwindung der Folgen der SED-Diktatur im Prozess der deutschen Einheit"(1995–1998)*, vol. III.2 (Baden-Baden: Nomos, 1999), 1726–1791, here 1727.

2. Wolfgang Presber and Rolf Löther quoted in Heinrich Behr, "Marxistisch-Leninistische Aussagen zu Fragen des Wertes und der Erhaltung des Lebens," *Fröhlich helfen: Handreichung des Diakonischen Werkes—Innere Mission und Hilfswerk—der Evangelischen Kirche in der DDR* 1 (1986), 75–76, here 76. The thematic focus on Nazi "euthanasia" of this special issue of the East German Protestant church welfare journal *Fröhlich helfen* was inspired by the groundbreaking "confession of guilt" over inadequate Christian opposition to Nazi abuse and murder of people with disabilities published at the fortieth anniversary of war's end the prior year by the West German Protestant church in the Rhineland.

3. "Resolution der IX. Konferenz der Gesundheitsminister der sozialistischen Länder (Prag 21.-24.11.1967)," quoted in the sidebar to Peter Uibe, "Mit dem Defekt leben," *Deine Gesundheit* 9 (September 1977), 262–265, here 263.

4. Gisela Helwig, "Frauen im SED-Staat," in Deutscher Bundestag, ed., *Materialien der Enquete-Kommission "Aufarbeitung von Geschichte und Folgen der SED-Diktatur in Deutschland"*

(1992–1994) (Baden-Baden: Nomos, 1995), 1223–1274; Dorothee Wierling, "Work, Workers, and Politics in the German Democratic Republic," *International Labor and Working-Class History* 50 (Fall 1996), 44–63; Christoph Klessmann, *Arbeiter im "Arbeiterstaat" DDR: Deutsche Traditionen, sowjetisches Modell, westdeutsches Magnetfeld (1945–1971)* (Bonn: Dietz, 2007); Donna Harsch, "Between State Policy and Private Sphere: Women in the GDR in the 1960s and 1970s," *Clio* 41 (2015), 85–105.

5. Hanns Schwarz, "Gedanken zu einem Jubiläum," *Deine Gesundheit* 5 (May 1970), 132–133, here 133.

6. On the durability of the fiction, see Kohnert, "Pflege," 1729–1731.

7. Sebastian Barsch, *Geistig behinderte Menschen in der DDR: Erziehung—Bildung—Betreuung,* 2nd ed. (Oberhausen: Athena, 2013), 56–59.

8. Uwe Körner, Rolf Löther, and Achim Thom, "Sozialistischer Humanismus und geschädigtes Leben," in Wolfgang Presber and Rolf Löther, eds., *Sozialistischer Humanismus und die Betreuung Geschädigter* (Jena: G. Fischer, 1981), 11–33, here 12.

9. Verfassung der Deutschen Demokratischen Republik vom 7. Oktober 1949, https://www.verfassungen.de/ddr/verf49.htm.

10. Horst Groschopp, *"Der Ganze Mensch": Die DDR und der Humanismus—Ein Beitrag zur deutschen Kulturgeschichte* (Marburg: Tectum Verlag, 2013), 18.

11. In 1947, even before the GDR was founded, the future Minister of Education Paul Wandel told a congress of pedagogues why remedial schools had to be reestablished quickly. It was, he said, because "we had strongly to dissociate ourselves from the Nazi disregard for those who have been so severely affected by fate. The mastery of this very task appeared to us in this respect also as a proof of the sincerity and reality of our new humanism." Wandel quoted in Klaus-Peter Becker, *Rehabilitationspädagogik* (Berlin: Verlag Volk und Gesundheit, 1979), 14.

12. Schwarz, "Gedanken," 133.

13. Klaus-Peter Becker, *Rehabilitationspädagogik,* 2nd ed. (1984), 22, quoted in Falk Bersch, *Kinder und Jugendliche in sonderpädagogischen, psychiatrischen und Behinderteneinrichtungen in den DDR-Nordbezirken. Teil 1: Die historische Entwicklung* (Schwerin: Die Landesbeauftragte für Mecklenburg-Vorpommern für die Aufarbeitung der SED-Diktatur, 2020), 27.

14. As he put it: "Not all physicians of the time realized that, under pseudo-scientific cover, it [the law] was a racial-political regulation, and believing themselves to be the 'appointed hereditary guardians of their people,' they issued slapdash diagnoses [*Pauschalurteile*] and strove to put record numbers under the knife." Schwarz, "Gedanken," 133.

15. Karla Nitsch, "Damit sie nicht hilflos bleiben," *Für Dich* 4 (April 1977), 24–27, here 26–27. The photographs were by Wilfried Glienke. See also the influential subsequent book by Gerda Jun, *Kinder, die anders sind* (Berlin: VEB Verlag Volk und Gesundheit, 1981); and the retrospective report: Gerda Jun, "'Kinder, die anders sind' in der DDR—Erfahrungen aus der Dispensaire-Betreuung in der Kinder- und Jugendneuropsychiatrie u. Psychotherapie," in Christa Grosch, ed., *Kinder mit Behinderungen: Früherkennung und Rehabilitation im Kindes- und Jugendalter—DDR* (Berlin: Interessengemeinschaft Medizin und Gesellschaft, 2002), 54–59.

16. Sigmar Eßbach, "Fähig durch Geduld," *Deine Gesundheit* 9 (September 1977), 266–267, here 266.

17. Honecker quoted in Karlheinz Renker, "Rehabilitation," *Deine Gesundheit* 9 (September 1977), 260–261, here 261. Yet a further essay devoted to the topic of physical disabilities once again made a point of invoking "the generous support of our state." Uibe, "Mit dem Defekt," 263. In a different issue, the journal was pleased to announce on the government's behalf that "joyous vacations are no longer reserved only for healthy schoolchildren. It has become possible also for numerous mentally disabled children to recuperate excellently through shared experiences and develop their personalities." R. Bunge, "Frohe Ferien," *Deine Gesundheit* 6 (June 1977), 178–180, here 178.

18. Uibe, "Mit dem Defekt," 263. A concession made in passing: "In conclusion, it must be stated that sometimes there are bureaucratic obstacles standing in the way of such a positive development" (264). Or, from a different essay: "As of yet not all impaired children can be cared for in a special facility, as there are not enough placements available." Nitsch, "Damit," 26.

19. "Verordnung zur weiteren Verbesserung der gesellschaftlichen Unterstützung schwerst- und schwerbeschädigter Bürger vom 29. Juli 1976" (sidebar), *Deine Gesundheit* 9 (September 1977), 267, 270–271, 279, here 267.

20. For one of countless typical calls for everyone to pitch in, see Renker, "Rehabilitation," 261: "Our socialist state takes special responsibility for the impaired citizen. But every citizen is called upon to assist." However ironically, and while these essays directed at the general public regularly asserted a great contrast with the capitalist system—where "the human being is obliged to sell his labor power" and any fateful encounter with disability would diminish the worth of that labor power, whereas socialism had already realized "emancipation from exploitation" (261)—nonetheless, the frequent concluding message was that the person with disabilities should pull themselves up by their own bootstraps. The goal enjoined, and repeated for emphasis, was that the disabled person should "accept her fate and recognize that, with active participation, positive sides to life can be found. . . . [numerous people] learned to live with their suffering and to discover a positive side to life [*mit ihrem Leid zu leben und dem Leben eine positive Seite abzugewinnen*]" (Uibe, "Mit dem Defekt," 264). Above all, the person with disabilities should as soon as possible get back to work.

21. On reluctant but resigned acceptance, see Kohnert, "Pflege," 1731, 1752.

22. "Verordnung über die Beschulung und Erziehung von Kindern und Jugendlichen mit wesentlichen physischen oder psychischen Mängeln" (October 1951), discussed in Barsch, *Geistig behinderte Menschen*, 76–77, 82; Tobias Niemann, *Geistigbehindertenpädagogik in der DDR: Die Entwicklung einer Pädagogik zwischen Entwicklungsfähigkeit und Ausgrenzung* (Hamburg: DiplomicaVerlag, 2015); Laura Hottenrott, "'Der Kern der Gesundheit ist Anpassung': Medizinische Aspekte der DDR-Heimerziehung," in Anke Dreier-Horning and Karsten Laudien, eds., *Jugendhilfe und Heimerziehung im Sozialismus: Beiträge zur Aufarbeitung der Sozialpädagogik in der DDR* (Berlin: Berliner Wissenschafts-Verlag, 2016), 83–102. See also Eckhard Rohrmann, "Das Unerziehbarkeitsdogma der Deutschen Heil- und Sonderpädagogik in der Theorie und Praxis der Rehabilitationspädagogik der DDR," *Behindertenpädagogik* 31.2 (1992), 138–149; and Ute Geiling, "Schulfähigkeit und Einschulungspraxis in der DDR: Ein Rückblick—im Spannungsfeld von Förderung und Ausgrenzung," in Annedore Prengel, *Vielfalt durch gute Ordnung im Anfangsunterricht* (Wiesbaden: Springer, 1999), 161–219.

23. Sigmar Eßbach was from 1972–1990 professor of "Rehabilitation Pedagogy for the Ineducable [but] Developable Intellectually Impaired" (*Rehabilitationspädagogik der schulbildungsunfähigen förderungsfähigen Intelligenzgeschädigten*) at the Humboldt University in Berlin. He was the individual most responsible for creating a space within the GDR for training professionals in pedagogic-therapeutic approaches for children with significant (though not the most severe) intellectual disabilities. Eßbach, himself the father of a son with cognitive impairments, played a crucial role within the GDR, probably most comparable to the West German special pedagogue Heinz Bach, the promoter of the concept of "practical educability" there, albeit against innumerably greater obstacles than Bach faced in the West. Although rebuffed, harshly, by Minister of Education Margot Honecker when he sought to create schools for "developable" children, between 1970 and 1988 Eßbach succeeded in creating, under the auspices of the Ministry of Health, 14,750 placements for children in "rehabilitation-pedagogy"-oriented day programs and residential institutions. Martin Th. Hahn, "Zum 80. Geburtstag von Sigmar Eßbach—Wegbereiter der Pädagogik von Menschen mit geistiger Behinderung in der Deutschen Demokratischen Republik (DDR)," *Vierteljahresschrift für Heilpädagogik und ihre Nachbargebiete* 4 (2009), 342–345, here 343.

24. Christine Fraas, *Leben mit Hermine* (Erfurt: UNZ-Verlag, 1996), 78; Barsch, *Geistig behinderte Menschen*, 163–188; Nils Löffelbein, "Die institutionelle Landschaft zur Unterbringung von Minderjährigen in der Kinder- und Jugendpsychiatrie und der stationären Behindertenhilfe," in Heiner Fangerau et al., eds., *Leid und Unrecht: Kinder und Jugendliche in Behindertenhilfe und Psychiatrie der BRD und DDR 1949 bis 1990* (Köln: Psychiatrie-Verlag, 2021), 36-80, here 61.

25. Bersch, *Kinder und Jugendliche*; Kohnert, "Pflege," 1736.

26. Kohnert, "Pflege," 1731, 1732, 1736. In meticulous and devastating detail, scholars associated with the Stiftung Anerkennung und Hilfe (Foundation Recognition and Assistance)—funded jointly by the German federal government and the Protestant and Catholic churches—between 2017 and 2021 investigated historical conditions in the institutions in both West (1949–1975) and East (1949–1990) and recorded the pervasiveness of mistreatment: overcrowded wards, insufficient and utterly underqualified staff, physical and emotional violence at the hands of staff as well as from other residents that created an atmosphere of constant tension and fear, unremunerated exploitation of labor, humiliations and restrictions on freedom (including physical restraints, from straitjackets and bed shackles to padded cells), and overmedication for purposes either of experimentation or of control. The authors of the study, finally, while calling attention both to significant asynchronicity in the uptake of reform trends from institution to institution and noting that also in the West there were institutions in which improvements were delayed until the 1980s, nonetheless joined prior scholars in observing that, precisely because there was no free press and no public sphere in the East that permitted scandalization, the most truly horrendous conditions persisted longer in the East than in the West. See "Fazit und abschließende Bewertung," in Fangerau et al., *Leid und Unrecht*, 269–299, here 293–296.; and cf. Siv Stippekohl, "Eingesperrt, fixiert, gequält: Kinderschicksale in der DDR," *ndr.de*, January 3, 2023, https://www.ndr.de/geschichte/schauplaetze/Eingesperrt-fixiert-gequaelt-Kinderschicksale-in-der-DDR,lievalleen112.html.

27. "Beschluß über Maßnahmen zur Förderung, Beschulung und Betreuung geschädigter Kinder und Jugendlicher sowie psychisch behinderter Erwachsener," August 20, 1969, Ministerrat der DDR, Bundesarchiv (Berlin), quoted in Kohnert, "Pflege und Umgang," 1736.

28. Nitsche, "Damit," 25–27.

29. Helwig, "Frauen."

30. S. M. from Schwerin, quoted in Bersch, *Kinder und Jugendliche*, 82.

31. Ulrike Winkler, *Mit dem Rollstuhl in die Tatra-Bahn. Menschen mit Behinderungen in der DDR: Lebensbedingungen und materielle Barrieren* (Halle: Mitteldeutscher Verlag, 2023). Winkler describes, for example, the impressive successes of self-advocacy groups like the "Multiple Sclerosis Patient Support Group." Nonetheless, a network comparable to the militant "cripple movement" in the West could not develop under GDR conditions. Carol Poore, "Disability and Socialist Images of the Human Being in the Culture of the German Democratic Republic," in *Disability in Twentieth-Century German Culture* (Ann Arbor: University of Michigan Press, 2007), 231–272; Barsch, *Geistig behinderte Menschen*; Bertold Scharf, Sebastian Schlund, and Jan Stoll, "Segregation oder Integration? Gesellschaftliche Teilhabe von Menschen mit Behinderungen in der DDR," in *Geschichte in Wissenschaft und Unterricht* 70.1-2 (2019), 52–70, here 66–68.

32. Bettina Westfeld, *Innere Mission und Diakonie in Sachsen 1867–2017* (Leipzig: Evangelische Verlagsanstalt, 2017), 232–233.

33. Kohnert, "Pflege," 1753; Bersch, *Kinder und Jugendliche*.

34. Uta König and Sabine Sauer, "Gefangen, gequält, vergessen," *Stern* 24 (June 7, 1990), 26–34, 36.

35. *Die Hölle von Ueckermünde* (film, dir. Ernst Klee, 1993). All three parts are available on YouTube.

36. Uta König, "Die Kinder von Lüneburg," *Stern* 49 (November 27, 1980).

37. Klee's "Laudatio" was reprinted in Ernst Klee, *Behindert: Über die Enteignung von Körper und Bewußtsein* (Frankfurt / Main: Fischer, 1980), http://bidok.uibk.ac.at/library/klee-behindert.html.

38. E.g., see Klaus Weise, "Zur Besichtigung freigegeben," *Symptom: Leipziger Beiträge zu Psychiatrie und Verrücktheit* 2 (1993), 61–62; Helga Wegner, "Beklemmend," *Leipziger Volkszeitung* (April 16, 1993). Although unfair specifically to Klee, the more general perception of Western condescension was of course accurate. See Sophinette Becker and Hans Becker, "Die Wiedervereinigung der Schuld," *psychosozial* 45 (1991), 64–75.

39. Staatsanwaltschaft b. d. Landgericht Frankfurt / Main to Ernst Klee, March 24, 1994, Gedenkstätte Hadamar, Sammlung, NL Klee, HR-Hölle.

40. Description of special session on Ueckermünde of the Sozialausschuß des Landtags Mecklenburg-Vorpommern, April 20, 1993, in Ernst Klee, letter to Heinz Schwarz, May 1, 1993, Gedenkstätte Hadamar, Sammlung, NL Klee, HR-Hölle. The same folder contains numerous related letters and media clippings.

41. See especially the powerful and differentiated statement by Heike Bernhardt, "'Der ihnen beistehe, sei ein Engel des Zorns': Anmerkungen zum Film 'Die Hölle von Ueckermünde'," *Mabuse* 85 (August / September 1999), 29.

42. Jürgen Reuter, "Entsetzen, Beklemmung, Wut," *Die Lebenshilfe-Zeitung* 14.3 (June 1993), 1, 5.

43. Kathleen Haack, "'Im Grunde gibt es … keine Chance zu Veränderungen zu kommen': Zur Lage der Anstaltspsychiatrie in der DDR in den 1980er Jahren—Das Beispiel Ueckermünde," in Ekkehardt Kumbier, ed., *Psychiatrie in der DDR II* (Berlin: be.bra, 2020), 377–392; Bersch, *Kinder und Jugendliche*, 230–240.

44. Späte in a letter, October 13, 1986, to a Dr. Rohland in the Ministry of Health in the GDR, quoted in Sascha Topp, *Geschichte als Argument in der Nachkriegsmedizin: Formen der Vergegenwärtigung der nationalsozialistischen Euthanasie zwischen Politisierung und Historiographie* (Göttingen: V&R Unipress, 2013), 286.

45. Joachim S. Hohmann, *Der "Euthanasie"-Prozeß Dresden 1947: Eine zeitgeschichtliche Dokumentation* (Frankfurt / Main: Peter Lang, 1993), 80–81.

46. Topp, *Geschichte als Argument*, 288–300; Christian Dirks, *Die Verbrechen der anderen: Auschwitz und der Auschwitz-Prozess der DDR. Das Verfahren gegen den KZ-Arzt Dr. Horst Fischer* (Paderborn: Schöningh, 2006); Annette Weinke, "Fritz Bauer und Friedrich Karl Kaul—zwei Juristen im Kalten Krieg," in Martin Sabrow, ed., *Das Jahrhundert der Parallelbiographien* (Göttingen: Akademische Verlagsanstalt, 2017), 139–155; Katharina Rauschenberger, "Friedrich Karl Kaul: Ein DDR-Anwalt in westdeutschen 'Euthanasie'-Prozessen," in Jörg Osterloh and Jan Erik Schulte, eds., *"Euthanasie" und Holocaust: Kontinuitäten, Kausalitäten, Parallelitäten* (Paderborn: Schöningh, 2021), 385–406.

47. Friedrich Karl Kaul, *Nazimordaktion T4: Ein Bericht über die erste industriemässig durchgeführte Mordaktion des Naziregimes* (Berlin: Verlag Volk und Gesundheit, 1973).

48. Kaul, undated note, quoted in Rauschenberger, "Friedrich Karl Kaul," 398.

49. Kaul, final court statement, November 28, 1968, at the Landgericht Frankfurt / Main, quoted in Rauschenberger, "Friedrich Karl Kaul," 401.

50. Thom was soon in regular exchange with Dörner and other co-founders of the West German "Working Group for Research on National Socialist 'Euthanasia' and Coercive Sterilization" (*Arbeitskreis zur Erforschung der nationalsozialistischen "Euthanasie" und Zwangssterilisation*). Thom was an SED-affiliated Marxist by conviction; for testimonials to the integrity with which he interacted with colleagues of differing views, see the obituaries by Klaus Weise ("Achim Thom, 14. August 1935–19. September 2010") and Sonja Süß ("Nachruf auf meinen Doktorvater") in *Sozialpsychiatrische Informationen* 41.1 (2011), 47–48.

51. Wolf-Dieter Talkenberger, "Vorwort," in *"Euthanasie"—Familienerinnerungen aus Ost-deutschland an die Verbrechen der Nazi-Zeit* (Evangelischer Pressedienst, Dokumentation Nr. 52 (December 7, 1992), 1, Evangelisches Landesarchiv Berlin 55.5 / 468. The three dozen testimonies he subsequently published are themselves cumulatively devastating.

52. Thomas Schilter, *Unmenschliches Ermessen: Die nationalsozialistische "Euthanasie"-Tötungsanstalt Pirna-Sonnenstein 1940 / 41* (Weimar: Gustav Kiepenheuer Verlag, 1999), 7–8. As it turned out, citizens who had lived through the Third Reich near the Pirna-Sonnenstein T4 center as children knew, as did all the residents of the Pirna area who saw the thick dark-brown clouds of smoke billowing from the Sonnenstein's crematorium, that it had been a murder site. But in the decades of the GDR, silence about this shared knowledge of the past had been the norm. See the post-reunification video interview with Pirna resident Wolfgang Schumann, Gedenkstätte Pirna-Sonnenstein. Schumann movingly reports the story of a disappeared former playmate who had been moderately mentally disabled, as well as the comment made to him and his young peers by a soldier guarding the terrain around the Sonnenstein: "Yeah, don't you all know that they're finishing off the crazies now, those are useless eaters" (*Ja wisst Ihr denn nicht das nun mit den Verrückten Schluss gemacht wird, das sind unnütze Esser*). But when the interviewer gently inquires about why these memories were never discussed among the townspeople during the postwar decades, Schumann demonstratively evades the question.

53. Helmut F. Späte and Achim Thom, "Die Verantwortung der sozialistischen Gesellschaft für ihre geistig schwer behinderten Mitglieder," in Uwe Körner, Karl Seidel, and Achim Thom, eds., *Grenzsituationen ärztlichen Handelns* (Jena: VEB Gustav Fischer Verlag, 1981), 153–165, here 153–54; Roswitha Geppert, *Die Last, die du nicht trägst* (Halle: Mitteldeutscher Verlag, 1978).

54. Thus, on the one hand, the future had already arrived: "The attitude of the surrounding world toward seriously psychically and severely disabled people is transformed from one of revulsion, rejection and indifference to tolerance, understanding and active helping to the extent that the social consciousness in general is increasingly given shape." On the other hand, Späte and Thom noted that if one were to start excluding from personhood those people who lack speech, communication- and work-capacity, then one would also quickly be raising the questions of dementia and chronic illness and at what point people could be denied the quality of "personality" (*Persönlichkeit*) they had once been known to possess. Späte and Thom, "Die Verantwortung," 160, 163.

55. Späte and Thom, "Die Verantwortung," 153, 158, 160–161.

56. Späte and Thom, "Die Verantwortung," 158, 161. Emphasis added. They did go on to say: "Admittedly the creation of a personal relationship to the most severely intellectually disabled people is a difficult and sometimes also unsolvable task, whereby the complications lie both in the psychological defenses active in all of us in response to incomprehensible ways of responding and surely also frequently in the pronounced autistic reactions on their parts, which can make many expressions of caring appear futile. But since on the other hand we also know little about the vulnerable aspects of their sensations and about the spontaneously emerging reactions of satisfaction which they can show, it is above all a matter of shaping social interactions in such a way that they could in principle be suited to preventing feelings of exclusion, experiences of devaluation and of isolation in the first place" (161–162).

57. Topp, *Geschichte als Argument*, 286.

58. Helmut Späte, "Faschistische Massenvernichtung psychisch Kranker—Traditionspflege als Mahnung," in Achim Thom and Horst Spaar, eds., *Medizin im Faschismus: Symposium über das Schicksal der Medizin in der Zeit des Faschismus in Deutschland 1933–1945. Protokoll* (Berlin: VEB Verlag Volk und Gesundheit, 1983), 333–340, here 335, 337.

59. Topp, *Geschichte als Argument*, 284–287; Ute Hoffmann, "'Das ist wohl ein Stück verdrängt worden…': Zum Umgang mit den 'Euthanasie'-Verbrechen in der DDR," in Annette

Leo, ed., *Vielstimmiges Schweigen: Neue Studien zum DDR-Antifaschismus* (Berlin: Metropol, 2001), 51–66.

60. Literary scholar Carol Poore, who reviewed all the major texts written on disability during the years of the GDR, noted that Fühmann "is the only GDR writer I know of who cultivated contacts with disabled people and incorporated the insights he gained from these experiences into his writing." Poore, *Disability*, 245.

61. Dietmar Riemann, "'Was für eine Insel in was für einem Meer': Die Geschichte eines Bildbandes mit Franz Fühmann," *Palmbaum* 58 (Bucha bei Jena, 2014), 129–138, here 129–130. Fühmann died in 1984, before the book saw the light of day, but not before he had delivered meditative radio programs in which he further explored how much his meetings at the Samariteranstalten and at other institutions for the disabled had meant to him, and how they had changed him; he had begun in Fürstenwalde by coming to give story readings, then wrote a fairy tale on demand for one of the residents (*Anna die Humpelhexe*), and later returned to discuss with residents their interpretations of a cycle of woodcuts made by the artist and leftist pacifist anti-dictatorship activist HAP Grieshaber, a 1960s update on a late medieval "dance of death"— and Fühmann was unmistakably bowled over by the residents' creative and profound responses. The Samariteranstalten remain to this day an extraordinary place. It is surely relevant that the institution, under new leadership in the late 1960s, had initiated earlier than many peer institutions in the GDR an internal paradigm shift in therapeutic approaches, concretized as well in a certification program launched in 1969, the "Seminar für Psychiatriediakonie." The key conceptual change lay in a move away from a unidirectional model of caregiver-to-recipient provision of services and toward a model of "reciprocal giving and receiving," in which people with disabilities were "no longer only objects of therapeutic action," but seen as "communication-capable and themselves active subjects." Wolfgang Rose, "Die Samariteranstalten in der SBZ und DDR (1945–1990)," in Jens C. Franze and Paul-Gerhardt Voget, eds., *Die Samariteranstalten Fürstenwalde: Eine diakonische Stiftung zwischen Kaiserreich und Bundesrepublik* (Berlin: be.bra, 2012), 105–140, here 121–122. See also the essay collection—including reflections on advocacy, theology, and memorialization of the Samariteranstalten's own losses to the "euthanasia" murder program: Wolfgang Matzke, ed., *Entfaltung* (Leipzig: Evangelische Verlagsanstalt, 1991).

62. Franz Fühmann and Dietmar Riemann, *Was für eine Insel in was für einem Meer: Leben mit geistig Behinderten* (Frankfurt am Main: Büchergilde Gutenberg, 1985), 11, 14, 15, 19. The photos have just been reprinted in high quality in a new English translation: Franz Fühmann, *What Kind of Island in What Kind of Sea*, transl. Elizabeth C. Hamilton; photog. Dietmar Riemann (Ann Arbor, MI: Lever Press, 2021).

63. Fühmann and Riemann, *Was für eine Insel*, 9–10.

64. Fühmann and Riemann, *Was für eine Insel*, 12–13.

65. Fühmann and Riemann, *Was für eine Insel*, 12.

66. Fühmann and Riemann, *Was für eine Insel*, 19, 21.

67. Fühmann and Riemann, *Was für eine Insel*, 19–21.

68. Fühmann and Riemann, *Was für eine Insel*, 22.

69. Fühmann and Riemann, *Was für eine Insel*, 22.

70. Ewald Meltzer, *Das Problem der Abkürzung "lebensunwerten" Lebens* (Halle / Saale: Marhold, 1925); J. Thomas Hörnig, "Ewald Meltzer—der Grenzgänger zwischen Nächstenliebe und Eugenik, Apologetik und Zwangssterilisation," in *Herr, höre meine Stimme—Stimmen aus dem Katharinenhof Großhennersdorf* (Diakoniewerk Oberlausitz, 2021), 29–41.

71. "Zwischen großem Berg und Lindenallee. Der Katharinenhof im sächsischen Großhennersdorf während der Zeit des Nationalsozialismus" (exhibit flyer, 2010), http://www .augenauf.net/de/dnl/ssl_flyer_ausstellungzgbul_01-2010.709.pdf?PHPSESSID=2f84e535c 3ada8bfe89fb74c72654114 (accessed January 22, 2023); Boris Böhm, "Abriss zur Geschichte des Katharinenhofs 1721 bis 1945," in *"Nun liesse sich viel erzählen von all den Tagesereignissen…":*

Kommentierte Chronik des Katharinenhofes Großhennersdorf 1934–1941 (Dresden: Stiftung sächsische Gedenkstätten, 2017), 11–21, here 19.

72. See the timeline, "Zur Geschichte des Katharinenhofs," at Diakoniewerk Oberlausitz, https://www.diakoniewerk-oberlausitz.de/im-wandel-der-zeit.html.

73. Jürgen Trogisch, conversation, March 1, 2021; Uta Trogisch, conversation, March 11, 2021.

74. Uta Elisabeth Trogisch and Jürgen Trogisch, "'Wir sind alle Quereinsteiger!' Als Arztehepaar in Verantwortung für rund 400 Menschen mit Behinderungen von 1971 bis 1990," in *Herr, höre meine Stimme*, 95–110, here 100.

75. Trogisch and Trogisch, "'Wir sind alle,'" 96.

76. Uta Trogisch, conversation, March 11, 2021.

77. Jürgen Trogisch and Uta Trogisch, "Sind Förderungsunfähige 'nur' Pflegefälle?," *Zeitschrift für ärztliche Fortbildung* 71, no. 15 (1977): 720–722, here 720, 722. See also the report on the success, both of the concept and the therapeutic approach it stood for, in Manfred Hellmann, "Förderpflege im Katharinenhof: Ein komplizierter Weg wurde zurückgelegt," *Der Ring* (June 1987), 14–17. A noteworthy echo with the views of the radical disability pedagogue Georg Feuser in West Germany was the Trogischs' adamant endorsement of the value of parental involvement and love. As Hellmann with striking frankness acknowledged on behalf of Bethel and West German "experts" more generally (and this in 1987!), the Trogischs' pro-parent perspective was "in contrast to the widespread view, even in professional circles in the Federal Republic, that parents are often a disruptive factor because of their emotional attachment" (17).

78. "*Health* is a state of complete physical, mental and social *well-being* and not merely the absence of disease or infirmity." World Health Organization, "Constitution of the World Health Organization," https://www.who.int/about/governance/constitution.

79. With regard to "special goals," the Trogischs highlighted "relative independence in the most basic realms: of *self-care*, for example independent eating and drinking, orderly behavior at table, independent management of excretion, walking and climbing stairs, undressing and dressing, assistance with washing; of *social integration*, for example responsiveness, need for contact, ability to follow simple rules of daily shared living, e.g. when eating, going to the toilet, taking a walk; and of *orientation in the environment*, e.g. familiarity with regard to objects in the nearest surroundings. In some instances also the *most simple monotechnical tasks* are learnable and the *most simple aesthetic needs* can be awakened, for example joy in music and movement." But in their conclusion they above all emphasized the importance of redefining what would count as learning: "The *capacity [to benefit from] developmental care [Förderpflegefähigkeit]* is not limited to the achievement of these *maximal* goals," they stressed. "Thus for a most severely disabled individual it is already to be seen as a *success* and a *goal* of developmental care, if an otherwise impassive, constantly bedridden disabled person through years of intentional exercises learns to smile at the sight of his caregiver or when hearing an evening song." Trogisch and Trogisch, "Sind Förderungsunfähige 'nur' Pflegefälle?," 721–722.

80. Uta Trogisch, conversation, March 11, 2021. On the awfulness of receiving the label "carecase" and the hope that the term would be replaced by "human," see also Jürgen Trogisch, "Offener Brief an Gott," *Die Union* 10 (January 12–13, 1991).

81. Trogisch and Trogisch, "'Wir sind alle,'" 101.

82. Discussed in Jürgen Trogisch, "Vortrag auf der Gedenkveranstaltung am 17.11.2020 im Katharinenhof Großhennersdorf" (n.d.), 2–3. Archiv Jürgen und Uta Trogisch.

83. "Bundesbesuchtage im Katharinenhof Großhennersdorf: Begegnungen" (newspaper clipping, no source, no date, 1981). Archiv Jürgen und Uta Trogisch.

84. Trogisch and Trogisch, "'Wir sind alle,'" 101–106, here 103. For reflections (from a staff member at the affiliated Martinshof institution) on the meaningfulness of an adapted worship service with adults with significant impairments, see also Annelore Larsen, "Überprüfen, ergänzen und erproben Sie Inhalte und Formen des geistlichen Lebens für eine Gruppe geistig

schwerstbehinderter Erwachsener." Hausarbeit, Heilerziehungspflege, 1981, Archiv Katharinenhof Großhennersdorf.

85. Heinz Reimann and Jürgen Trogisch, "Zur Sexualität Imbeziller," *Zeitschrift für ärztliche Fortbildung* 71.4 (1977), 188–193; Heinz Reimann, Jürgen Trogisch, and Uta Trogisch, "Zur Problematik der Partnerbeziehungen bei imbezillen Jugendlichen und Erwachsenen," Vortrag gehalten an der XI. Tagung der Medizinischen Gesellschaft der DDR zum Studium der Lebensbedingungen und der Gesundheit 24.-26.11.1977 in Berlin (Manuskript). Archiv Jürgen und Uta Trogisch.

86. Georg Kanig, "Die Heilerziehungspflege: Ausbildung im Katharinenhof," in *Herr, höre meine Stimme*, 141–159, here 145, 158. Wonderful examples of "individualized development and accompaniment" are given in Eva-Maria Franke, "Die planmäßige Förderung geistig Schwerstbehinderter erfolgt im wesentlichen im Vollzug der alltäglichen pflegerischen Verrichtungen. . . ." Hausarbeit, Heilerziehungspflege, 1984, Archiv Katharinenhof Großhennersdorf.

87. See the entry for "1979" in "Zur Geschichte des Katharinenhofs." Technically, it was absolutely forbidden to provide education to those deemed "undevelopable"; the Trogischs and Tippelt went ahead anyway and therewith "broke the taboo of the GDR educational doctrine."

88. Winfried Tippelt and Uta Tippelt, conversation, March 15, 2021.

89. *Das Wunder vom Katharinenhof* (film, dir. Dinah Münchow and Stephan Liskowsky, Mitteldeutscher Rundfunk, 2012). Uta Trogisch—characteristically—to this day gives the credit for the idea of the launch of that program to the residents themselves, who had asked for the help so that they would be independently able to, for instance, decipher train schedules, or a newspaper. Uta Trogisch, conversation, March 11, 2021.

90. E.g., see Henning Heide, "Welche Bedeutung haben äussere Bedingungen für den Erfolg der Einzelförderung geistig schwerstbehinderter Kinder?" Hausarbeit, Heilerziehungspflege, 1981, Archiv Katharinenhof Großhennersdorf.

91. Especially moving testimonies of three resident women who worked in the laundry and in childcare: Susanne Nebe, "Wohnen, arbeiten und alt werden innerhalb der Mauern des Katharinenhofs: Erinnerungen von Marlene Kempe, Sieglinde Schloßbauer und Ursula Hahnel," in *Herr, höre meine Stimme*, 86–93.

92. Arnaud Liszka, *Versuche, in der Wahrheit zu leben: DDR Südost - Nichtanpassung und Opposition in der Oberlausitz. Interviews* (Dresden: Neisse Verlag, 2010); Kerstin Engelhardt and Norbert Reichling, *Eigensinn in der DDR-Provinz: Vier Lokalstudien über Nonkonformität und Opposition* (Frankfurt / Main: Wochenschau Verlag, 2011).

93. Trogisch and Trogisch, "'Wir sind alle,'" 106.

94. See for instance the rather hostile remarks by Andreas ("Frieder") Friedrich, "Opposition in der Provinz: Die Aktivisten von Großhennersdorf," MDR.de (2017), https://www.mdr .de/geschichte/ddr/deutsche-einheit/mauerfall/umweltbibliothek-grosshennersdorf -friedensaktivisten-friedliche-revolution-100.html; Jürgen Trogisch, conversation in Dresden, June 14, 2021.

95. Hans-Georg Matthes, conversation in Großhennersdorf, May 4, 2022.

Afterword: The Legacy of Antipostfascism

1. In *Sex after Fascism*, I used the term antipostfascist to describe the generation of 1968 in West Germany. New Left and sex rights activists in that generation frequently described themselves as antifascist, but could better be designated as anti*post*fascist, because what they were rebelling against was not Nazism per se, but rather the conservative sexual-political culture of the 1950s in which they had been raised and which they (as it turns out, quite mistakenly) believed was a watered-down continuation of the sexual politics of the Third Reich. Unbeknownst to the young, however, the traditionalist-normative postwar settlement was less a continuity

than itself a strategic memory-political invention, constructed in partial backlash against Nazism's numerous and (once-notorious, but soon avidly forgotten) sexual incitements, even as Nazism's homophobic and eugenic agendas were perpetuated in new forms. By contrast, here in this book tracing the history of attitudes and practices with regard to intellectual disability, the intergenerational dynamics were completely reversed: The antipostfascist activists of the 1970s–1980s understood—on an at once cognitive and emotional, indeed even corporeal level—a profound truth about Nazism that had eluded, or was being denied by, their elders. See Dagmar Herzog, *Sex after Fascism: Memory and Morality in Twentieth-Century Germany* (Princeton, NJ: Princeton University Press, 2005), esp. 7, 139–140, 182–183.

2. See for instance the remarkable memorandum, with its comprehensive catalogue of considerations for advancing disability rights and equality and reciprocity between people with and without disabilities developed by representatives of the Protestant church and the Inner Mission in the GDR in conjunction with the World Council of Churches and guests from fifteen other nations at a gathering in Bad Saarow, GDR, in 1978: "Leben und Zeugnis der Behinderten in der christlichen Gemeinde," *Evangelischer Pressedient Dokumentation* 36a (August 28, 1978).

3. Dan Diner, "On the Ideology of Antifascism," *New German Critique* 67 (Winter 1996), 123–132; Antonia Grunenberg, *Antifaschismus, ein deutscher Mythos* (Reinbek: Rowohlt, 1993).

4. Worth noting as well are the echoes between what Jantzen meant by "the fascism in the heads" and the ways in which related ideas were expressed by his French contemporary Félix Guattari in his counterculture manifesto cowritten with Gilles Deleuze, *Anti-Oedipus* (1972). See Dagmar Herzog, *Cold War Freud: Psychoanalysis in an Age of Catastrophes* (New York: Cambridge University Press, 2017), 159–174.

5. Helmut Späte, "Faschistische Massenvernichtung psychisch Kranker—Traditionspflege als Mahnung," in Achim Thom and Horst Spaar, eds., *Medizin im Faschismus: Symposium über das Schicksal der Medizin in der Zeit des Faschismus in Deutschland 1933–1945. Protokoll* (Berlin: VEB Verlag Volk und Gesundheit, 1983), 333–340, here 337.

6. Cf. for the US context—with its quite differently tangled interrelations between fantasies and fears around intellectual disability, "race," and class—Michael E. Staub, *The Mismeasure of Minds: Debating Race and Intelligence between Brown and The Bell Curve* (Chapel Hill: University of North Carolina Press, 2018).

7. Gerhard Schmidt, *Selektion in der Heilanstalt 1939–1945* (Stuttgart: Evangelisches Verlagswerk, 1965), 30, 35.

8. On the rapidity of uptake, see, e.g., Michael Burleigh and Wolf Wippermann, *The Racial State: Germany, 1933–1945* (New York: Cambridge University Press, 1991); David Crew, "The Pathologies of Modernity: Detlev Peukert on Germany's Twentieth Century," *Social History* 17.2 (1992), 319–328; Stefan Kühl, *The Nazi Connection: Eugenics, American Racism, and German National Socialism* (New York: Oxford University Press, 1994). On the durable impact, see, e.g., Jürgen Matthäus, "'The Axis around which National Socialist Ideology Turns': State Bureaucracy, the Reich Ministry of the Interior, and Racial Policy in the First Years of the Third Reich," in Devin Pendas et al., eds., *Beyond the Racial State: Rethinking Nazi Germany* (New York: Cambridge University Press, 2017), 241–271.

9. Sometimes the connections between anti-Jewishness and antidisability can seem more incidental or more circuitous, but the linkages that are expressed by contemporaries in diverse eras are not therefore any less affectively potent, on the contrary. Scenes of intensity that demand further research include: in the early 1900s, the heated debates over (apparently) higher rates of intellectual disability and mental illness among Jews, in comparison with Protestants or Catholics (see the long footnote 19 in chapter 1); in the 1920s, the indirect causation perceived between (supposedly) Jewish-encouraged sexual liberalization and the rising number of births of children with intellectual impairments (see Hermann Büchsel's comments in chapter 2); and in the late 1960s, the deployment of antisemitic idiom both in the violence and in the more

"reasoned" objections to the establishment of a home for boys with intellectual impairments at the Aumühle in Bavaria (see chapter 4, footnote 7, and—for the acquittals in the ensuing trial for incitement (*Volksverhetzung*) against the priest and a prominent businessman—see "Eh hinten dran," *Der Spiegel* 22 (May 27, 1973). In the 2010s (discussed below), the AfD's insidious argumentation that Muslim migrants' (purported) higher tendency toward marriage among blood relatives produced an increased proportion of children with disabilities was, arguably, grafted onto older tropes making similar claims about Jews, "incest," and preponderance of instances of mental disability. See, e.g., Ernst Mann [Gerhard Hoffmann], *Die Wohltätigkeit als aristokratische und rassenhygienische Forderung* (Weimar: Fritz Fink, 1924), 116: "Contributing to the emergence of this inferior type of human was excessive inbreeding in Jewish circles."

10. Theodor Adorno, "Freudian Theory and the Patterns of Fascist Propaganda" (1951), in Andrew Arato and Eike Gebhardt, eds., *The Essential Frankfurt School Reader* (New York: Continuum, 1977), 118–137 and 177–180, here 130. Emphasis in the original. Written in English, the essay was translated into German only in 1970: "Die Freudsche Theorie und die Struktur der faschistischen Propaganda," *Psyche* 24.7 (July 1970), 486–509, here 500. Adorno is said to have been the first to draw attention to the theretofore underappreciated Nazism-narcissism connection. See Klaus Horn, "Gesellschaftliche Produktion von Gewalt: Vorschläge zu ihrer politpsychologischen Untersuchung," in Otthein Rammstedt, ed., *Gewaltverhältnisse und die Ohnmacht der Kritik* (Frankfurt / Main: Suhrkamp, 1974), 59–106, here 99.

11. An indicative example from a public health physician from Dortmund, sharing with his colleagues the persuasive effectiveness of sweet-talking compliments: "I see a particularly favorable opportunity for influence in the examination for suitability for marriage and marriage loans. Here a particularly trusting atmosphere, admittedly at first often fear-filled, between the doctor and the applicant, is present, must be present. As I said above, I usually ask the women about the number of siblings and their own desire for children, and then in the case of the fully high-value ones, I add: 'From such couples, as from you and your husband, we must have quite a lot of children. Otherwise, even the Führer will not be able to lift up Germany in the long run, if in 20 years there are not many healthy young people. You, as well as every capable German woman, must help him. We don't want to have any children from the drunkards, the mentally ill and the feeble-minded, they are after all being made infertile. But from people who are like you and your husband, there must be many children.' The response to this on the spot is always good, in some cases ecstatic." Med.-Rat. Dr. Wollenweber, "Das Gesundheitsamt im Kampf gegen den Geburtenschwund," *Der öffentliche Gesundheitsdienst* 5 (1939–1940), 447–459, here 454.

12. On the libidinally inciting sexual politics and the addressing of yearnings for happiness, see Herzog, *Sex after Fascism*, 10–63.

13. For those members of the antipostfascist cohorts who had in their therapeutic practice met survivors of the murders in person—and let themselves be transformed by those encounters—the intrinsic connection between pasts and presents was tangible and often overwhelming. See, e.g., Gerhard Kneuker and Wulf Steglich, *Begegnungen mit der Euthanasie in Hadamar* (Rehburg-Loccum: Psychiatrie-Verlag, 1985).

14. David H. Thurn, review of *Cold War Freud*, in *Contemporary Psychoanalysis* 55.3 (2019), 306–320. Or, as the French analysts Jean Laplanche and Jean-Bertrand Pontalis phrased their explication of "après-coup" decades ago: "It is not lived experience in general that undergoes a deferred revision but, specifically, whatever it has been impossible in the first instance to incorporate fully into a meaningful context. The traumatic event is the epitome of such unassimilated experience." Jean Laplanche and Jean-Bertrand Pontalis, "Deferred Action," in *The Language of Psychoanalysis* (New York: Norton, 1974), 111–114, here 112.

15. It is no coincidence, for instance, that it was the deinstitutionalization activist and member of the Fachausschuß geistig Behinderte Christian Bradl who wrote the first (and to this day still the best) history of Catholic charity care for people with intellectual disabilities in Germany, organized around the research question of the astonishingly tenacious durability of the

mega-institutions. Christian Bradl, *Anfänge der Anstaltsfürsorge für Menschen mit geistiger Behinderung ("Idiotenanstaltswesen"): Ein Beitrag zur Sozial- und Ideengeschichte des Behindertenbetreuungswesens am Beispiel des Rheinlands im 19. Jahrhundert* (Frankfurt / Main: AFRA, 1991).

16. Ernst Klee, *"Euthanasie" im NS-Staat: Die "Vernichtung lebensunwerten Lebens"* (Frankfurt / Main: Fischer, 1983).

17. Jonathan Judaken, "Rethinking Anti-Semitism: Introduction," *American Historical Review* 124.4 (October 2018), 1122–1138, here 1129. With regard to "chimerical" and "functional" hostilities, Judaken is referencing: Gavin Langmuir, *Toward a Definition of Antisemitism* (Berkeley: University of California Press, 1990), 311–352; and Theodor Adorno, "Prejudice in the Interview Material," in Theodor Adorno et al., *The Authoritarian Personality* (New York: Harper & Bros., 1950), 605–653, esp. 609–623.

18. For theorizations of contempt for weakness and / or of vulnerability as exceedingly threatening, see Johannes Klevinghaus, "Der geistig behinderte Mensch in der heutigen Gesellschaft," *Hundert Jahre Dienst an Geistesschwachen in Alsterdorf* (Hamburg: Alsterdorfer Anstalten, 1963), 12–17; Kurt R. Eissler, "Perverted Psychiatry?," *American Journal of Psychiatry* 123.11 (1967), 1352–1358; Julia Kristeva, "Liberty, Equality, Fraternity, and . . . Vulnerability," *WSQ* 38.1-2 (Spring 2010), 251–268.

19. Significant interventions: Marius Turda and Paul J. Weindling, eds., *Blood and Homeland: Eugenics and Racial Nationalism in Central and Southeast Europe, 1900–1940* (New York and Budapest: CEU Press, 2007); Alison Bashford and Philippa Levine, eds., *The Oxford Handbook of the History of Eugenics* (New York: Oxford University Press, 2010); Stefan Kühl, *For the Betterment of the Race: The Rise and Fall of the International Movement for Eugenics and Racial Hygiene* (New York: Palgrave Macmillan, 2013); Angelo Matteo Caglioti, "Race, Statistics and Italian Eugenics: Alfredo Niceforo's Trajectory from Lombroso to Fascism (1876–1960)," *European History Quarterly* 47.3 (2017), 461–489; Paul-André Rosental, *A Human Garden: French Policy and the Transatlantic Legacies of Eugenic Experimentation* (New York: Berghahn, 2019); Volker Roelcke, "International and German Eugenics from ca. 1880 up to the Post-World War II Period: Medical Expertise—Political Ambition—Relations to Euthanasia in the Nazi Context," in Sheldon Rubenfeld and Daniel P. Sulmasy, eds., *Physician-Assisted Suicide and Euthanasia* (London: Rowman & Littlefield, 2020), 45–58. On inter-ideological comparisons within Germany, and the fundamentally important point that German Social Democrats also favored eugenics, see the groundbreaking work of Michael Schwartz, "'Proletarier' und 'Lumpen': Sozialistische Ursprünge eugenischen Denkens," *Vierteljahresheft für Zeitgeschichte* 42.4 (1994), 537–570. For the important news that the much-revered Italian physician Maria Montessori—long celebrated as an inspiration in alternative educational circles—had a strong attachment to eugenics and actually held deeply hostile views towards children with disabilities, see "'Exklusion war ihre pädagogische Leitlinie'" (interview with Montessori-scholar Sabine Seichter by Andreas Frey), *Neue Zürcher Zeitung*, February 16, 2024.

20. On the precociousness, see esp. Warren Rosenblum, "The Romance of the Institution: Educational Optimism and the Confinement of the 'Feebleminded' in Modern Germany," in Linda Leskau et al., eds., *Disability in German-Speaking Europe: History, Memory, Culture* (Rochester, NY: Boydell & Brewer, 2022), 89–109.

21. Wilhelm Wittneben, "Was muß der evangelische Erzieher von der Rassenpflege wissen und wie kann er sich in ihren Dienst stellen?," *Evangelische Jugendhilfe* 10.7-8 (July–August 1934), 171–185, here 175.

22. The manipulative cleverness of the techniques—as espoused very frankly by Walter Groß—is analyzed especially well by Hans-Walter Schmuhl, *Rassenhygiene, Nationalsozialismus, Euthanasie: Von der Verhütung zur Vernichtung "lebensunwerten Lebens," 1890–1945* (Göttingen: Vandenhoeck und Ruprecht, 1987), 173–177.

23. For a moving and sorrowful assessment, see Theodor Strohm, "Diakonie im 'Dritten Reich'—Versuch einer Bilanz," in Theodor Strohm and Jörg Thierfelder, eds., *Diakonie im "Dritten Reich": Neuere Ergebnisse zeitgeschichtlicher Forschung* (Heidelberg: HVA, 1990), 15–33. Strohm

appreciatively cites the pioneering analysis of Kurt Nowak, *"Euthanasie" und Sterilisierung im "Dritten Reich": Die Konfrontation der evangelischen und katholischen Kirche mit dem Gesetz zur Verhütung erbkranken Nachwuchses und die "Euthanasie"-Aktion* (Göttingen: Vandenhoeck & Ruprecht, 1978).

24. A crucial shift occurred in April 1979, when *Die Zeit* in its weekly magazine published a dramatic cover story—titled "Snake Pits in Our Land"—divulging in detail the atrocious conditions persisting at the venerable Protestant charity institution Alsterdorfer Anstalten in Hamburg; the story had been set in motion by a conscientious objector doing his service stint in the institution, who happened to have connections at *Die Zeit*. Although notably, a group of engaged young staffers had already started publicly scandalizing the grotesqueries of the situation the prior year—deliberately deploying impious vulgarity—the coup was getting *Die Zeit* involved. Reporter Renate Just's at once empathic and horrified account of her visit included: the sensory assault of noise and acrid stench; a summary of the typical cocktail of side-effect-packed psychopharmaceuticals daily pumped into residents; her incredulity at the infantilizing decorations of adult living spaces and dismay at the torn and stained clothing in which the residents were carelessly dressed; and her shock at the fact that only the "help-boys" (*Hilfsjungs*)—i.e., "more moderately disabled" adult residents, who earned small change assisting the staff with daily cleaning of the houses and care of their less independent peers—had the slightest amount of private storage space for personal items. The red thread of her analysis was made unmistakable in the pull quotes: "Mass custodial internment in psychiatric mega-clinics exacerbates and produces the very afflictions that are supposed to be cured there." She recorded as well the affecting remark of a conscientious objector working at the institution who observed with regard to the way "they [the residents] assist each other with tender devotion. 'From them one can learn what solidarity means.'" No less dramatically, the cover story was supplemented with an account of the travails of longtime resident Albert Huth and his descriptions of what he had survived and seen of the deportations of hundreds of his fellow residents during the years of Nazi "euthanasia"—including the role of then-pastor-director Friedrich Lensch and his head physician in permitting and facilitating the deportations. (Huth had already managed to alert a local prosecutor in the late 1960s, but at that time the case had been successfully quashed by Hamburg municipal elites, and this despite the prosecutor's strong willingness to pursue the matter; the institution had continued to develop its effective counternarrative. A dozen years later, the power constellation had been rearranged.) The *Die Zeit* author's sympathies for Huth's perspective were evident, with skepticism verging on sarcasm implicit in his recording of administrators' confident declarations that Huth was "schizophrenic," "feebleminded," "a liar," and "unable"—as the then-current director, Hans-Georg Schmidt, like his predecessors a pastor, baldly declared—"to distinguish between fiction and truth." *Die Zeit*'s version of events, by contrast, suggested that it was the *director* who was having significant trouble with that particular distinction. See Renate Just, "Versteckt, verdrängt, vergessen . . . ," and Reimar Oltmanns, "In der Pflegeanstalt zerbrochen," both in *ZEITMagazin* 17 (April 20, 1979), 6–18, here 7 and 9, and 19–22, the latter reprinted with very slight variations on Oltmanns' website: https://reimaroltmanns.blogspot.com/1979/04/in-der-pflegeanstalt-zerbrochen.html; Ernst Klee, "Der lange Weg zur Wahrheit," *Die Zeit* 2 (January 8, 1988); and Gerda Engelbracht and Andrea Hauser, "Das Ende der Verwahranstalt, 1968–1979," in *Mitten in Hamburg: Die Alsterdorfer Anstalten, 1945–1979* (Stuttgart: Kohlhammer, 2013), 231–299. For former prosecutor Dietrich Kuhlbrodt's retrospective accounts of the events of the 1960s–1970s, see *Die Alsterdorfer Passion* (film, dir. Bertram Rotermund and Rudolf Simon, 2018), https://www.rotermundfilm.de/?page_id=792; and Dietrich Kuhlbrodt (interviewed by Marc Widmann and Hauke Friederichs), "'Ich war ein Nestbeschmutzer,'" *Die Zeit*, October 21, 2019. Kuhlbrodt was an absolutely crucial contact person for many of the earliest authors of studies on Nazi "euthanasia," including Ernst Klee, Götz Aly, Henry Friedlander, and Wulf Steglich and Gerhard Kneuker. For the protest-kickstarting and deliberately, earnestly offending cover image on the "black brochure" produced

by the critical young staffers in September 1978, see Uwe Gleßmer und Alfred Lampe, *Mit-Leiden an Alsterdorf und seinen Geschichtsbildern von den Anstalten* (Norderstedt: Books on Demand, 2019), 149.

25. Elisabeth Kunz, email, June 3, 2022.

26. Kunz was recently honored for her decades of service. See "Elisabeth Kunz" in "Thüringer Rose verliehen" (July 7, 2022), Mühlhausen, Ritterliche Reichsstadt, https://www.muehlhausen.de/home/?tx_news_pi1%5Baction%5D=detail&tx_news_pi1%5Bcontroller%5D=News&tx_news_pi1%5Bnews%5D=6573&cHash=3ebdc3371a58883432fbf6f02539d05b.

27. On the disrespect and the incapacity to recognize even very significant East German innovations, see Sigmar Eßbach, "Die Rehabilitationspädagogischen Förderungseinrichtungen des Gesundheits- und Sozialwesens," in Christa Grosch, ed., *Kinder mit Behinderungen: Früherkennung und Rehabilitation im Kindes- und Jugendalter—DDR* (Berlin: Interessengemeinschaft Medizin und Gesellschaft, 2002), 79–90, here 85–89; Christin Seifert, "Rehabilitationspädagogik und Qualifizierung in der Behindertenhilfe—Professionelle Herausforderungen und Veränderungen vor und nach dem Mauerfall," *Erwachsenenbildung und Behinderung* 20.1 (April 2009), 9–14.

28. Sieglind Ellger-Rüttgardt, *Geschichte der Sonderpädagogik: Eine Einführung* (Stuttgart: UTB, 2019), 336; Werner Brill, "Sonderpädagogik und Behinderung im Nationalsozialismus: Spezifika der Situation in Berlin," in Rüdiger vom Bruch and Rebecca Schaarschmidt, eds., *Die Berliner Universität in der NS-Zeit*, vol. 2 (Stuttgart: Franz Steiner, 2005), 229–241, here 241.

29. Dagmar Herzog, "Moral Reasoning in the Wake of Mass Murder: Disability and Reproductive Rights in 1980s–1990s Germany," *Bulletin of the German Historical Institute* 66 (Spring 2020), 9–29.

30. On overlap with the Green Party, as well as West-East and global cripple-movement connections post-1989, see the photographs of Lothar Sandfort, Nati Radtke, Udo Sierck, Judy Heumann, Horst Frehe, Ilja Seifert and others at the website of the Institut zur Selbstbestimmung: http://www.isbbtrebel.de/wir-%C3%BCber-uns-kontakt/.

31. Gabriele Lingelbach, "Konstruktionen von 'Behinderung' in der Öffentlichkeitsarbeit und Spendenwerbung der Aktion Sorgenkind seit 1964," in Elsbeth Bösl et al., eds., *Disability History: Konstruktionen von Behinderung in der Geschichte: Eine Einführung* (Bielefeld: transcript, 2010), 127–150; Elsbeth Bösl, "The Contergan Scandal: Media, Medicine, and Thalidomide in 1960s West Germany," in Susan Burch and Michael Rembis, eds., *Disability Histories* (Urbana: University of Illinois Press, 2014), 136–162; Thomas Großbölting and Niklas Lenhard-Schramm, eds., *Contergan: Hintergründe und Folgen eines Arzneimittel-Skandals* (Göttingen: Vandenhoeck & Ruprecht, 2017).

32. With regard to periodization, see the thoughtful reflections in Michael Wunder, "Paradigmenwechsel in Alsterdorf" (2005), https://www.alsterdorf.de/fileadmin/user_upload/images/geschichte/Paradigmenwechsel_1_.pdf. For insight into the practical mechanisms by which activists, with dedicated perseverance, gradually succeeded in making concrete improvements in government policy on behalf of individuals with intellectual impairments, see the work of the Deutsche Gesellschaft für seelische Gesundheit bei Menschen mit geistiger Behinderung, founded 1995 and led for more than twenty years by the physician Michael Seidel (former East German, subsequent medical director at the v.Bodelschwinghsche Anstalten Bethel) as well as the Arbeitskreis Behindertenrecht (for lawyers) and Arbeitskreis Gesundheitspolitik (for healthcare workers) of the Fachverbände für Menschen mit Behinderung: https://dgsgb.de/stellungnahmen/; https://www.diefachverbaende.de/arbeitskreise.html#AKGesundheitspolitik.

33. E.g., see the presentation by Sebastian Urbanski in "NS-Gedenken: Erstmals spricht ein Mensch mit Downsyndrom im Bundestag," *ZEIT Online*, January 27, 2017, https://www.youtube.com/watch?v=033TpUJ66Kk. Two years later, Urbanski has become the first person with Down syndrome to join the executive board of the Lebenshilfe: Frank Odenthal, "The Sky's the

Limit for Sebastian Urbanski," *Fair Planet*, February 7, 2019, https://www.fairplanet.org/story/the-skys-the-limit-for-sebastian-urbanski/.

34. Ludwig Hermeler, *Die Euthanasie und die späte Unschuld der Psychiater: Massenmord, Bedburg-Hau und das Geheimnis rheinischer Widerstandslegenden* (Essen: Klartext, 2002); Sigrid Falkenstein, "Erinnerungsarbeit: Gegen das Vergessen der 'Euthanasie' Opfer," (2012), https://www.euthanasie-gedenken.de/bedburg_hau_2.htm#2009%20-%202012.

35. See Gunter Demnig's website: https://www.stolpersteine.eu/chronik/2003; and "Gunter Demnig verlegt seinen 100.000. Stolperstein," *Evangelische Zeitung*, May 26, 2023, https://www.evangelische-zeitung.de/gunter-demnig-verlegt-seinen-100-000-stolperstein.

36. See the compelling and beautiful statements by Hagai Aviel, "Durch ihre Namen die Würde der Opfer wiederherstellen," https://www.psychiatrie-erfahren.de/explanation.html; Götz Aly, "Henry K. und Louise S.—Tote ohne Namen," *Die Belasteten: 'Euthanasie' 1939–1945: Eine Gesellschaftsgeschichte* (Frankfurt / Main: Fischer, 2013), 9–18; "Rede von Sigrid Falkenstein, Tag des Gedenkens an die Opfer des Nationalsozialismus" (January 27, 2017), https://www.bundestag.de/resource/blob/490396/97b4b8f30bfd514073082bf2483534c0/kw04_de_gedenkstunde_sfalk-data.pdf; Andreas Hechler, "Diagnoses That Matter: My Great-Grandmother's Murder as One Deemed 'Unworthy of Living' and Its Impact on Our Family," *Disability Studies Quarterly* 37.2 (Spring 2017), https://dsq-sds.org/article/view/5573/4651.

37. "Bundesarchiv erleichtert Recherche nach Opfern der NS-'Euthanasieverbrechen'" (August 30, 2018), https://www.bundesarchiv.de/DE/Content/Pressemitteilungen/nennung-opfernamen-euthanasie.html.

38. See Uta George, *Kollektive Erinnerung bei Menschen mit geistiger Behinderung* (Bad Heilbrunn: Klinkhardt, 2008); and "Gedenkstätten und Menschen mit Lernschwierigkeiten," *Online-Handbuch Inklusion als Menschenrecht*, https://www.inklusion-als-menschenrecht.de/nationalsozialismus/materialien/behinderung-krankheit-und-euthanasie-im-nationalsozialismus/euthanasie-gedenkstaetten-und-menschen-mit-lernschwierigkeiten/.

39. "Menschen mit Behinderung führen durch die Euthanasie-Gedenkstätte," *Aktion Mensch*, https://www.aktion-mensch.de/menschen-und-geschichten/aus-dem-leben/gedenkstaetten-fuehrer. The guides began their preparation in 2016.

40. See, e.g., "Das Leid anerkennen," *Kobinet-Nachrichten*, March 27, 2017, https://kobinet-nachrichten.org/2017/03/27/das-leid-anerkennen/; "Das Leid anerkennen: Stiftung 'Anerkennung und Hilfe' zieht erste Bilanz," *Evangelische Stiftung Alsterdorf*, March 22, 2019, https://www.alsterdorf.de/presse-downloads/pressemeldung/das-leid-anerkennen-stiftung-anerkennung-und-hilfe-zieht-erste-bilanz.html; "Über 3,5 Millionen Euro für Opfer von Behinderteneinrichtungen," *NDR*, September 17, 2021, https://www.ndr.de/nachrichten/hamburg/Ueber-35-Millionen-Euro-fuer-Opfer-von-Behinderteneinrichtungen,stiftung388.html. On the relocation of the Nazi-era altar painting from the back wall of the St. Nicolaus church into a permanent memorial to the Alsterdorfer Anstalten's 511 victims of the "euthanasia" murders, see: "Versetzen des Altarbildes aus der Kirche St. Nicolaus," *Evangelische Stiftung Alsterdorf*, May 27, 2021, https://www.alsterdorf.de/presse-downloads/pressemeldung/versetzen-des-altarbildes-aus-der-kirche-st-nicolaus.html; "Tonnenschwere Altarwand aus der Kirche gehievt," *evangelisch.de*, May 27, 2021, https://www.evangelisch.de/inhalte/186679/27-05-2021/tonnenschwere-altarwand-aus-der-kirche-gehievt; Petra Schellen, "Kirchenbild tiefergelegt," *taz*, May 9, 2022, https://taz.de/NS-Gedenken-in-Hamburg/!5850515/.

41. Already in its 2016 party platform, the AfD had railed against the "ideologically motivated inclusion" of children with learning difficulties into mainstream classrooms (claiming it cost "'significant expenses'" and would "hamper other children in their 'learning successes'"). In subsequent years, AfD politicians self-profiled as demanding the reinstatement of the "achievement-principle" (*Leistungsprinzip*) and an end to what they derisively labeled a "cuddle-curriculum" (*Kuschelunterricht*). See Oliver Georgi, "So radikal will die AfD Deutschland

umbauen," *Frankfurter Allgemeine Zeitung*, May 2, 2016; and, e.g., "Markus Frohnmaier—AfD," Facebook, January 17, 2018, https://www.facebook.com/frohnmaier/posts/leistungsprinzip -statt-kuschelunterrichtseit-2011-sinkt-das-bildungsniveau-in-ba/1965846260332184/. See also "Wie die AfD gegen die Inklusion hetzt," *News4Teachers* (April 23, 2018), https://www .news4teachers.de/2018/04/wie-die-afd-gegen-die-inklusion-hetzt-sie-setzt-behinderungen -in-zusammenhaenge-mit-inzest-und-krankheit/; Ute Kirch, "Empörung im Landtag: AfD vergleicht Förderschüler mit ansteckenden Patienten," *Saarbrücker Zeitung*, April 19, 2018; and—on the cost to taxpayers of fellow citizens with psychiatric disorders—Bundestag-Drucksachen, 19. WP, Drucksache 19/12218, Kleine Anfrage der Abgeordneten René Springer, Jörg Schneider, Martin Sichert, Jürgen Pohl und der Fraktion der AfD, 7 August 2019, https:// dip21.bundestag.de/dip21/btd/19/122/1912218.pdf. For the most recent iteration of antidisability commentary from AfD leader Björn Höcke, see Ann-Katrin Müller and Maik Baumgärtner, "Höcke sorgt mit Äußerungen zu Schülern mit Behinderungen für Entsetzen," *Der Spiegel*, August 9, 2023. Critical responses were rapid: Martin Bernstein, "Ex-OB Ude warnt vor 'Rückfall in die Barbarei,'" *Süddeutsche Zeitung*, August 12, 2023, https://www.sueddeutsche.de/muenchen /behinderte-menschen-demonstration-muenchen-randgruppenkrawall-hoecke-afd-1.6122043.

42. See Bundestag-Drucksachen, 19. WP, Drucksache 19/1444, Kleine Anfrage der Abgeordneten Nicole Höchst, Franziska Gminder, Jürgen Pohl, Verena Hartmann und der Fraktion der AfD, 22 March 2018, 1, http://dip21.bundestag.de/dip21/btd/19/014/1901444.pdf.

43. Der Paritätische Gesamtverband, Projekt Vielfalt ohne Alternative, "Es geht uns alle an: Wachsam sein für Menschlichkeit," https://www.der-paritaetische.de/schwerpunkte/vielfalt -ohne-alternative/es-geht-uns-alle-an-wachsam-sein-fuer-menschlichkeit/.

44. Domradio, "AfD-Anfrage zu Menschen mit Behinderung," Facebook, April 13, 2018, https://ms-my.facebook.com/domradio.de/videos/afd-anfrage-zu-menschen-mit -behinderung/10156547286413311/; "Outrage of AfD 'incest' query," *Deutsche Welle*, April 13, 2018, https://www.dw.com/en/afd-disability-query-slammed-by-churches-ethics-council/a -43382621AfD Disability Query Slammed By Churches, Ethics Council," https://www.dw.com /en/afd-disability-query-slammed-by-churches-ethics-council/a-43382621; "Kirche hält AfD-Anfrage zu Behinderten für 'menschenverachtend'" (2018), https://www.sonderpaedagogik.uni -uerzburg.de/fileadmin/06040300/2018/Kirche_ha__lt_AfD-Anfrage_zu_Behinderten_fu __r_menschenverachtend.pdf.

45. Ilja Seifert and Markus C. Schulte, "Die AfD wertet das Leben von Behinderten als nicht lebenswert ab," *Süddeutsche Zeitung*, April 23, 2018, https://www.sueddeutsche.de/politik /sozialverbaende-die-afd-wertet-das-leben-von-behinderten-als-nicht-lebenswert-ab-1 .3956029.

46. From the *Ohrenkuss* online magazine (https://ohrenkuss.de/ohrenblog/page-1.html) to the many projects of Raúl Krauthausen (e.g., *Sozialhelden* and *Leidmedien*, https:// sozialhelden.de/en/social-heroes/and https://leidmedien.de/) to the blog of Rebecca Maskos (https://rebecca-maskos.net/) to older disability news sites like *Kobinet-Nachrichten* (https:// kobinet-nachrichten.org/) to the recent debate over disability politics between Kübra Sekin and EU politician Katrin Langensiepen (https://www.youtube.com/watch?v=xoBSHa6BjPc): self-representation and self-advocacy have become baseline.

47. Dusel quoted in Hauptschwerbehindertenvertretung im Geschäftsbereich des Niedersächsischen Ministeriums für Wissenschaft und Kultur, "DGUV-Interview mit Jürgen Dusel," *Info-Brief* 32 (November 2018), 6, https://www.uni-goettingen.de/de/document/download /3fd784dd3313104bdb089e4280e88a59.pdf/Textversion_Infobrief_November_2018.pdf.

48. See, e.g., Theresia Degener, "Die UN-Behindertenrechtskonvention: Grundlage für eine neue inklusive Menschenrechtstheorie," *Vereinte Nationen* 2 (2010), 57–63; "Leidmedien im Gespräch mit Theresia Degener" (interview conducted by Raúl Krauthausen, November 25, 2019), https://www.bizeps.or.at/leidmedien-im-gespraech-mit-theresia-degener/.

49. "Bundesteilhabegesetz" (March 23, 2020), https://www.bmas.de/DE/Soziales/Teilhabe-und-Inklusion/Rehabilitation-und-Teilhabe/bundesteilhabegesetz.html.

50. "Experten in eigener Sache," *Alle Inklusive*, https://www.alle-inklusive.de/experten-in-eigener-sache/.

51. Anke Langer, "Advokatorische Assistenz," *Inklusion-Lexikon.de* (August 2009), http://www.inklusion-lexikon.de/Assistenz_Langner.php; Sigrid Graumann, *Assistierte Freiheit: Von einer Behindertenpolitik der Wohltätigkeit zu einer Politik der Menschenrechte* (Frankfurt / Main: Campus, 2011); Tatjana Sorge, "Unterstützte Entscheidungsfindung gehört in die Eingliederungshilfe," *Neue Caritas*, October 29, 2020, https://www.caritas.de/neue-caritas/heftarchiv/jahrgang2020/artikel/unterstuetzte-entscheidungsfindung-gehoert-in-die-einglieder; "Barrierefreiheit in Deutschland," *Lebenshilfe*, https://www.lebenshilfe.de/informieren/wohnen/barrierefreiheit-fuer-menschen-mit-behinderung; Kerrin Stumpf, "'Nur ein kleiner Pieks': Bessere medizinische Versorgung von Menschen mit Behinderung durch unterstützte Entscheidungsfindung," *Inklusive Medizin* 17.1 (October 2020), 5–12.

52. Karina Ulrike Sturm, "Wahlprogramme im Check: Was die Parteien in Sachen Inklusion und Teilhabe versprechen," *Aktion Mensch* (2021), https://www.aktion-mensch.de/inklusion/bundestagswahl/analyse-der-wahlprogramme.

53. For a sampling of current projects working at the intersection of migration and disability – both in self-advocacy and in service provision – see the offerings at: Mina (http://mina-berlin.eu/), Lebenshilfe (https://www.lebenshilfe.de/informieren/arbeiten/interkulturelle-oeffnung), Der Paritätische (https://www.der-paritaetische.de/themen/migration-und-internationale-kooperation/projekte/perspektivwechsel-interkulturelle-oeffnung-der-behindertenhilfe/), Bundesverband für Körper- und Mehrfachbehinderte e.V. (https://bvkm.de/unsere-themen/migration-und-behinderung/), and Aktion Mensch, in "easy-to-understand" language (https://www.familienratgeber.de/leichte-sprache/beratung-hilfen/beratungsangebote/flucht-und-behinderung). On migration and disability, and an illuminating analysis of both the remarkably belated and the still uneven uptake of intersectional concerns in the Lebenshilfe, see Helen Baykara-Krumme and Vanessa Rau, "Dynamische Zeiten, Zögerlicher Wandel: Migrationsbezogene Vielfalt in der Lebenshilfe," in Hella von Unger et al., eds., *Organisationaler Wandel durch Migration? Zur Diversität in der Zivilgesellschaft* (Bielefeld: transcript, 2022), 33-66. Meanwhile, the age-old class-stratified tracking system in which the children of the poor were relatively scarce in Gymnasium and Realschule and instead predominantly landed in the lower-tier Hauptschule or even in a segregated school for the "learning-disabled" has over the past decades become most evident in a triangular correlational overlap between diagnoses of disability, conditions of poverty, and a background of familial flight or migration. Although there is tremendous regional variation across Germany, scholars, journalists, and politicians concur that the tracking system persists. Thus, whether they hail from the classic guestworker-supplying countries (Turkey, Italy, Greece) or, more recently, a succession of war zones (first ex-Yugoslavia, then Lebanon, Afghanistan, Syria, Russia, Ukraine), and even as the explanatory theories proffered range from the challenges of bilinguality to trauma, culture clash, or economic stress and social marginalization – or racism – statistically, children with migratory background are in almost all locales disproportionately more likely to be deemed to require special education services, whether in inclusive or segregated facilities. See Thomas Kemper and Horst Weishaupt, "Zur Bildungsbeteiligung ausländischer Schüler an Förderschulen - unter besonderer Berücksichtigung der spezifischen Staatsangehörigkeit," *Zeitschrift für Heilpädagogik* 62/10 (2011), 419-431; "Förderschule – die Schule für Einwanderer? Interview der Integrationsagenturmitarbeiterin Mercedes Pascual Iglesias mit dem Sozialwissenschaftler Dr. Wolfgang Zaschke" (14.6.2011), NRWGegenDiskriminierung, http://nrwgegendiskriminierung.de/files /pdf /Foerderschule_die_Schule_fuer_Einwanderer.pdf; Wolfgang Dworschak, "Kinder und Jugendliche mit einer geistigen Behinderung und Migrationshintergrund: Überrepräsentation an Förderschulen in Bayern," *Schweizerische Zeitschrift für Heilpädagogik*, 22/1 (2016), 34-40; Renate Allgöwer, "Zu viele Migrantenkinder auf der Förderschule," *Stuttgarter Zeitung*, January 2, 2019, https://www

.stuttgarter-zeitung.de/inhalt.ungleiche-bildungschancen-zu-viele-migrantenkinder-auf-der-foerd
erschule.43bcf7f7-o6aa-4a2b-b9c2-oca71fec63ca.html; Johannes Mand, "Je mehr Migranten desto
mehr Förderschüler" (May 18, 2020), https://johannes-mand.de/blog/2020/05/18/mehr
-migranten-mehr-foerderschueler/; Santina Battaglia, "Bildungsausschluss durch Inklusion: bev-
orzugt nach Herkunft," *Migazin*, July 3, 2023, https://www.migazin.de/2023/07/03/regelschulen
-bildungsausschluss-durch-inklusion-bevorzugt-nach-herkunft/.

54. E.g., see "Bremer Grundschullehrer kritisieren Bildungsbehörde scharf," *Weser-Report*,
June 9, 2015, https://weserreport.de/2015/06/bremen-bremen/panorama/bremer
-grundschullehrer-kritisieren-bildungsbehoerde-scharf/. For an early analysis of how things already began to go wrong and how the integration movement lost momentum, unexpectedly, after
reunification in 1990, see Ulf Preuss-Lausitz, "Separation oder Inklusion—Zur Entwicklung der
sonderpädagogischen Förderung im Kontext der allgemeinen Schulentwicklung" (2010), reprinted in Frank J. Müller, ed., *Blick zurück nach vorn—WegbereiterInnen der Inklusion. Band 1*
(Gießen: Psychosozial, 2018), 245–269. For examples of the precious creative disobedience with
which teachers determined to maintain islands of inclusion despite a lack of interest or support
from administrators in the 1990s and early 2000s, see the interview with Gerhard Sennlaub,
"Gegen amtlich angeordnete Kinderschädigung-ein Schulrat erzählt," in Reinhard Stähling and
Barbara Wenders, eds., *Ungehorsam im Schuldient: Der praktische Weg zu einer Schule für alle* (Balt-
mannsweiler: Schneider Verlag Hohengehren, 2009).

55. Helmut Rau quoted in Anna Lehmann and Christian Füller, "Die UN kann uns nichts
vorschreiben," *taz*, December 30, 2009, https://taz.de/!5150230/?goMobile2=1580860800042.

56. For example Niedersachsen, where a petition campaign launched by the Free Democratic Party is urging citizens to support the maintenance of the special schools (in the meantime renamed, almost everywhere, as "developmental schools" [*Förderschulen*]): Nadine Conti,
"Volksbegehren zur Förderschule," *taz*, July 28, 2022, https://taz.de/Wahlkampf-in
-Niedersachsen/!5867362/; Lars Laue, "Wie die FDP in Niedersachsen die Förderschulen
erhalten will," *Noz*, August 28, 2022, https://www.noz.de/deutschland-welt/niedersachsen
/artikel/wie-die-fdp-in-niedersachsen-die-foerderschulen-erhalten-will-42961651; FDP, "Offene Förderschulen. Offene Chancen," https://www.fdp-nds.de/offene-foerderschulen-offene
-chancen; https://taz.de/!5150230/?goMobile2=1580860800042. Meanwhile, in the Rhineland, further "developmental schools" are being built, despite prior resolutions to the contrary:
"LVR plant neue Förderschulen: Inklusion bleibt Lippenbekenntnis," *mittendrin e.V.*, September
21, 2022, https://www.mittendrin-koeln.de/aktuell/nrw. And in metropolitan Berlin alone—
although it actually counts as one of the centers in which rates of inclusion are generally higher
than elsewhere—800 spots at the "developmental schools with an emphasis on mental development" (*Förderschulen mit dem Schwerpunkt geistige Entwicklung*) are, as of 2022, being created:
Lisa Reimann, "Verkaufsschlager Förderschule? Warum weiterhin in ein gescheitertes System
investiert wird," *Inklusionsfakten.de*, January 16, 2020, https://inklusionsfakten.de/was-ist-das
-gute-an-foerderschulen/. As Reimann notes: "The expansion of an inclusive educational system was only ever half-heartedly implemented." Meanwhile, the blogosphere is filled with reports of parental distress at the relentless advocacy required to garner a suitably supported
setting for a child with a disability within a regular school.

57. Degener quoted in "Wissenschaftlerin: Bei der Inklusion liegt Deutschland weit
hinten," *Unsere Kirche*, April 2, 2019, https://chrismon.evangelisch.de/nachrichten/43824
/wissenschaftlerin-bei-der-inklusion-liegt-deutschland-weit-hinten#.

58. Otto Speck, "Inklusive Missverständnisse," *Süddeutsche Zeitung*, January 26, 2015, https://
www.sueddeutsche.de/bildung/inklusions-debatte-inklusive-missverstaendnisse-1.2182484.

59. Bertelsmann Stiftung, Jacob Muth-Preis, https://www.bertelsmann-stiftung.de/de
/unsere-projekte/abgeschlossene-projekte/jakob-muth-preis/preistraeger.

60. Jutta Schöler, "Interview," in Müller, *Blick zurück nach vorn*, 115–139, here 131. Disability
pedagogue Georg Feuser, still one of the most prominent veterans of the battles of the

1970s–1980s, had become caustic already six years ago in his summary assessments that what passes for "inclusion" in the contemporary German school system is nothing but a perverse, insidiously mendacious "false labeling" (*Etikettenschwindel*). ("[A] bottle filled with vinegar remains vinegar, even if we stick the label of a superior wine on the bottle.") Indeed, Feuser has become convinced that all the post-UNCRPD talk about fostering "inclusion" is concealing what is actually an ongoingly "selectionist" (*selektierenden*) and "exclusionary" (*exkludierendes, ausgrenzendes*) system. Georg Feuser, "Interview," in Frank J. Müller, ed., *Blick zurück nach vorn—WegbereiterInnen der Inklusion. Band 2* (Gießen: Psychosozial, 2018), 57–145, here 79, 83, 106, 127. For Feuser, as he had insisted consistently for decades, the maintenance of deliberate isolation of children with disabilities in segregated special settings deprives them of necessary opportunities for relationally interactive development and thereby actually *worsens* whatever their original vulnerability was that got them labeled as disabled in the first place. Yet, too, just as he has argued all along, no less appalling in his view is the damage being done to *everyone's* capacities for developing empathic and critical thinking abilities and learning early in life to act in solidarity with others. See also Georg Feuser, "Inklusion - das Mögliche, das im Wirklichen nicht sichtbar ist" (lecture delivered at the TU Darmstadt, January 16, 2019), https://www.georg-feuser.com/wp-content/uploads/2019/06/Feuser-V-Inklusion-Das-M%C3%B6gliche-im-Wirklichen-Transformation-der-Relativit%C3%A4t-16-01-2019.pdf; and – for the most up-to-date lucid critical analysis of the growing rollback on matters of inclusion – see Georg Feuser, "Inklusion," *vpod bildungspolitik* 233 (2023), 16–19. The headline summarizes forthrightly: "The implementation of inclusive education oscillates between arbitrary decision-making, populist distortions, rebuffed rights, and contempt for child welfare." Feuser is hardly alone in his convictions about euphemistic and mendacious "false labeling." In December 2022, the popular satiric TV cabaret *Die Anstalt* dedicated its Christmas show to a crushingly mocking critique of what it identified as massive evasiveness and hypocrisy in the German states' programmatic plans for schooling of children with disabilities (the state of Bremen, with 91 percent of its pupils with disabilities enrolled in regular schools, was praised as the sole laudable exception—compared, for instance, to only 33 percent in Baden-Württemberg or 32 percent in Bayern). See *Die Anstalt*, December 20, 2022, https://www.zdf.de/comedy/die-anstalt/die-anstalt-vom-20-dezember-2022-100.html. A month later, the serious TV news show *Monitor* ran a program that confirmed one of the more scandalous points identified by *Die Anstalt*. Under the headline "Inclusion in Schools: How Children Are Made 'Disabled,'" *Monitor* reiterated the finding that children having the slightest trouble in school were being officially re-categorized as "learning-disabled"—with damaging effects both on their self-understanding and their future prospects—simply so that the schools could *appear* as more compliant with UNCRPD-mandated standards and hence, in many cases, also receive desirable extra funding for additional staffing. Lara Straatmann, "Inklusion an Schulen: Wie Kinder 'behindert' gemacht werden," *Monitor*, January 19, 2023, https://www1.wdr.de/daserste/monitor/sendungen/inklusion-154.html.

61. "FDP-Kommunalpolitiker sehen Menschen mit Behinderung als Tourismusbremse," *Hessenschau*, May 4, 2022, https://www.hessenschau.de/politik/fdp-kommunalpolitiker-sehen-menschen-mit-behinderung-als-tourismusbremse,tann-flugblatt-100.html.

62. One significant recent scandal involving apparently routine violence at the Wittekindshof in Westphalia first came to light in 2019 (as the sister of one man with cognitive impairments discovered her brother had been locked in his room of 9 square meters for several months, at times heavily medicated and tied down with restraints, and it was ultimately—over the next two years—revealed that there were 32 victims of illegal confinement and restraint use, as 145 of 3,500 staff remained under investigation). Another scandal concerned the horrifying murders of four residents by a psychologically ill staff member at the Oberlinhaus in Potsdam in April 2021 (deaths that would not have been possible had the staff-to-resident ratio been better). Reiner Burger, "Anklagen nach schwerer Misshandlung von behinderten Heimbewohnern," *Frankfurter*

Allgemeine Zeitung, September 23, 2022, https://www.faz.net/aktuell/gesellschaft/kriminalitaet
/behinderte-schwer-misshandelt-anklagen-im-fall-wittekindshof-erhoben-18337908.html;
Christian Bradl, "Systemische Risiken für Gewalt und mangelnden Gewaltschutz in Einrichtungen der Behindertenhlfe bei erheblich herausforderndem Verhalten," *Behindertenpädagogik* 61.4
(2022), 358–383; "Vier Heimbewohner getötet: Schuldfähgkeit wird geprüft," *Morgenpost,*
April 30, 2021, https://www.morgenpost.de/berlin/polizeibericht/article232163859/oberlinhaus
-potsdam-4-tote-leichen-polizei.html; Julia Latscha, "Dieser Tod ist keine Erlösung," *Die Zeit,*
May 11, 2021, https://www.zeit.de/kultur/2021-05/behindertenfeindlichkeit-mord-potsdam
-pflegerin-inklusion-ableismus-erloesung?utm_referrer=https%3A%2F%2Fwww.google
.com%2F; "Ableismus Tötet," https://ableismus.de/toetet/de.

63. "Gewaltschutz in Einrichtungen der Behindertenhilfe ausbauen," *Deutsches Institut für
Menschenrechte,* May 12, 2021, https://www.institut-fuer-menschenrechte.de/aktuelles/detail
/gewaltschutz-in-einrichtungen-der-behindertenhilfe-ausbauen.

64. "Anteil der Leistungsbeziehenden von Assistenzleistungen mit Wohnbezug nach Wohnform und nach primärer Behinderung Ende 2021," *Statista,* https://de.statista.com/statistik
/daten/studie/1261057/umfrage/leistungsbeziehende-im-ambulanten-und-stationaeren
-wohnen-nach-primaerer-behinderung/; "Zentrale Ergebnisse Soziale Teilhabe," BAGüS-
Kennzahlenvergleich. Eingliederungshilfe 2022—Berichtsjahr 2020, 6, https://www.lwl.org
/spur-download/bag/Bericht_2020_final.pdf. This persisting impasse and the failure to move
forward with comprehensive deinstitutionalization—as well as the pretexts used for not moving forward—have been expressly criticized by the UN commission tasked with evaluating
Germany's compliance with the UNCRPD and by the German Institute for Human Rights in
2023. See "Parallel Report to the UN Committee on the Rights of Persons with Disabilities for
Germany's 2nd/3rd State Party Review Procedure," *Deutsches Institut für Menschenrechte,*
July 2023, https://www.institut-fuer-menschenrechte.de/das-institut/abteilungen/monitoring
-stelle-un-behindertenrechtskonvention/staatenberichtsverfahren; UNCRPD, "Concluding
observations on the combined second and third periodic reports of Germany," October 3, 2023,
https://tbinternet.ohchr.org/_layouts/15/treatybodyexternal/Download.aspx?symbolno
=CRPD%2FC%2FDEU%2FCO%2F2-3&Lang=en; and "Selbstbestimmt leben: Umfassender
Wandel der Unterstützungssysteme notwendig," *Deutsches Institut für Menschenrechte,* October 25, 2023, https://www.institut-fuer-menschenrechte.de/aktuelles/detail/selbstbestimmt
-leben-umfassender-wandel-der-unterstuetzungssysteme-notwendig.

65. The Evangelische Stiftung Alsterdorf now provides employer-employee matching
services, as newly passed guidelines at the federal level pressure businesses to hire workers with
disabilities: "Bundesrat stimmt über inklusiven Arbeitsmarkt ab," *Evangelische Stiftung Alsterdorf,*
May 12, 2023, https://www.alsterdorf.de/presse-downloads/pressemeldung/bundesrat-stimmt
-ueber-inklusiven-arbeitsmarkt-ab.html; the University of Bielefeld Medical School sponsored
a conference on improved inclusive provision of therapeutic and medical services together with
the v. Bodelschwingsche Stiftungen Bethel, June 15–16, 2023, https://bethel.de/teilhabekon
gress2023; and since June 2022, the organization "reha" in the city of Saarbrücken opened the
doors on a new initiative in which people with and without disabilities live side by side, with
both self-determination and supports ("Wohnen in der City," Lampertshof), https://rehagmbh
.de/unternehmen/historie.

INDEX

Note: Page numbers followed by an *f* refer to figures. Page numbers followed by an *n* refer to notes.